AF883159

Fibrinogen
Fibrin Formation and Fibrinolysis
Volume 4

Fibrinogen

Fibrin Formation and Fibrinolysis

Volume 4

Proceedings
Workshop on Fibrinogen
April 2–3, 1985, London, England

Editors
D. A. Lane · A. Henschen · M. K. Jasani

Walter de Gruyter · Berlin · New York 1986

Editors

Dr. David A. Lane
Department of Haematology
Charing Cross and Westminster Hospital
Medical School
Fulham Palace Road
Hammersmith
London W6 8RF
Great Britain

Dr. M. Kris Jasani
Ciba-Geigy Pharmaceuticals
Wimblehurst Road
Horsham
West Sussuex, RH12 4AB
Great Britain

Dr. Agnes Henschen
Max-Planck-Institute of Biochemistry
8033 Martinsried
Federal Republic of Germany

Library of Congress Cataloging in Publication Data

Workshop on Fibrinogen (1985 : Queen Elizabeth College, London, England)
Fibrinogen, fibrin formation and fibrinolysis.
Bibliography: p.
Includes index.
1. Fibrinogen--Congresses. 2. Fibrin--Congresses. 3. Fibrinolysis--Congresses. I. Lane, D. A. (David A.) 1949- II. Henschen, A. (Agnes), 1935- . III. Jasani, M. K. IV. Title.
QP93.5.W67 1985 612'.115 85-29304
ISBN 0-89925-152-8 (U.S.)

CIP-Kurztitelaufnahme der Deutschen Bibliothek

Fibrinogen : proceedings / Workshop on Fibrinogen. - Berlin ; New York : de Gruyter. 1 ohne Kongressbenennung
NE: Workshop on Fibrinogen
Vol. 4. Fibrin formation and fibrinolysis. - 1986

Fibrin formation and fibrinolysis : proceedings / Workshop on Fibrinogen, April 2-3, 1985, London, England. Ed. D. A. Lane . . . - Berlin ; New York : de Gruyter, 1986
(Fibrinogen ; Vol. 4)
ISBN 3-11-010597-7
NE: Lane, David A. [Hrsg.]; Workshop on Fibrinogen <1985, London>

Copyright © 1986 by Walter de Gruyter & Co., Berlin 30.
All rights reserved, including those of translation into foreign languages. No part of this book may be reproduced in any form – by photoprint, microfilm or any other means nor transmitted nor translated into a machine language without written permission from the publisher. Printing: Gerike GmbH, Berlin. – Binding: D. Mikolai, Berlin. – Printed in Germany.

PREFACE

This volume contains the proceedings of a workshop entitled "Fibrinogen, fibrin formation and fibrinolysis" that was held on April 2-3 1985 at Queen Elizabeth College, London. The workshop was attended by approximately 100 basic and clinical researchers and its aim was to encourage informal interchange of ideas about the fibrinogen molecule, its involvement in normal haemostasis and in pathology. Previous workshops have been held at Martinsried, Leiden and Stockholm. Their proceedings have been published as earlier volumes in a series of which this volume constitutes the 4th:

Fibrinogen - Recent Biochemical and Medical Aspects; A. Henschen, H. Graeff and F. Lottspeich, editors. Vol. 1, W. de Gruyter, Berlin and New York, 1982.

Fibrinogen - Structure, Functional Aspects and Metabolism; F. Haverkate, A. Henschen, W. Neiuwenhuizen and P.W. Straub, editors. Vol. 2, W. de Gruyter, Berlin and New York, 1983.

Fibrinogen - Structural Variants and Interactions; A. Henschen, B. Hessel, J. McDonagh and T. Saldeen, editors. Vol. 3, W. de Gruyter, Berlin and New York, 1985.

The meeting at Queen Elizabeth College was judged a success by the participants who found time in between a packed scientific programme to mix informally in the pleasant environment of the College. Dr. Neville Marsh of the Department of Physiology, Queen Elizabeth College, is warmly thanked by the Editors for arranging this aspect of the meeting.

Finally, the Editors wish to thank Dr. Alan White of Ciba Geigy Pharmaceuticals Division, Horsham for arranging financial support that made the workshop possible.

London, München and Horsham, September 1985

D.A. Lane
A. Henschen
M.K. Jasani

CONTRIBUTORS

Beck, E.A.
Central Haematology Laboratory, Inselspital, CH-3010 Berne, Switzerland

Bernadou, A.
Hôtel-Dieu, Paris, France

Bertrand, O.
Laboratoires Centraux d'Hématologie et de Biochemie, Hôtel-Dieu, Paris, France

Blobel, H.
Institut für Bakteriologie und Immunologie, Justus Liebig-Universität, Frankfurter Strasse 107, 6300 Giessen, FRG

Bode, W.
Max-Planck-Institut für Biochemie, D-8033 Martinsried, FRG

Bonnet, P.
Hôpital Lariboisière, Paris, France

Bouchieux, C.
Hôtel-Dieu, Paris, France

Brommer, E.J.P.
Gaubius Institute, Health Research Division TNO, Herenstraat 5d, 2313 AD Leiden, The Netherlands

Caen, J.P.
Hôpital Lariboisière, Paris, France

Chhatwal, G.S.
Institut für Bakteriologie und Immunologie, Justus Liebig-Universität, Frankfurter Strasse 107, 6300 Giessen, FRG

Coccheri, S.
Department of Angiology and Blood Coagulation, University Hospital S. Orsola, 40138 Bologna, Italy

Colella, S.
Istituo di Ricerche Farmacologiche Mario Negri, via Eritrea 62, 20157 Milano, Italy

Dejana, E.
Istituo di Ricerche Farmacologiche Mario Negri, via Eritrea 62, 20157 Milano, Italy

Delvos, U.
Clinical Research Unit for Blood Coagulation and Thrombosis of the Max-Planck-Gesellschaft at the Justus-Liebig-University, Giessen, FRG

Desvignes, P.
Hôpital Lariboisiere, Paris, France

Douglas, J.T.
University Department of Medicine, Royal Infirmary, Glasgow, G31 2ER, UK

Dunn, F.W.
Laboratoires Centraux d'Hématologie et de Biochemie, Hôtel-Dieu, Paris, France

Eastham, R.
Frenchay Hospital, Bristol, BS16 1LE, UK

Elwood, P.C.
MRC Epidemiology Unit, 4 Richmond Road, Cardiff CF2 3AS, UK

Engbers, J.
TNO Gaubius Institute for Cardiovascular Research, Herenstraat 5d, 2313 AD Leiden, The Netherlands

Errol, A.
Istituo di Richerche Farmacologiche Mario Negri, via Eritrea 62, 20157 Milano, Italy

Etherington, M.D.
Central Laboratory, St. Mary's Hospital, Portsmouth, PO3 6AG, UK

Forbes, C.D.
University Department of Medicine, Royal Infirmary, Glasgow, G31 2ER, UK

Fuhge, P.
Behringwerke AG, Marburg, FRG

Furlan, M.
Central Haematology Laboratory, Inselspital, CH-3010 Berne, Switzerland

Gabrijelčič, D.
Max-Planck-Institut für Biochemie, D-8033 Martinsried, FRG

Gaffney, P.J.
National Institute for Biological Standards and Control, Holly Hill, Hampstead, London, NW3 6RB, UK

Gilmour, R.A.
Frenchay Hospital, Bristol, BS16 1LE, UK

Ginsberg, M.H.
Research Institute of Scripps Clinic, La Jolla, CA 92037, USA

Gollwitzer, R.
Max-Planck-Institut für Biochemie, D-8033 Martinsried, FRG

Graeff, H.
Frauenklinik der Technischen Universität, D-8000 München, FRG

Hafter, R.
Frauenklinik der Technischen Universität, D-8000 München, FRG

Handley, D.A.
Department of Medicine, College of Physicians and Surgeons, Columbia University, New York, NY 10032, USA

Haverkate, F.
Gaubius Institute, Health Research Division TNO, Herenstraat 5d, 2313 AD Leiden, The Netherlands

Heimburger, N.
Behringwerke AG, Marburg, FRG

Henschen, A.
Max-Planck-Institute for Biochemistry, D-8033 Martinsried, FRG

Hugo, R. von
Frauenklinik der Technischen Universität, D-8000 München, FRG

Huijsmans, C.M.G.
TNO Gaubius Institute for Cardiovascular Research, Herenstraat 5d, 2313 AD Leiden, The Netherlands

Ireland, H.
Department of Haematology, Charing Cross and Westminster Medical School, Hammersmith, London, W6 8RP, UK

Jasani, M.K.
Ciba Geigy Pharmaceuticals, Horsham, West Sussex, RH12 4AB, UK

Jayson, M.I.V.
Rheumatic Diseases Centre, University of Manchester, Hope Hospital, Salford, UK

Kaudewitz, H.
Max-Planck-Institute for Biochemistry, D-8033 Martinsried, FRG

Keegan, A.
Rheumatic Diseases Centre, University of Manchester, Hope Hospital, Salford, UK

Kehl, M.
Max-Planck-Institute for Biochemistry, D-8033 Martinsried, FGR

Keyser, J.
TNO Gaubius Institute for Cardiovascular Research, Herenstraat 5d, 2313 AD Leiden, The Netherlands

Knight, I.
Department of Haematology, Charing Cross and Westminster Medical School, Hammersmith, London, W6 8RP, UK

Koopman, J.
Gaubius Institute, Health Research Division TNO, Herenstraat 5d, 2313 AD Leiden, The Netherlands

Koppert, P.W.
TNO Gaubius Institute for Cardiovascular Research, Herenstraat 5d, 2313 AD Leiden, The Netherlands

Kudryk, B.
Lindsley F. Kimball Research Institute, New York Blood Center, New York, NY 10021, USA

Kulbe, G.E.
Max-Planck-Institut für Biochemie, D-8033 Martinsried, FRG

Lane, D.A.
Department of Haematology, Charing Cross and Westminster Medical School, Hammersmith, London, W6 8RP, UK

Languino, L.R.
Istituo di Ricerche Farmacologiche Mario Negri, via Eritrea 62, 20157 Milano, Italy

Leeksma, O.C.
Central Laboratory of the Netherlands Red Cross Blood Transfusion Service, Amsterdam, The Netherlands

Lijnen, H.R.
Center for Thrombosis and Vascular Research, University of Leuven, Campus Gasthuisberg, Herestraat 49, B-3000 Leuven, Belgium

Linke, R.P.
Institut für Immunologie der Universität München, D-8000 München, FRG

Liu, C.Y.
Department of Medicine, College of Physicians and Surgeons, Columbia University, New York, NY 10032, USA

Lowe, G.D.O.
University Department of Medicine, Royal Infirmary, Glasgow, G31 2ER, UK

Maes, L.
Faculty of Medicine, VUB, Brussels, Belgium

Mantovani, A.
Istituo di Ricerche Farmacologiche Mario Negri, via Eritrea 62, 20157 Milano, Italy

Manucci, P.M.
Centro Angelo Bianchi Bonomi, 1-20122 Milano, Italy

Marguerie, G.
Inserm U 217, Centre d'Etude Nuclèaire, Grenoble, France

Meijer-Huizinga, F.M.
Central Laboratory of the Netherlands Red Cross Blood Transfusion Service, Amsterdam, The Netherlands

Million, R.
Rheumatic Diseases Centre, University of Manchester, Hope Hospital, Salford, UK

Mirshahi, M.
Laboratoires Centraux d'Hématologie et de Biochemie, Hôtel-Dieu, Paris, France

Miyada, D.
Department of Pathology, College of Medicine, University of California, Irvine, CA 92717, USA

Mourik, J.A. van
Central Laboratory of the Netherlands Red Cross Blood Transfusion Service, Amsterdam, The Netherlands

Müller, E.
Max-Planck-Institute for Biochemistry, D-8033 Martinsried, FRG

Müller-Berghaus, G.
Clinical Research Unit for Blood Coagulation and Thrombosis of the Max-Planck-Gesellschaft at the Justus-Liebig-University, Giessen, FRG

Nieuwenhuizen, W.
TNO Gaubius Institute for Cardiovascular Research, Herenstraat 5d, 2313 AD Leiden, The Netherlands

O'Brien, J.R.
Central Laboratory, St. Mary's Hospital, Portsmouth, PO3 6AG, UK

Palareti, G.
Department of Angiology and Blood Coagulation, University Hospital S. Orsola, 40138 Bologna, Italy

Perry, M.J.
National Institute for Biological Standards and Control, Holly Hill, Hampstead, London, NW3 6RB, UK

Perrot, J.Y.
Laboratoires Centraux d'Hématologie et de Biochemie, Hôtel-Dieu, Paris, France

Peters, R.F.
Ciba Geigy Pharmaceuticals, Horsham, West Sussex, RH12 4AB, UK

Pirkle, H.
Department of Pathology, College of Medicine, University of California, Irvine, CA 92717, USA

Plow, E.F.
Research Institute of Scripps Clinic, La Jolla, CA 92037, USA

Poggi, M.
Department of Angiology and Blood Coagulation, University Hospital S. Orsola, 40138 Bologna, Italy

Pountain, G.
Rheumatic Diseases Centre, University of Manchester, Hope Hospital, Salford, UK

Preissner, K.T.
Clinical Research Unit for Blood Coagulation and Thrombosis of the Max-Planck-Gesellschaft at the Justus-Liebig University, Giessen, FRG

Prydz, H.
Research Institute for Internal Medicine, University of Oslo, Rikshospitalet, Oslo, Norway

Rampling, M.W.
Department of Physiology and Biophysics, St. Mary's Hospital Medical School, London, W2 1PG, UK

Reber, P.
Central Haematology Laboratory, Inselspital, CH-3010 Berne, Switzerland

Redman, C.
Lindsley F. Kimball Research Institute, New York Blood Center, New York, NY 10021, USA

Rötker, J.
Clinical Research Unit for Blood Coagulation and Thrombosis, Max-Planck-Gesellschaft at the Justus-Liebig-University, Giessen, FRG

Rupp, C.
Central Haematology Laboratory, Inselspital, CH-3010 Berne, Switzerland

Samama, M.
Hôtel-Dieu, Paris, France

Scheefers-Borchel, U.
Clinical Research Unit for Blood Coagulation and Thrombosis of the Max-Planck-Gesellschaft at the Justus-Liebig-University, Giessen, FRG

Schröck, R.
Frauenklinik der Technischen Universität, D-8000 München, FRG

Schubring, C.
Department of Obstetrics and Gynaecology, Evangelisches Krankenhaus, Giessen, FRG

Selmayr, E.
Clinical Research Unit for Blood Coagulation and Thrombosis, Max-Planck-Gesellschaft at the Justus-Liebig-University, Giessen, FRG

Smith, E.
Department of Chemical Pathology, University of Aberdeen, Foresterhill, Aberdeen, AB9 2ZD, UK

Soria, C.
Laboratoires Centraux d'Hématologie et de Biochemie, Hôpital Lariboisière, Paris, France

Soria, J.
Laboratoires Centraux d'Hématologie et de Biochemie, Hôtel-Dieu, Paris, France

Southan, C.
Department of Haematology, Charing Cross and Westminster Medical School, Hammersmith, London, W6 8RP, UK

Svenson, E.
Laboratoires Centraux d'Hématologie et de Biochemie, Hôtel-Dieu, Paris, France

Sweetnam, P.M.
MRC Epidemiology Unit, 4 Richmond Road, Cardiff, CF2 3AS, UK

Talbot, M.D.
Ciba Geigy Pharmaceuticals, Horsham, West Sussex, RH12 4AB, UK

Takada, A.
Department of Physiology, Hamamatsu University, School of Medicine, Hamamatsu-shi, Shizuoka 431-31, Japan

Takada, Y.
Department of Physiology, Hamamatsu University, School of Medicine, Hamamatsu-shi, Shizuoka 431-31, Japan

Theodor, I.
Department of Pathology, College of Medicine, University of California, Irvine, CA 92717, USA

Thiel, W.
Clinical Research Unit for Blood Coagulation and Thrombosis, Max-Planck-Gesellschaft at the Justus-Liebig-University, Giessen, FRG

Thomaidis, A.
Hôpital Lariboisière, Paris, France

Thompson, E.
Department of Haematology, Charing Cross and Westminster Medical School, Hammersmith, London, W6 8RP, UK

Tomlinson, I.
Rheumatic Diseases Centre, University of Manchester, Hope Hospital, Salford, UK

Tweed, M.F.
Ciba Geigy Pharmaceuticals, Horsham, West Sussex, RH12 4AB, UK

Vukasin, P.
Department of Pathology, College of Medicine, University of California, Irvine, CA 92717, USA

Walker, J.E.
Department of Chemical Pathology, University of Aberdeen, Foresterhill, Aberdeen, AB9 2ZD, UK

Wallen, P.
Department of Physiological Chemistry, University of Umea, S-90187, Umea, Sweden

Weimar, B.
Clinical Research Unit for Blood Coagulation and Thrombosis of the Max-Planck-Gesellschaft at the Justus-Liebig-University, Giessen, FRG

Werf, W.G.C. van der
Gaubius Institute, Health Research Division TNO, Herenstraat 5d, 2313 AD Leiden, The Netherlands

Yarnell, J.W.G.
MRC Epidemiology Unit, 4 Richmond Road, Cardiff, CF2 3AS, UK

Yu, S.
Lindsley F. Kimball Research Institute, New York Blood Center, New York, NY 10021, USA

CONTENTS

I. SYNTHESIS AND ASSEMBLY

II. STRUCTURE AND FUNCTION

III. CONGENITAL VARIANTS

I. Synthesis and Assembly

A SCHEME FOR THE INTRACELLULAR ASSEMBLY OF HUMAN FIBRINOGEN.

Sharon Yu, Bohdan Kudryk and Colvin Redman
Lindsley F. Kimball Research Institute,
New York Blood Center New York, N.Y., 10021

Introduction

Human plasma fibrinogen is a dimer with each half-molecule composed of three non-identical chains (Aα, Bβ and γ). The half-molecules of the dimer are held together by symmetrical disulfide bonds between two Aα chains and two γ chains. In addition, fibrinogen contains a number of inter- and intrachain disulfide linkages. It is our aim to elucidate how this multichain protein is assembled and secreted and to understand how the process is regulated.

Molecular cloning of cDNA for each of the chains and translation of fibrinogen mRNA have established that the three component chains are synthesized by separate mRNA's (1-5). In vivo studies have indicated that the three chains are assembled into dimeric fibrinogen at an early stage of the secretory process, in the rough endoplasmic reticulum (ER) (6), but that assembly is not immediate and perhaps involves a series of intermediate steps. Analysis of the time course of secretion of rabbit fibrinogen showed that the specific radioactivity of the component chains of secreted fibrinogen differed and that the Bβ chain is first incorporated into fibrinogen followed nearly simultaneously by the Aα and γ chains (7). This suggested that intracellular pools of Aα and γ chains existed within the hepatocyte. We now present a hypothetical scheme for the assembly of fibrinogen from its component chains. For the most part, our proposal is based on interpretations of previously published results obtained by studying fibrinogen biosynthesis in Hep G2 cells, a human hepatocellular carcinoma (8,9).

Methods

Hep-G2 cells were "pulse" labelled with L-[^{35}S]methionine and "chase"

Fibrinogen - Fibrin Formation and Fibrinolysis, Vol. 4
© 1986 Walter de Gruyter & Co., Berlin · New York - Printed in Germany.

incubated with non-radioactive L-methionine. At various times, the cells and the incubation medium were separated and fibrinogen and other fibrinogen-related materials were isolated from each fraction by immunoprecipitation with a polyclonal antibody recognizing the intact molecule as well as its component chains. The radioactive proteins were separated by SDS-polyacrylamide gel electrophoresis (SDS-PAGE) and radioactivity determined. Prior to immunoprecipitation the cells were homogenized in the presence of 0.2M iodoacetamide, in order to block free sulfhydryl groups and minimize further disulfide interactions during the isolation procedure, and with detergents (to solubilize membranes and release membrane-enclosed fibrinogen). In some experiments the fibrinogen-related compounds, separated by SDS-PAGE, were excised, reduced and re-electrophoresed in order to determine the chain composition and the radioactivity of each component. These methods have been described in detail in previous studies (8,9).

Results and Discussion.

Intracellular forms of fibrinogen. Hep-G2 cells incubated with L-[^{35}S]methionine incorporate radioactivity into fibrinogen and seven other fibrinogen-related compounds. The fibrinogen-related compounds, which have smaller molecular sizes than intact fibrinogen, appear to be precursors of fibrinogen, since during a "chase" incubation with non-radioactive L-methionine, there is little or no change in the radioactivity of the total proteins in the immunoprecipitate, but there is a decline in the radioactivity of some of these compounds and an increase in that of fibrinogen. (See figure 1).

The identities of the various fibrinogen-related compounds in the immunoprecipitate were deduced by calculating the molecular sizes, based on migration on SDS-PAGE, and by reducing each of the isolated compounds, re-electrophoresing and identifying the component fibrinogen chains. The total immunoprecipitate, when reduced, only yields radioactive Aα, Bβ and γ chains of fibrinogen (8). It should be noted that under non-reducing conditions proteins may migrate aberrantly on SDS-PAGE. The chain composition of the various fibrinogen-related compounds was determined not only during the pulse-chase periods shown in figure 1, but also after 2 h of continous incubation with L-[^{35}S]methionine, a time at which all fibrinogen precursors and pools have been radiolabeled. A summary of the results is presented in Table I. The following intracellular radioactive compounds were identified: 1. Fibrinogen (band A); 2. Half-molecule of fibrinogen (band B); 3. An Aα - γ complex (band C); 4. A mixture of Bβ - Aα and Bβ - γ complexes (band D); 5. A complex of incomplete Bβ chains with complete Aα chains (band E); 6. Incomplete Bβ chains with complete γ chains; 7. Free Aα chains; 8. Free γ chains.

Table I

Size and Chain Composition of Intracellular Fibrinogen Precursors.

Bands on SDS-PAGE	Estimated Mr	Chain Composition
A	340,000	Aα, Bβ, γ
B	214,000	Aβ, Bβ, γ
C	140,000	Aα, γ
D	125,000	Mixture Bβ,γ & Bβ,Aα
E	113,000	Aα, Incomplete Bβ
F	102,000	γ, Incomplete Bβ
Aα	65,000	Aα
γ	45,000	γ

The Mr of the fibrinogen-related compounds were calculated based on the electrophoretic mobilities of the non-reduced materials. The chain compositions were deduced by excising each of the bands, reducing and re-electrophoresing them on SDS-PAGE as previously described (9).

Pools of Aα and γ chains. There are several lines of evidence which indicate that hepatocytes contain intracellular pools of Aα and γ chains. 1.) Rabbits injected with [^{75}Se]methionine, secrete fibrinogen whose component chains have different specific radioactivities. A kinetic analysis of secreted fibrinogen indicated that radioactive Bβ chain is first incorporated into rabbit fibrinogen and that nascent Aα and γ chain are added at a later time (7). 2) Pulse-chase studies with Hep G2 cells confirmed the above studies and also showed that within the cell pulse-labeled fibrinogen is first composed of radioactive Bβ chain and unlabelled Aα and γ chain and that later radioactive Aα chains followed by nascent γ chains are incorporated into fibrinogen (8). 3) More direct evidence was obtained by incubating Hep G2 cells with, L-[^{35}S]methionine and demonstrating the intracellular presence of an excess of free γ chains and of an Aα - γ complex (8,9). 4) At the end of a 6 h chase incubation, a time at which radioactive fibrinogen has virtually ceased to be secreted, Hep G2 cells still contain radioactive Aα - γ complex (9). 5) Western blot analysis, using a rabbit antibody to human fibrinogen, also showed that the three most abundant endogenous fibrinogen-related compounds are the Aα-γ complex, free γ chains and fibrinogen (10).

The pools of Aα and γ chain are probably produced by unequal synthesis of the fibrinogen chains since, in Hep G2 cells, the initial rates of synthesis are unequal with that of the Bβ chain being less than that of the Aα and γ chains(9). These data clearly indicate the presence of a pool of Aα and γ chains but we do not yet understand the interrelationship between the free Aα and γ chains and the Aα - γ complex.

Sequence of Assembly. The postulated order in which the individual polypeptide chains enter into fibrinogen is depicted in figs 2 and 3. The initial sequence by which the three components chain of fibrinogen interact with each other to form fibrinogen was determined by following the order in which the radioactivities of the pulse-labeled precursor forms of fibrinogen decrease during the "chase" incubation period. Following a 3 min pulse period, the radioactivities of bands E and F, which are composed of incomplete Bβ chains and preformed Aα chains (band E) and incomplete Bβ chains and γ chains (band F), are the first to decline(see Fig 1). These precursors are only found in polysomes and not in the lumen of the ER. In addition, treatment of Hep G2 cells with cyclohexamide arrests the further processing of these compounds, indicating that incomplete polypeptide chains are involved in fibrinogen assembly. Bands E and F, in addition to containing radioactive incomplete Bβ chains, were also shown to be comprised, during the pulse-period and at the earlier chase times, of unlabelled Aα or γ chains. Later during the chase period, when the incomplete Bβ chains are no longer radiolabeled, radioactive Aα and γ chains appear in these compounds. This suggests that preformed Aα and γ chains obtained from the intracellular pool, react with incomplete Bβ chains while they are still attached to polysomes (Step 2, Fig 3). In order for incomplete Bβ chains to react with preformed Aα and γ chains the incomplete Bβ chains would have to be of sufficient length to span both the large

Figure 1.

Pulse-chase incubation of Hep G2 cells with L-[^{35}S]methionine

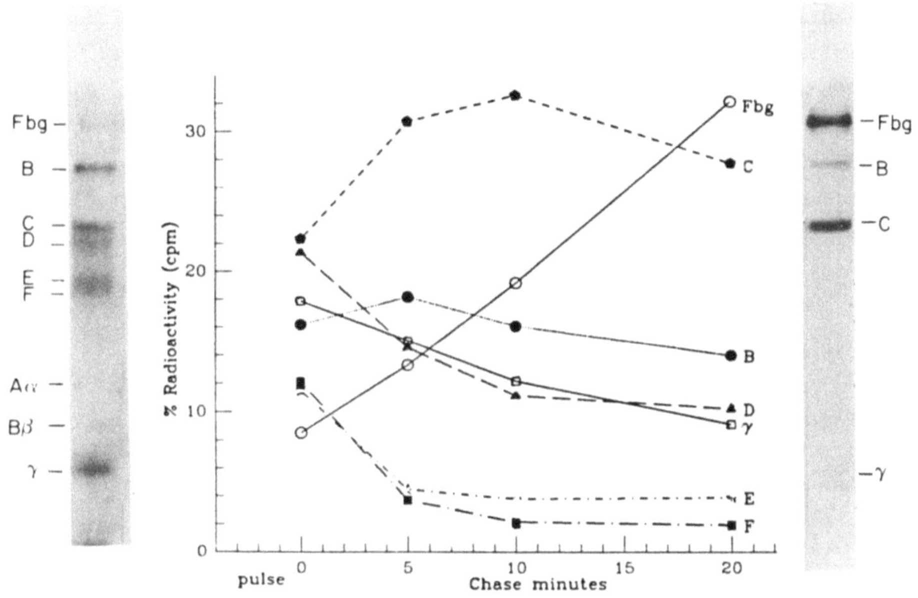

On the left is an autoradiogram of fibrinogen-related material, separated by SDS-PAGE at the end of a 3 min pulse period and on the right that at the end of a 20 min chase period. The radioactivities of the various fibrinogen-related compounds at various times of the incubation is given.

----

ribosomal subunit and the width of the ER membrane and to expose the N-terminal cysteine residues to the luminal surface of the ER. The first N-terminal cysteine residues of the Bβ chain are in positions 65, 76 and 80. In this regard it is of interest to note that polypeptides of less than 26,000 daltons were not detected as components of bands E and F, and that most incomplete Bβ chains found in bands E and F were between 27,000 and 32,000 daltons. These are sizes which are sufficiently large to meet the above criteria.

On completion of Bβ chain synthesis the Bβ - Aα and Bβ - γ complexes are released into the luminal side of the ER (step 3, fig 3) and the remainder of the assembly process occurs within this organelle. Fibrinogen assembly is rapid and some nascent fibrinogen can be noticed even at the end of a 3 min pulse period. In vivo we have shown the presence of the dimeric form of fibrinogen in the rough ER (6) and recent cell fractionation studies with Hep G2 cells also demonstrate the presence of nascent fibrinogen in this cell fraction (unpublished data).

Within the lumen of the rough ER the Bβ - Aα and Bβ - γ complexes are the earliest precursors. These compounds migrate together as a broad band on SDS-PAGE with an estimated molecular size of about 125,000 daltons (band D). During the "chase" incubation period the decline of their radioactivity closely follows that of the polysome-bound precursors (see fig 1). An analysis of their radioactive chain composition shows that at the end of the 3 min pulse period and at 5 min. of chase incubation only the Bβ chain is radioactive. The Aα and γ chains are unlabeled and are incorporated into these complexes from a pool of preformed chains. At later times of the chase period, radioactive Aα and γ chains appear and by 20 min. of chase incubation nearly all of their radioactive components have been replaced by nascent unlabeled chains, indicating that they are intermediates which are quickly converted to another form.

The next step in fibrinogen assembly appears to be the formation of a half molecule by the addition of a γ chain to the Bβ-Aα complex and an Aα chain to the Bβ-γ complex. (Step 4 Fig 3). The putative half-molecule (band B) is formed quickly (it is present at the end of a 3 min pulse), its radioactivity increases slightly at 5 min of the chase period and then declines slowly during the remainder of the chase period (Fig 1). An analysis of the radioactive chain composition of the half-molecule shows that it only contains radioactive Bβ chains at the end of the 3 min. pulse period, followed by increasing amounts of radioactive Aα, starting at 5 min of the chase period and continuing at 10 to 20 min. Finally, a radioactive γ chain appears in the half-molecule at 30 min. If the cells are incubated for 2 h with L-[^{35}S]methionine, to label the pool of Aα and γ chain, then band B contains equal amounts of radioactivity in all 3 chains. The estimated size of band B (based on its migration on SDS-PAGE) of 214,000 daltons (Table I) is higher than the 170,000 expected of a half-molecule, but as mentioned earlier non-reduced protein often migrate aberrantly on SDS-PAGE.

We suggest that the final step in fibrinogen assembly is the joining of two half-molecules by the formation of symmetrical bonds between two Aα and two γ chains(step 5, Fig 3). An indication that band B (the putative half-molecule) is an immediate precursor to fibrinogen was obtained by comparing the specific radioactivities of band B and fibrinogen at different times of the pulse-chase incubation. The radioactive chain composition of bands B and fibrinogen are similar but it appears that the nascent radioactive chains enter band B a few minutes before they appear in fibrinogen. For example, at the end of the pulse period the only radioactive component of both the half-molecule and fibrinogen is the Bβ chain. At 5 mins of the chase period radioactive Aα enters the half-molecule, but does not yet appear in fibrinogen. At 10 mins of the chase period radioactive Aα enters into fibrinogen. Similarly, radioactive γ chain enters into the half-molecule before it enters fibrinogen. There is a 30 min lag, following pulse incubation, before radioactive γ chains enter the half-molecule and the lag period is longer (40 to 50 mins) for fibrinogen.

Figure 2

Paths of individual fibrinogen chains

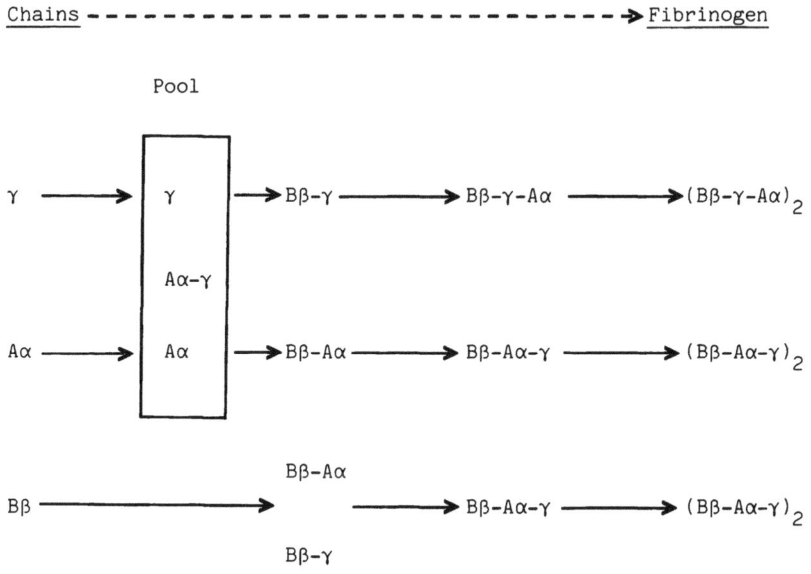

Sequential paths of individual chains. The fate of the individual chains, was determined by measuring at various times of the pulse-chase period, the radioactivities of each of the chains in the various fibrinogen-related compounds. This allowed us to calculate not only the sequence of events but what percent of each nascent chain is incorporated into each of the fibrinogen-related compounds at different times. An interpretation of the results is presented in Fig 2.

At the end of the pulse period over 80% of the γ chain radioactivity occurs as the free chain. During a 20 min chase period the percent radioactivity in the free γ chain drops to 50% and there is a concomitant increase in the radioactivity of γ chain in the Aα-γ complex. At the end of 20 min of the chase period about 80% of the γ chain radioactivity can be accounted for in these two forms, (free γ chain and the Aα-γ complex). These are thought to be the intracellular "pool" forms of the γ chain. γ chain radioactivity also appears in the incomplete Bβ-γ and the Bβ-γ complexes at early times, but in low amounts, less than 5% of the total γ chain radioactivity. Radioactive γ chains are not part of the half-molecule and of dimeric fibrinogen until 30 to 40 min of the chase period.

Radioactive Aα chains also quickly enters the pool of free chains and Aα-γ complex. At the end of the pulse period 20% of Aα chain radioactivity exists as the free chain and 60% is as the Aα-γ complex. This distribution is different to that of the γ chain, which as mentioned above was 80% as the free chain and only 5% as the Aα-γ chain complex at the same incubation period. This indicates that the Aα chain is more quickly converted to the Aα-γ complex than is the γ chain. This also suggests that Hep G2 cells may contain an an excess amount of γ chains. During a 20 min chase incubation period the amount of Aα chain radioactivity in the Aα-γ complex is relatively constant, but a number of other events are noticed. There is a sequential decline in free Aα chain radioactivity,quickly followed by a similar decline in Aα radioactivity of the Bβ-Aα complex. This leads to an increase Aα chain radioactivity of the half-molecule and then in Aα chain radioactivity of fibrinogen. This sequence of events is shown in Fig 2.

In marked contrast to the Aα and γ chains, nascent Bβ chains do not appear intracellularly as free chains. Radioactive Bβ chain is from the onset complexed to other fibrinogen chains. The majority(40%) of Bβ chain radioactivity, at the end of the pulse period, is in Bβ-Aα, and Bβ-γ complexes. During the chase period the Bβ radioactivity of these complexes quickly declines and appears sequentially in the half-molecule and in fibrinogen (9).

Figure 3

Scheme for the assembly of fibrinogen

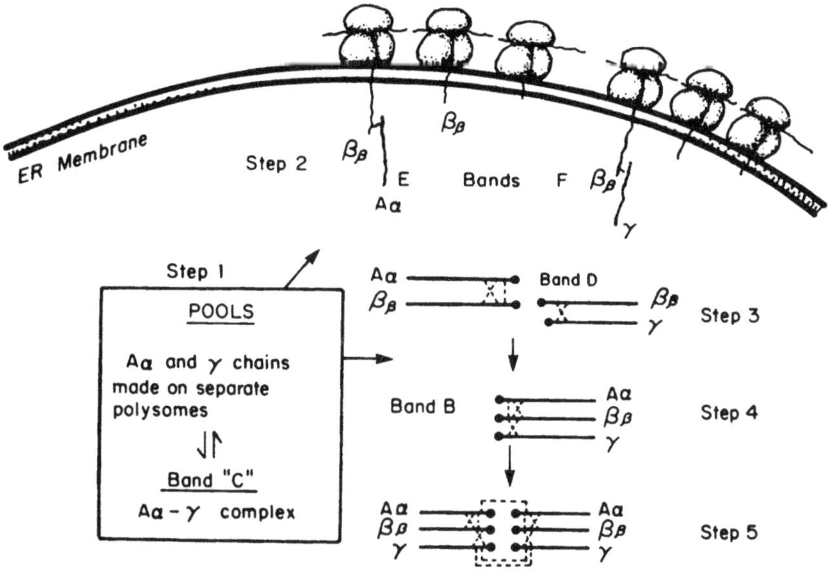

The above hypothetical scheme is based on studies of fibrinogen assembly in Hep G2 cells (8,9).

The mechanisms by which interchain disulfide bonds are formed need to be clarified. Fibrinogen assembly appears to be well ordered. For this to occur the correct segments of the 3 polypeptides chains have to be exposed and aligned in order to obtain the proper disulfide interactions. Doolittle has suggested that the driving force in assembly is the formation of coiled coils and disulfide rings (11). In order to determine whether the fibrinogen precursors contain free sulfhydryl groups we added [^{14}C]iodoacetamide to Hep G2 cell homogenates and isolated fibrinogen related materials. Most of the incorporation of radioactivity occurred in the Aα-γ complex with smaller amounts in the free γ chain. Free sulfhydryl groups were not detected in the other fibrinogen-related compounds (10). We do not know however whether this is a reflection of the fact that the cell contains large amounts of Aα-γ and free γ chains (as we have determined by Western blots) and that the other fibrinogen intermediates, which turn over rapidly, are only present in small amounts and therefore go undetected. A relatively weak incorporation of [^{14}C]iodoacetamide into free γ chain was observed and this may be because the free γ chain is folded by intrachain disulfide bonds. This is suggested by the observation that under non-reducing conditions the free γ chain migrates faster on SDS-PAGE than does the reduced γ chain. It is possible that just prior to its interaction with another chain, the free γ chain undergoes an enzyme mediated rearrangement allowing interchain disulfide reactions to occur. The same argument may be used to explain the lack of detection of free sulfhydryl groups, by [^{14}C]iodoacetamide incorporation, in the other fibrinogen related compounds.

The synthesis of the Bβ chain appears to be the limiting factor in the assembly of fibrinogen. It is the only component chain of fibrinogen which does not exist in "pool" form . This suggest that fibrinogen assembly may be easily regulated by modifying the rate of synthesis of the Bβ chains. However it should be noted that stimulation of rabbit fibrinogen synthesis did not change the relationship of the specific radioactivity of the component chains of secreted fibrinogen (7) and that studies by Crabtree and Kant (12) have shown an increase in the levels of mRNA for all 3 chains following the acute-phase response.

The Bβ and γ chains of fibrinogen are glycosylated and the oligosacclaride moieties are of the biantennary type (13,14). It is assumed that glycosylation of fibrinogen occurs in the same manner as described for other secretory glycoproteins and that processing is not completed in the endoplasmic reticulum and that the final touches such as terminal glycosylation, phosphosylation of the Aα chain and sulfation of the Bβ chain occurs in the Golgi complex. Previously we showed that nascent fibrinogen present in the rough endoplasmic reticulum of dog liver is not phosphorylated nor sulfated (6). Fibrinogen probably undergoes other processing steps whose cellular location has not yet been determined. For example, cDNA cloning studies indicate the Aα chain is first synthesized as a precursor with an extension at the carboxyl terminus (15) and since this Aα form is not detected in the plasma it is assumed that it is cleaved intracellularly.

References

1. Yu, S., Redman C. M., Goldstein, J., and Blomback, B. (1980) Biochem. Biophys. Res. Commun. 96, 1030-1038

2. Chung, D. W., MacGillivray, R.T.A., and Davie, W. E. (1980) Ann. N.Y. Acad. Sci. 343, 210-215

3. Nickerson, J. M., and Fuller, G. M. (1981) Proc. Natl. Acad. Sci. U.S.A. 78, 303-307

4. Crabtree, G. R., and Kant, J.A. (1981) J. Biol. Chem. 256, 9718-9723

5. Chung, D. W., Rixon, M. W., MacGillivray, R.T.A., and Davie, E. W. (1981) Proc. Natl. Acad. Sci. U.S.A. 78, 1466-1470

6. Kudryk, B., Okada, M., Redman, C. M., and Blomback, B. (1982) Eur. J. Biochem., 125, 673-682

7. Alving, B. M., Chung, S. I., Murano, G., Tang, D. B., and Finlayson,, J. S. (1982) Arch. Biochem. Biophys. 217, 1-9

8. Yu, S., Sher, B., Kudryk, B., and Redman, C. M. (1983) J. Biol. Chem. 258, 13407-13410

9. Yu, S., Sher, B., Kudryk, B. and Redman, C. M. (1984) J. Biol. Chem. 259, 10574-10581

10. Yu, S., and Redman C. M., (1985) Amer. Soc. Cell Biol; Abstracts.

11. Doolittle, R. F. (1984) In: Annual Review of Biochemistry, (C. R. Richardson, P.D. Boyer and A. Meister, eds.) Annual Reviews Inc., 195-229.

12. Crabtree, G. R., and Kant, J. A. (1982) J. Biol. Chem. 257, 7277-7279

13. Townsend, R.R., Hilliker, E., Li, Y.-T., Laine, R. A., Bell, W. R., and and Lee, Y.C. (1982) J. Biol. Chem. 257, 9704-9710

14. Mizuochi, T., Taniguchi, T., Asami, Y., Takamatsu, J., Okade, M., Iwanaga, S., and Kobata, A. (1982) J. Biochem. (Tokyo) 92, 283-293

15. Rixon, M. W., Chan, W. -Y., Davie, E. W., and Chung, D. W. (1983) Biochemistry 22, 3237-3244

EVIDENCE THAT PLATELET AND PLASMA FIBRINOGEN HAVE THE SAME A-ALPHA CHAIN GENE PRODUCT

Christopher Southan, Irina Knight, Helen Ireland and David A. Lane.

Department of Haematology, Charing Cross and Westminster Medical School, Hammersmith, London W6 8RP, UK.

Introduction

The fibrinogen circulating in plasma at a concentration of approximately 2.5 mg/ml, is synthesised in the hepatocytes. However, a separate intra cellular pool of fibrinogen exists within the alpha storage granules of the platelet. At a concentration of approximately 100 ug per 10^9 cells this has been estimated to be 12% of the total platelet protein and 3% of the total blood fibrinogen (1). Platelet fibrinogen may be functionally important in haemostasis because of the high local concentrations provided when stimulated platelets release their alpha granule contents.

Both the genetic origin and site of synthesis of platelet fibrinogen have been open questions because of many conflicting reports in the literature. Genetic variants of fibrinogen, where the heterozygous phenotype is readily detectable, are particularly suitable to confirm or disprove the hypothesis that plasma and platelet fibrinogen arise from the same set of structural genes. Fibrinogen Manchester (2) is a recently characterised variant with an Aα 16 Arg -> His substitution (3). Thrombin can release a variant form of fibrinopeptide A (FPA) with a C-terminal Histidine residue, [His^{16}]FPA, from fibrinogen purified from the plasma of patients who are heterozygous for this abnormality. Because this variant peptide can be detected by high performance liquid chromatography (HPLC) the possibility arose of establishing the presence or absence of this variant phenotype within the platelet fibrinogen pool and thereby addressing the question of the genetic origin of the two fibrinogen pools.

Methods

Although fibrinogen can be purified from the intraplatelet pool, this is associated with low yields, proteolytic degradation and co-purifying contaminants. We have been able to avoid all these problems by developing a method to directly analyse the fibrinopeptides derived from platelet fibrinogen (4). Platelets were prepared from plasma by differential centrifugation (5) and several methods were used to measure

Fibrinogen - Fibrin Formation and Fibrinolysis, Vol. 4
© 1986 Walter de Gruyter & Co., Berlin · New York - Printed in Germany.

the almost complete removal of plasma fibrinogen. The washed platelets were then lysed by freezing and thawing to release intracellular fibrinogen. After treating the lysate with thrombin, high molecular weight substances were removed by boiling, centrifugation and filtration. Samples were then injected onto an analytical reverse-phase HPLC column fitted with a pre-column. The HPLC conditions were basically those described by Kehl et al. (6). The fibrinopeptides from normal platelets and platelets from an affected family member of fibrinogen Manchester were analysed by this method together with plasma-derived fibrinopeptides as controls. The identity of FPA-related peaks was confirmed by analysing HPLC fractions with a specific FPA radioimmunoassay (RIA) (7).

Results

The HPLC analysis of a normal platelet lysate without thrombin treatment is shown in Fig 1(a). The general profiles including the large peaks eluting at 12 and 24 min were similar between preparations of platelets. The affect of adding thrombin to the platelet lysate is shown in (b) and new peaks can be seen eluting in identical positions to the fibrinopeptide standards (c). A clearer illustration of the thrombin-releasable peaks is shown in Fig.2 which is a sectional enlargement of two traces from Fig.1. The lower trace shows the platelet lysates without thrombin treatment and the upper trace the same lysate which has been treated with thrombin. Fibrinopeptides AP, A, AY and B were all clearly identifiable by their co-elution with fibrinopeptide standards. The peak eluting at 18.5 mins in trace (b) was shown by co-elution experiments not to be Des-Arg B and is therefore probably a thrombin releasable peptide unrelated to the fibrinopeptides.

From measurements of peak areas on chromatograms we were able to compare the proportions between the three types of A peptides derived from platelet fibrinogen and plasma fibrinogen of normal individuals. The % proportion of the total FPA of AY from platelets (mean $\pm$ SD, n=5) was 14.6$\pm$2.4% compared with 13.2$\pm$3.7% (n=18) for plasma fibrinogen. To check the completeness of fibrinopeptide release the FPA:FPB ratios were determined and found to be 1.10 $\pm$ 0.13 for platelet compared with 1.03 $\pm$ 0.09 for plasma fibrinogen. The only suggested difference for platelet fibrinogen was an increase in the phosphorylated form of FPA, 28.2$\pm$2.5% compared with 18.9$\pm$4.2% for plasma fibrinogen. Quantitative HPLC analysis also provided a new method of determining platelet fibrinogen content. The FPB peak sizes were compared with those released from a standard fibrinogen solution. From the platelet counts we obtained a result (mean$\pm$SD, n=5) of 90$\pm$30 ug per 10^9 platelets. This was in good agreement with the value of 110$\pm$30 ug using a fragment E radioimmunoassay and both measurements fall within the wider range reported in the literature (1).

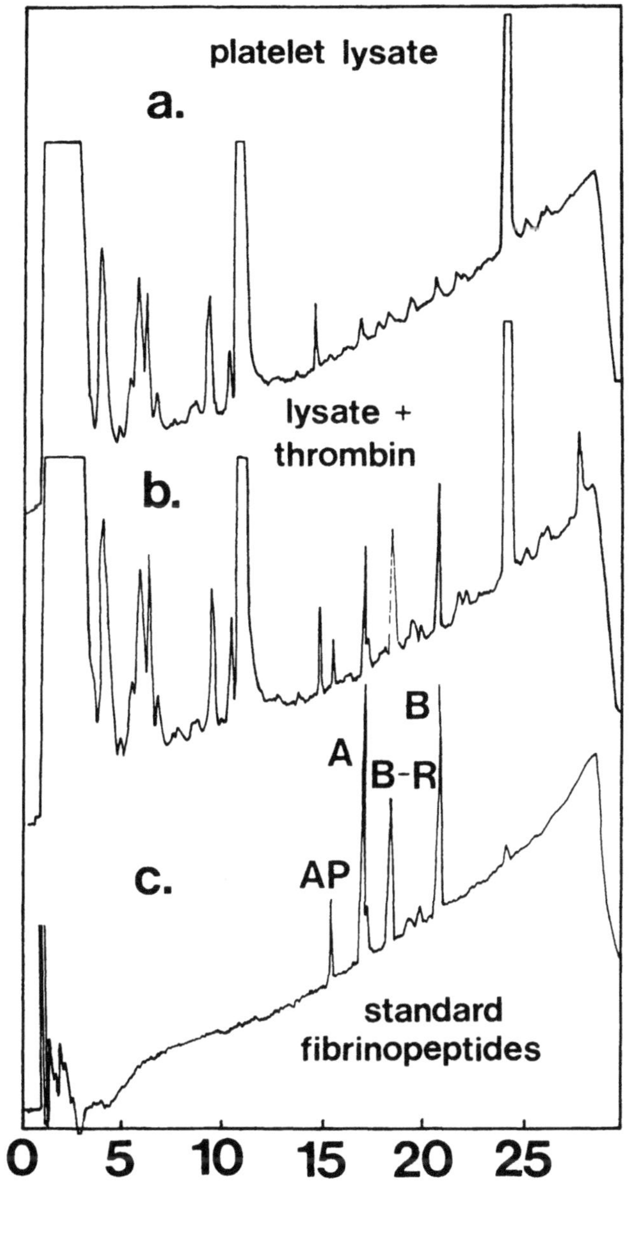

Figure 1: HPLC analysis of normal platelet extracts. These were analysed (a) before and (b) after thrombin treatment. The vertical axis is the absorbance at 210 nm and the horizontal axis the elution time in minutes. The injected sample of lysate was derived from 6 x 10^8 platelets. The gradient was 0% B increasing linearly to 40% B in 25 mins with a flow rate of 1.5 ml/min. The absorbance units full-scale was 0.08. Control fibrinopeptides (c) were 10 ul of supernatant from a 7.6 mg/ml plasma fibrinogen solution clotted with thrombin. The identity of each fibrinopeptide species is indicated according to Kehl et al. (6). [Reprinted by permission from The Biochemical Journal, Vol 229, pp 723-730. Copyright (c) 1985, The Biochemical Society, London]

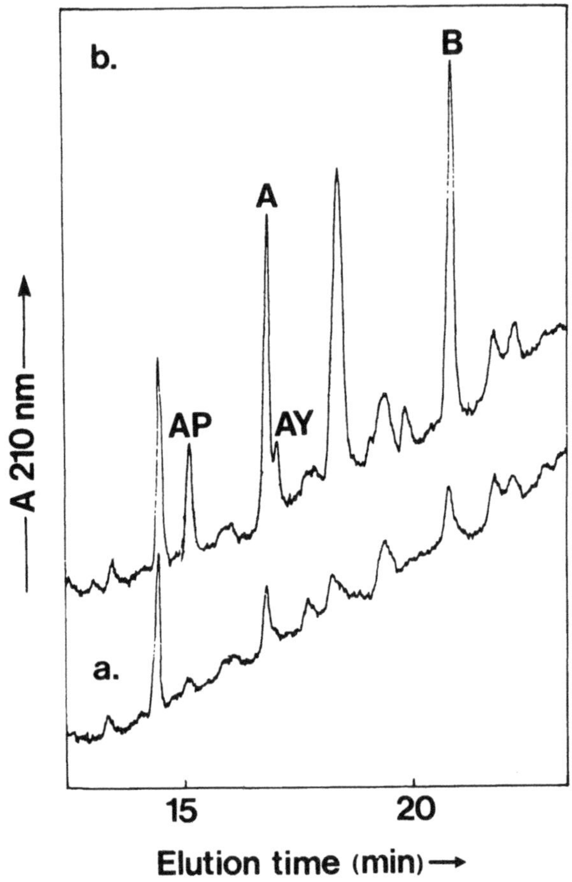

Figure 2: Sectional enlargements of HPLC traces of thrombin treated and non-treated platelet extracts. These are identical to traces in Fig. 1 (a) and (b) but are enlargements of the elution profiles between 12 and 22 min elution time. Thrombin treatment was 200 u/ml for 10 mins at room temperature. [Reprinted by permission from The Biochemical Journal, Vol 229, pp 723-730. Copyright (c) 1985, The Biochemical Society, London]

The HPLC analysis carried out with platelets from an affected family member with fibrinogen Manchester is shown in Fig.3a, together with control fibrinopeptides, derived from plasma fibrinogen Manchester, Fig. 3b. The general pattern of extra peaks for all the A peptides containing C-terminal histidine instead of arginine is the same as that already published for plasma fibrinogen Manchester (3). A similar pattern can be seen in the fibrinopeptides derived from the platelets. The presence of both normal and $[His^{16}]$FPA is indicated both by peaks with elution times corresponding to FPA and $[His^{16}]$FPA and by the area ratio between these two peaks.

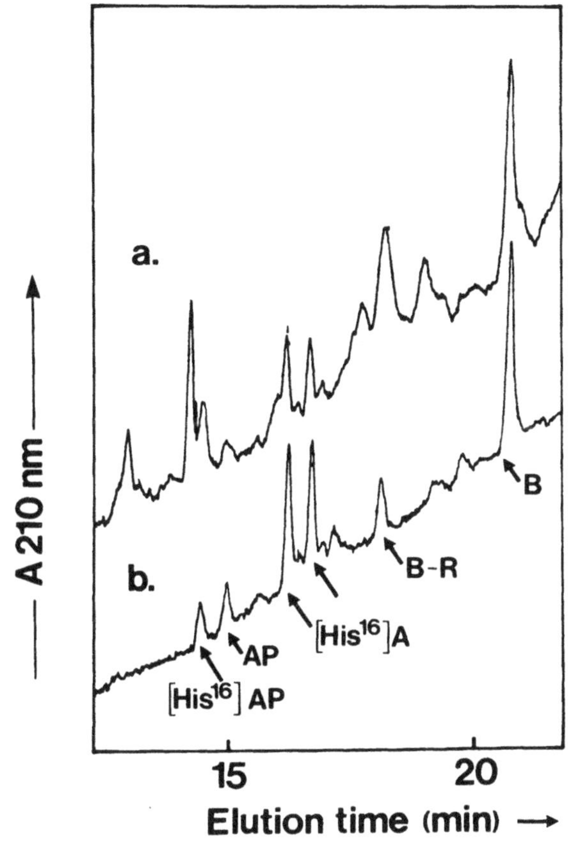

Figure 3: HPLC analysis of a thrombin treated platelet lysate from a family member with fibrinogen Manchester. This is shown in trace (a) and the fibrinopeptides released from a sample of plasma fibrinogen purified from a family member are shown in trace (b). These traces are sectional enlargements between 12 and 22 min elution time. The sample for trace (a) was derived from approximately 4 x 10^8 platelets and for trace (b) 10 ul of supernatant from thrombin treated plasma fibrinogen at a concentration of 3 mg/ml. [Reprinted by permission from The Biochemical Journal, Vol 229, pp 723-730. Copyright (c) 1985, The Biochemical Society, London]

In order to confirm the identities of the peaks released from the platelet we employed a radioimmunoassay specific for FPA where the immunological specificity is directed against the C-terminal end of the peptide (7). Our previous studies on fibrinogen Manchester have already shown that the presence of a C-terminal histidine residue in the abnormal FPA lowers the immunoreactivity towards some FPA antisera (8). From the results shown in Fig. 4 we were able to demonstrate the same differences in immunoreactivity in fibrinopeptides released from platelet lysates.

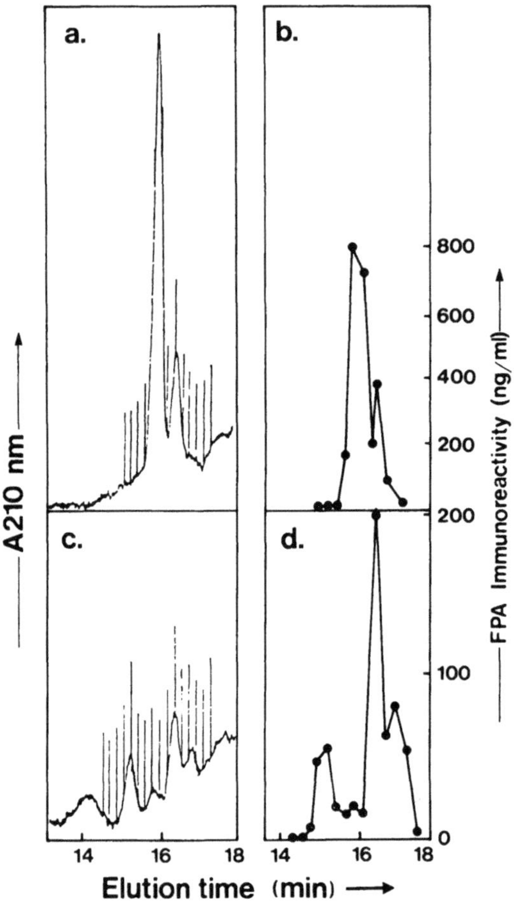

Figure 4: HPLC analysis of thrombin treated platelet lysates and parallel radioimmunoassay. The HPLC trace in (a) shows the FPA peak from normal platelets. The vertical lines mark the fractions collected at 20 second intervals. In (b) is illustrated a plot of FPA immunoreactivity in the HPLC fractions collected from the experiment (a). The corresponding analysis from the platelets of the family member of fibrinogen Manchester is shown in the trace (c) and the plot of FPA immunoreactivity from the HPLC fractions in (d). [Reprinted by permission from The Biochemical Journal, Vol 229, pp 723-730. Copyright (c) 1985, The Biochemical Society, London]

The normal platelet control HPLC trace of the FPA section, Fig.4a, clearly shows two immunoreactive peaks corresponding to the elution positions of FPA and AY, Fig. 4b. Analysis of peptides derived from platelets from the family with fibrinogen Manchester revealed that the peaks eluting prior to normal FPA and AY had the same reduced immunoreactivity as the [His^{16}]FPA and [His^{16}]AY obtained from plasma fibrinogen.

Discussion

This work demonstrates that fibrinopeptides derived from platelet fibrinogen can be quantitated by HPLC techniques using as little as 20 ml of platelet-rich plasma. The observed increased proportion of FPAP in the platelet has also been recently reported by Leeksma (9) and this may reflect some protection of the intracellular fibrinogen against phosphatase activity. Precise determinations of the normal and abnormal fibrinopeptides of plasma fibrinogens Manchester (2) and Sydney I (10), has established a symmetrical heterozygous phenotype (i.e. a normal:abnormal peptide ratio of 1:1) for both these cases of an Aa Arg->His substitution and this is consistant with a single genetic locus for the plasma Aa chain. The demonstration in this work of the same symmetrical phenotype in platelet fibrinogen is evidence that the plasma and platelet Aa chains are products of a single gene. Extension of this conclusion to all three genes is provided in a recent study of fibrinogen Oslo I (altered charge on Bb chain) and Oslo III (extended Y chain) which were detected in both the plasma and platelet pools (11). More direct evidence is provided by two studies that have mapped single copies of all three genes to a specific locus on human chromosome 4 (12,13).

Some earlier studies are in apparent contradiction with the single-gene hypothesis. In the homozygous case of fibrinogen Metz, an Aa16 Arg->Cys substitution (14), the failure to detect this abnormality in the platelet was based upon small differences in electrophoretic mobility which may have been caused by the problems of isolating platelet fibrinogen (15). Alternative explanations may also apply for the absence of the extended Y chains of fibrinogen Paris I from the platelet (16), including tissue-specific differences in mRNA processing or the exclusion of extended Y chains from packaging into alpha granules.

This work was supported by a grant from the Wellcome Trust to D.A.Lane. We would like thank Jill Bottomley of the Manchester Royal Infirmary for blood collection and the member of the fibrinogen Manchester family, S.J., for her cooperation.

References

1. Niewiarowski, S. 1977. Thrombos. Haemostas. 38, 924-934.

2. Lane D.A., Van Ross, M., Kakkar, V.V., Bottomley, J., Dhir, E., Holt L.P.J. and MacIver, J.E. 1980. Brit. J. Haematol. 46, 84-98.

3. Southan, C., Kehl, M., Henschen, A., and Lane, D.A. 1983. Brit. J. Haematol. 54, 143-151.

4. Southan, C., Knight, I., Ireland, H., Bottomley, J., and Lane, D.A. 1985. Biochemical Journal, 229, 723-730.

5. Broekman, M.J., Westmoreland, N.P. and Cohen, P. 1974. J. Cell Biol. 60, 507-519.

6. Kehl, M., Lottspeich, F. and Henschen, A. 1981. Hoppe-Seyler's Z Physiol. Chem. 362, 1661-1664.

7. Nossel, H.L., Yudelman, I., Canfield, R.E., Butler, V.P., Spandonis, K., Wilner, G.D. and Quereshi, G.D. 1974. J. Clin. Invest. 54 43-53.

8. Lane, D.A., Southan, C., Ireland, H., Thompson, E., Kehl, M. and Henschen, A. 1983. Brit. J. Haemtol. 53, 587-597.

9. Leeksma et al., this volume.

10. Southan, C., Lane, D.A. Bode, W. and Henschen, A. 1985. Eur. J. Biochem. 147, 593-600.

11. Teige, B., Gogstadt, G., Brosstadt, F. and Olaisen, B. 1985. Blood, 65, 120-126.

12. Henry,I., Uzan, G., Weil, D., Nicolas, H., Kaplan, J.C., Marguerie, G., Kahn, A. and Junien, C. 1984. Am. J. Hum. Genet. 36, 760-768.

13. Kant, J.A., Crabtree, G.R. and McBride, W. 1984. Cytogenet. Cell. Genet. 37, 503-510.

14. Southan, C., Henschen, A. and Lottspeich, F. 1982 In: Fibrinogen - Recent Biochemical and Medical Aspects. (Henschen, A., Graeff, H. and Lottspeich, F. eds.) Walter de Gruyter, Berlin.New York. pp. 153-166,

15. Soria, J., Soria, C., Samama, M., Poirot, E., and Kling, C. 1976. Path. Biol. 24, 15-17.

16. Jandrot-Perrus, N., Mosesson, M.W., Denninger, M.H. and Menache, D. 1979. Blood 54, 1109-1115.

FIBRINOPEPTIDE A AND THE PHOSPHORYLATION OF FIBRINOGEN

O.C. Leeksma, F.M. Meijer-Huizinga and J.A. van Mourik

Central Laboratory of the Netherlands Red Cross Blood Transfusion Service, Amsterdam, The Netherlands.

INTRODUCTION

Fibrinogen in normal human plasma is phosphorylated for about 30% at position Ser 3 of the Aα chain (1). We have observed that in patients with elevated fibrinopeptide A (FPA) levels as much as 80% of the fibrinogen molecules may be phosphorylated at this site (2). Since anticoagulant treatment resulted in a normalization of the extent of phosphorylation of fibrinogen in these patients (2), our results suggest that blood clotting activation may be associated with a high phosphate content of fibrinogen. High fibrinogen turnover rates in these clinical conditions could explain our observations, provided that newly synthesized fibrinogen is fully phosphorylated. Therefore, we examined the extent of phosphorylation of fibrinogen synthesized by hepatocytes as well as that of megakaryocyte-derived platelet fibrinogen. Since evidence was obtained that newly synthesized fibrinogen may indeed be highly phosphorylated, a formula is proposed which allows for an estimation of the t½ of fibrinogen by its AP peptide content.

TABLE I

Fibrinogen synthesis by cultured hepatocytes*

Concentration μg/ml	Percentage FPA-P / Total FPA
1.5 ± 1.4	87.7 ± 4.4

*24-h conditioned medium obtained on days 1 or 2 from four different primary cultures of normal human hepatocytes isolated as will be described in detail elsewhere (3), plated at a density of 10^6 cells/ml and cultured in Williams Medium E supplemented with 10% FCS, 2 mM L-glutamine, porcine insulin 20 mU/ml and dexamethason 50 nM (provided by Drs. Yap and Moshage, Dept. of Gastroenterology, University of Nijmegen, The Netherlands). Fibrinogen production and AP peptide content were quantitated by treating 5-ml aliquots of medium for 30 min at 37°C with 0.5 U of human thrombin per ml (3000 U/mg, Sigma) and analyzing the released A peptide material by HPLC combined with radioimmunoassay of FPA. Data are expressed as mean ± SD.

Fibrinogen - Fibrin Formation and Fibrinolysis, Vol. 4
© 1986 Walter de Gruyter & Co., Berlin · New York - Printed in Germany.

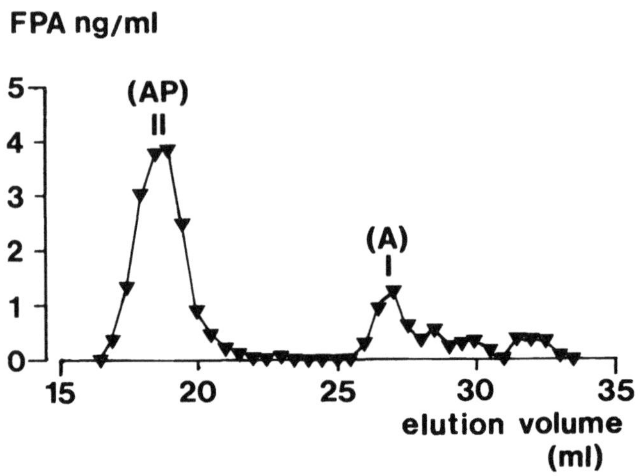

Fig. 1 - HPLC profile of fibrinopeptide A immunoreactivity released by thrombin from fibrinogen in 2 ml of medium conditioned for 24 h by normal human hepatocytes (Table I). Samples were processed for HPLC and run in an ammonium-acetate buffer on a reversed-phase C18 column. Peptides were eluted with a shallow acetonitrile gradient; fractions were tested by radioimmunoassay with anti-FPA antiserum R44656. Procedures are described in detail elsewhere (2).

AP peptide content in fibrinogen synthesized by hepatocytes in vitro

Fig. 1 shows an analysis by high-performance liquid chromatography (HPLC) of the AP peptide content of fibrinogen synthesized *in vitro* by primary cultures of normal human hepatocytes. Fibrinogen from hepatocyte-conditioned medium was found to be over 85% phosphorylated at position Aα Ser 3 (Table I).

AP peptide content in platelet fibrinogen

Fibrinogen in platelets is derived from megakaryocytes (4,5). As platelet α granules might therefore contain newly synthesized 'virgin' fibrinogen, we decided to analyze the fibrinopeptide AP content in platelet fibrinogen. Triton X-100 lysates of washed normal platelets were treated with thrombin and the released A peptide material was analyzed by HPLC combined with radioimmunoassays of fibrinopeptide A. An example of such an analysis is shown in Fig. 2A.

Fig. 2B shows the elution profile of material from the same washed platelet preparation incubated with thrombin without prior lysis with Triton. Triton had no effect on total FPA immunoreactivity recovered, but a significant effect on the FPA-P total FPA ratio, as illustrated in Table II.

A formula to estimate the $t_{1/2}$ of fibrinogen by its AP peptide content

Since our studies using hepatocytes and platelets suggested that newly syn-

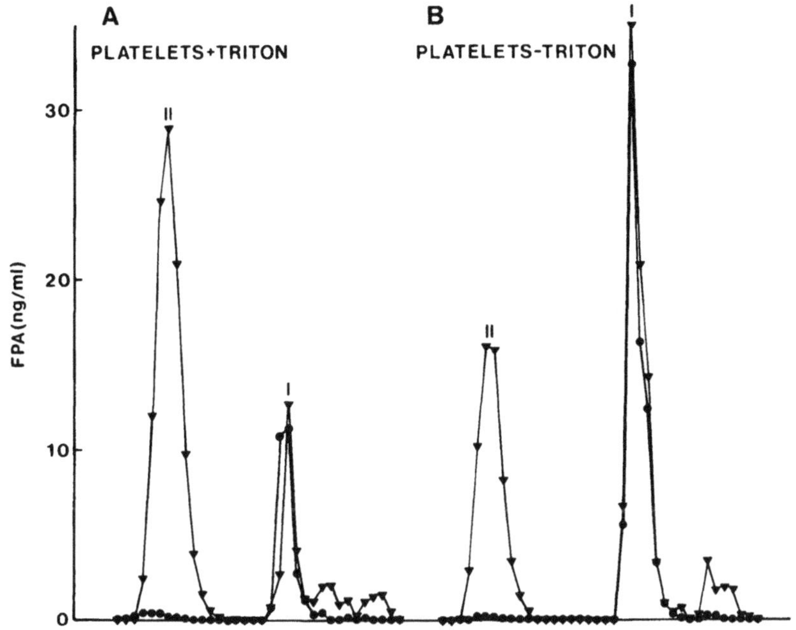

Fig. 2 - HPLC analysis of fibrinopeptide A immunoreactivity in extracts from thrombin-treated washed normal platelets. Platelets were obtained by differential centrifugation at 4°C from blood containing 4 mM EDTA and button washed 5 times in an ice-cold TENA buffer (0.01 M Tris, 0.01 M Na_2 EDTA, 0.15 M NaCl, pH 7.4). After the final wash, platelets were gently resuspended, and 150 µl of 0.1 M glycine, 0.038 M Tris, pH 8.7, with or without 0.5% Triton-X 100 (Koch--Light), were added to 50 µl of platelet suspension (usually about $5x10^9$/ml). Five µl of human thrombin (3000 U/mg, Sigma) were added (f.c. 12.5 U/ml). After a 5-min incubation period at 37°C, 0.025 ml β-glycerophosphate (Sigma, 100 mM, f.c.), and 0.025 ml of an anticoagulant mixture of citrate, heparin and Trasylol® were added. All further procedures (ethanol precipitation and processing) for HPLC as described (2) were performed in the cold. HPLC fractions were tested by radioimmunoassay with 2 different anti-FPA antisera R6216 (●–●) and R44656 (▼–▼), one of which (R6216) reacts poorly with FPA-P (2).

TABLE II

Effect of Triton-X 100 on the AP peptide content in platelet fibrinogen

	+	-
Fibrinogen (µg/10^9 platelets)*	66.3 ± 25.3	68.6 ± 27.2
Percentage AP/total A + AP	74.2 ± 7.6	33.3 ± 16

*As calculated from thrombin-released FPA immunoreactivity. Values are expressed as mean ± SD. Data are from 4 different donors. Difference in fibrinogen concentrations in platelets treated with or without Triton is not significant; the difference in AP peptide content is significant ($p < 0.005$, paired t test). From one of the 4 donors, the AP peptide content in platelet fibrinogen was tested in blood samples obtained on 3 different occasions. Values ranged from 56 to 80.4% (mean 65.8%)

thesized fibrinogen was fully phosphorylated at position Aα Ser 3, we wondered whether the AP peptide content in fibrinogen in plasma from a given individual was a reflection of the $t\frac{1}{2}$ of fibrinogen in that individual. In other words, we asked ourselves if one could estimate the turnover rate of fibrinogen in individuals based on the AP peptide content in their plasma fibrinogen.

A formula allowing for such an estimation was devised as follows. The total fibrinogen population (P) in any given individual can be considered to consist of an endless number of portions of fibrinogen each synthesized within the same arbitrary time period, for instance one hour. As fibrinogen has a certain half life ($t\frac{1}{2}$), the more time passes after this one-hour period of synthesis, the more fibrinogen molecules from a given portion will have disappeared. This phenomenon can be expressed mathematically as follows:

$$^{2}\log \frac{Po}{Pt} = \frac{\Delta t}{t\frac{1}{2}} \rightarrow Pt = Po.2^{-\Delta t/t\frac{1}{2}} \rightarrow Pt = Po\ (2^{-1/t\frac{1}{2}})^{\Delta t},$$

in which Po denotes the amount of fibrinogen originally synthesized in one hour (= fibrinogen synthesis per hour or p), and Pt the amount of fibrinogen that is left after a certain time period t has passed since the moment of synthesis. The total fibrinogen population at any given time will consist of:

$$P_0 = p.(2^{-1/t\frac{1}{2}})^0;\ P_1 = p.(2^{-1/t\frac{1}{2}})^1;\ P_2 = p.(2^{-1/t\frac{1}{2}})^2;\ \text{etc.}$$

$$P_\infty = p.(2^{-1/t\frac{1}{2}})^\infty.$$

Mathematics tells us that the sum of a given mathematical array $br^0+br^1+br^2+.....br^{n-1}$ is:

$$b.\ \frac{1-r^n}{1-r}$$

(provided $r < 1$). Therefore, the following equation can be applied for the fibrinogen population as a whole:

$$\text{sum} = p.\ \frac{1-(2^{-1/t\frac{1}{2}})^\infty}{1-2^{-1/t\frac{1}{2}}} = p.\ \frac{1}{1-2^{-1/t\frac{1}{2}}},\ \text{(formula I)},$$

introducing 96 h for the $t\frac{1}{2}$ of fibrinogen [a value well within the range generally accepted in the literature (6)]; total fibrinogen = 139 x p.

If one assumes that: 1 fibrinogen is synthesized as phosphorylated fibrinogen, 2 the transition of phosphorylated to unphosphorylated fibrinogen has a half life $T\frac{1}{2}$, and 3 phosphorylated and unphosphorylated fibrinogen have the same $t\frac{1}{2}$, the $T\frac{1}{2}$ of the phosphate groups can be determined as follows:

$$^{2}\log \frac{A_0}{At} = \frac{\Delta T}{T\frac{1}{2}} \rightarrow At = A_o.2^{-\Delta T}/T\frac{1}{2}$$

in which A_0 represents the phosphate in fibrinogen at the time of synthesis, which equals 1 (or 100%) and in which At denotes the phosphate in fibrinogen after a time period t has passed since the moment of synthesis. Because every fibrinogen "portion" P will have its own phosphate content:

$$P_0 = p.(2^{-1/t\frac{1}{2}})^0 .1.(2^{-1/T\frac{1}{2}})^0$$

$$P_1 = p.(2^{-1/t\frac{1}{2}})^1 .1.(2^{-1/T\frac{1}{2}})^1, \text{ etc.}$$

Total phosphate in the fibrinogen population as a whole can be expressed as follows:

$$\text{sum} = p. \frac{1 - \{ (2^{-1/t\frac{1}{2}}) (2^{-1/T\frac{1}{2}}) \}^{\infty}}{1 - (2^{-1/t\frac{1}{2}}) (2^{-1/T\frac{1}{2}})}, \text{ (formula II).}$$

As about 33% of the fibrinogen molecules in normals are phosphorylated at position Aα Ser 3 (1,2), total phosphate in fibrinogen (at position Aα Ser 3) can be calculated also by using formula I:

$$\frac{p}{1-2^{-1/t\frac{1}{2}}} .a$$

in which a represents the percentage phosphorylated fibrinogen as determined by HPLC (a will be between 0 and 1 = 0 and 100%). Normally, total phosphate =

$$\frac{p}{1-2^{-1/96}} .0.33 = 139.0.33.p$$

$$\rightarrow p. \frac{1-(2^{-1/96})^{\infty} (2^{-1/T\frac{1}{2}})^{\infty}}{1-(2^{-1/96}) (2^{-1/T\frac{1}{2}})} = 139.0.33.p \rightarrow$$

$$\frac{1}{1-(2^{-1/96}) (2^{-1/T\frac{1}{2}})} = 45.87 \rightarrow$$

$T\frac{1}{2} = 46.8$ h

A fourth assumption is now needed to determine the t½ of fibrinogen, in a given individual, based on its AP peptide content (a), namely that T½ (the half life of the phosphate groups) remains constant, i.e. is independent of t½. To illustrate this:

$$\text{total phosphate} = \frac{p}{1-2^{-1/t\frac{1}{2}}} .a = p. \frac{1}{1-(2^{-1/t\frac{1}{2}}) (2^{-1/T\frac{1}{2}})} \rightarrow$$

$$2^{-1/T\frac{1}{2}} = \frac{2^{-1/t\frac{1}{2}} + a-1}{a.2^{-1/t\frac{1}{2}}}$$

Fig. 3A shows a graphical display of this relationship between t½ and T½, using different values for a, whereas in Fig. 3B the relation between the degree of

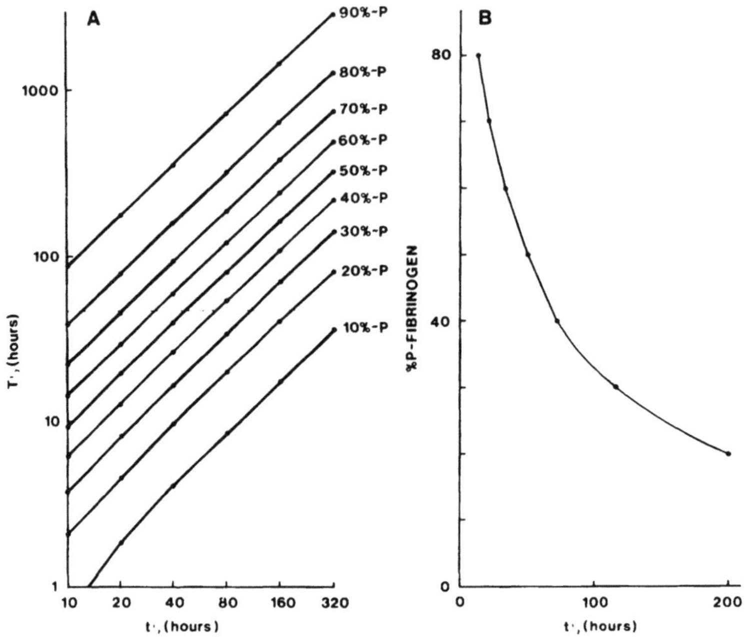

Fig. 3 - (A) Half life of the phosphate groups in fibrinogen (T½) as a function of the extent of phosphorylation of fibrinogen (expressed as percentage of P--fibrinogen) at different values for the half life (t½) of fibrinogen. (B) Relationship between the extent of phosphorylation of fibrinogen and the t½ of fibrinogen at a fixed half life of the phosphate groups (T½) of 46.8 h.

phosphorylation of total fibrinogen (as measured for instance by HPLC) and t½ of fibrinogen is depicted assuming that T½ is constant (= 46.8 h).

DISCUSSION

Our knowledge on the regulation of the degree of phosphorylation of fibrinogen in humans is still limited. In fact, although the data presented in this report are all in agreement with a concept proposed several years ago, in which a relationship between the phosphate content of fibrinogen and its half life in the circulation is suggested (7), they do not provide any proof for the actual existence of such a relationship. It is not excluded that factors which may cause a decrease in the t½ of fibrinogen, like *in-vivo* thrombin in activity (8), also have a stimulatory effect on fibrinogen phosphorylation, implying that an increased AP peptide content in plasma fibrinogen need not be caused by the presence of relatively more young fibrinogen in the circulation. It is evident that firm proof of a true relationship between the phosphate content of plasma fibrinogen and fibrinogen turnover is hard to obtain. Even studies currently performed in our laboratory, in which I^{125} fibrinogen kinetics are compared with the extent of phosphorylation of the protein, can only provide additional circumstantial evidence. The formula we propose to estimate the t½ of fibrinogen based on the phosphopeptide content of the protein may not be applicable to all patients, for instance because of large differences in the T½ of the phosphate groups.

The results of our studies using *in-vitro* cultures of normal human hepatocytes indicate that hepatocytes are indeed capable of synthesizing highly phosphorylated fibrinogen under certain experimental conditions. Interestingly, preliminary data from recent experiments using a human hepatoma cell line [Alexander PLC/PRF/5 (9)] suggest that this property may be lost upon transformation, because less than 1% of the fibrinogen molecules in medium conditioned by this hepatoma was found to be phosphorylated (unpublished observation).

As for our results with platelets, we feel that the data should still be interpreted with some caution as far as their proof that fibrinogen present within the platelet *in vivo* is really highly phosphorylated. Platelets are capable of actively phosphorylating fibrinogen (10) at position Aα Ser 3 (Leeksma and Meijer-Huizinga, unpublished observations). In spite of the efforts we have made in additional experiments (not shown here) to prevent such a reaction from occurring, it is difficult to fully exclude this possibility.

The positive effect of Triton-X 100 on the percentage phosphorylated FPA recovered from thrombin-treated washed platelets is poorly understood at the moment. Our working hypothesis is that this detergent at the concentration used impairs platelet β-glycerophosphatase activity. Although the mean percentage of FPA-P from total A peptide material released from non-detergent-treated washed platelets is still somewhat higher than that released from paired plasma, it is not clear at present whether *in-vivo* platelet fibrinogen reaches the platelet surface in its native, possibly highly phosphorylated state. Phosphorylated fibrinogen has been reported to clot faster (11), perhaps due to an enhanced binding of thrombin as a result of the phosphate group at position Aα Ser 3 (12). One could speculate therefore the presence of highly phosphorylated fibrinogen at the platelet surface, perhaps resulting from a selective release of α granules (that is without a concomittant release of acid hydrolases), to have an accelerating effect on clot formation. Validation of these and other considerations awaits further study.

Another issue which deserves attention is proteolysis of platelet fibrinogen (fibrinopeptides) by (platelet) proteases (13,14). It is very unlikely that proteolysis is responsible for the high AP peptide content in platelet fibrinogen observed in the present study, in view of the virtual absence of fragments of the A peptide in some analyses, as tested by radioimmunoassay with 2 different anti-FPA antisera (Fig. 2) and in view of the fairly good intra-individual reproducibility, which appeared to be independent of the extent of degradation of the A peptide seen on chromatograms (not shown). Proteolysis was observed under the conditions used however, and we have thus far been unable to get a firm grip on this phenomenon.

ACKNOWLEDGEMENTS

We gratefully acknowledge the "mathematical" help of Dr. H. van Heugten. This study was supported by grant no CLB 81-8 from the Netherlands Cancer Foundation (Koningin Wilhelmina Fonds).

REFERENCES

1. Blombäck, B., M. Blombäck, P. Edman and B. Hessel. 1966. Human fibrinopeptides. Isolation, characterization and structure. *Biochim. Biophys. Acta*. 115:371-396.
2. Leeksma, O.C., F.M. Meijer-Huizinga, E.A. Stoepman-van Dalen, C.J.W. van Ginkel, W.G. van Aken and J.A. van Mourik. 1985. Fibrinopeptide A and the phosphate content of fibrinogen in venous thromboembolism and disseminated intravascular coagulation. Submitted for publication.
3. Leeksma, O.C., H.J. Moshage, F. Meijer-Huizinga, J.A. van Mourik and S.M. Yap. 1985. Manuscript in preparation.
4. Belloc, F., P. Hourdille, P. Fialon, M.R. Boisseau and J. Soria. 1985. Fibrinogen synthesis by megakarocyte rich human marrow cell concentrates. *Thromb. Res.* 341:352.
5. Levene, R.M., P.K. Schick and A.Z. Budzynski. 1985. Fibrinogen biosynthesis in isolated guinea pig megakaryocytes. *Blood* 65:501-504.
6. Verstraete, M. and J. Vermylen. 1984. Blood Coagulation. in: *Thrombosis*, Pergamon Press, Oxford, pp 21-26.
7. Shainoff, J.R., P.G. Dyment, G.C. Hoffman and F.M. Bumpus. 1972. Fibrinopeptide composition in relationship to age of fibrinogen. *Circulation* 46 (Suppl. II), 52 (Abstr.).
8. Harker, L.A. and S.J. Slichter. 1972. Platelet and fibrinogen consumption in man. *New Engl. J. Med.* 287:999-1005.
9. Alexander, J.J., E.M. Bey, E.W. Geddes and G. Lecatasar. 1976. Establishment of a continuously growing cell line from primary carcinoma of the liver. *S. Afr. Med. J.* 50:2124-2128.
10. Krust, B., J. Galabru and A.G. Hovanessian. 1983. Phosphorylation of the α chain of fibrinogen by a platelet kinase activity enhanced by interferon. *Biochem. Biophys. Res. Commun.* 117:350-357.
11. Blombäck, B., M. Blombäck and J. Searle. 1963. On the occurrence of phosphorus in fibrinogen. *Biochim. Biophys. Acta* 74:148-151.
12. Hanna, L.S., H.A. Scheraga, Ch.W. Francis and V.J. Marder. 1984. Comparison of structures of various human fibrinogens and a derivative thereof by a

study of the kinetics of release of fibrinopeptides. *Biochemistry* 23:4681--4687.

13. Ganguly, P. 1969. Effect of proteolytic activity on the isolation and stability of platelet proteins. *Clin. Chim. Acta* 25:371-378.

14. Teige, B., G. Gogstad, F. Brosstad and B. Olaisen. 1985. Common structural genes for platelet and plasma fibrinogen. *Blood* 65:120-126.

II. Structure and Function

SIZE AND SHAPE OF THE FIBRINOGEN MOLECULE: CRYSTALLINE FORMS OF NATIVE AND MODIFIED HUMAN FIBRINOGEN

R. Gollwitzer, W. Bode
Max-Planck-Institut für Biochemie, D-8033 Martinsried, F.R.G.

Introduction

The three-dimensional structure of fibrinogen is still unknown. Several models have been discussed ranging from a pentagonal dodecahyder (1) to bent (2) and elongated forms (3). In the last years the trinodular model proposed by Hall and Slayter in 1959 (4) experienced a renaissance. It agrees with the domainal organization of the molecule derived from enzymatic and chemical fragmentation under reducing conditions (5).

The method of choice to obtain detailed information about the three-dimensional structure of a protein is X-ray analysis. But the prerequisite and the limiting factor of this technique is the availability of well ordered single crystals. 1974 Cohen and Tooney reported for the first time upon macrocrystals from modified bovine fibrinogen (6). Up to now a low resolution model has not been published. However, by comparison of electron micrographs from staining patterns of fibrin aggregates and of microcrystalline and crystalline forms a more detailed heptanodular model was presented by this group (7). Hewat et al. (8) proposed a multinodular model without a central domain by studying microcrystals also obtained from proteolytically modified bovine fibrinogen.

We started crystallization experiments with human fibrinogen several years ago, intrigued by the problem to grow crystals of such a long, jointed and hydrodynamically "swollen" molecule, which prefers to organize itself in extended aggregates. In this paper we describe the crystals and microcrystals obtained from native and modified human fibrinogen and their chemical properties.

Fibrinogen - Fibrin Formation and Fibrinolysis, Vol. 4
© 1986 Walter de Gruyter & Co., Berlin · New York - Printed in Germany.

Results and Discussion

Needle-like crystals with pointed ends (maximal length 0.5 mm, Ø 0.01 mm) were obtained from solutions of native human fibrinogen (Fig. 1). The crystals are not suitable for X-ray analysis. Laser light diffractograms of electron micrographs of negatively stained specimens show an orthogonal lattice of equatorial and meridional reflexions which can be indexed as the third and fourth order of a 225 Å periodicity and the first order of a 70 Å periodicity (9). One attractive feature of these crystals is that besides the fibrinopeptides (clottability: 88-95 %) the constituent molecules comprise the large carboxy-terminal α-chain fragments, which are not arranged in a compact tertiary structure (5). This could explain the rather weak order observed perpendicular to the long crystal axis. As shown by the ready integration into even macroscopic crystals, native fibrinogen can adopt a predominant, unique structure as far as intermolecular crystal contacts are concerned.

To obtain crystallizable fragments we studied the degradation of fibrinogen with various enzymes. According to these experiments (10) the C-terminal two thirds of the Aα-chain and a small part of the Bβ-chain, supposedly from the N-terminus, are easily cleaved off by most proteases, whereas the tightly structured core of the molecule comprising E-and D-domains is only accessible to

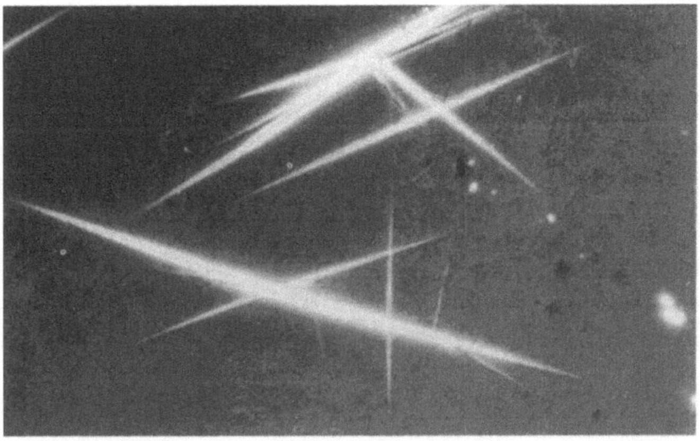

Figure 1. Crystalline needles of native human fibrinogen
Light optical magnification 200 x

plasmin and related enzymes like trypsin.
The trinodular structure of native fibrinogen is preserved in fibrin (11) and in plasminolysis fragment X, as shown by rotary shadowed samples of the native and the proteolytically modified protein (Table 1; Figure 2). The overall length of the extended trinodular particles is about 450 Å. The dimensions of both outer nodules (Ø 110 and 86 Å) and of the central nodule (Ø 73 and 59 Å) are preserved even in the separated D and E domains (Table 1: Cc; D). This suggests, that neither the C-terminal two thirds of the α-chain, nor N-terminal fragments (fibrinopeptides A and B, ß-chain residues 1-54) significantly contribute to the trinodular scaffold of the native molecule. One, rarely two satellite nodule(s) are observed frequently in samples of unmodified fibrinogen (Fig. 2a), especially after denaturating treatment (Fig. 2b). These satellites are never seen in samples of modified fibrinogen deprived of the C-terminal two thirds of its α-chain like plasminolysis fragment X (Figure 2c,d). Because of this fact and because of their displacement from central and outer nodules, the satellites are considered to contain the C-terminal fragments of the α-chains.

Table 1: Uncorrected Molecular Dimensions of native and modified Fibrinogen in Electron Micrographs of rotary shadowed Samples

S[+]	Overall Length[++]			Outer Nodules					Central Nodule				
					Length		Width			Length		Width	
	No	Å	SD[‡]	No	Å	SD	Å	SD	No	Å	SD	Å	SD
A	70	446	±15	114	110	±11	86	±11	57	73	± 9	59	±10
B	58	443	±18	108	115	± 8	94	±12	49	79	±10	66	±11
Ca	74	453	±15	78	122	±11	94	±10	42	81	± 9	67	± 9
b	65	451	±18	41	124	±11	96	±13	21	82	±13	68	± 9
c				124	121	± 8	105	± 9	39	79	± 7	69	± 8
D									82	72	±11	62	± 8
E	73	464	±16	84	124	±12	93	±11	51	77	±12	59	±12

[+]Sample; A native fibrinogen; B fibrin monomers; C native fibrinogen digested with plasmin (a) 30 minutes, (b) 60 minutes, (c) 120 minutes; D isolated, crystallized E-domains; E crystallized PAE modified fibrinogen; [++]the overall length was only determined from extended particles; [‡] No: number of particles analyzed, SD: standard deviation.

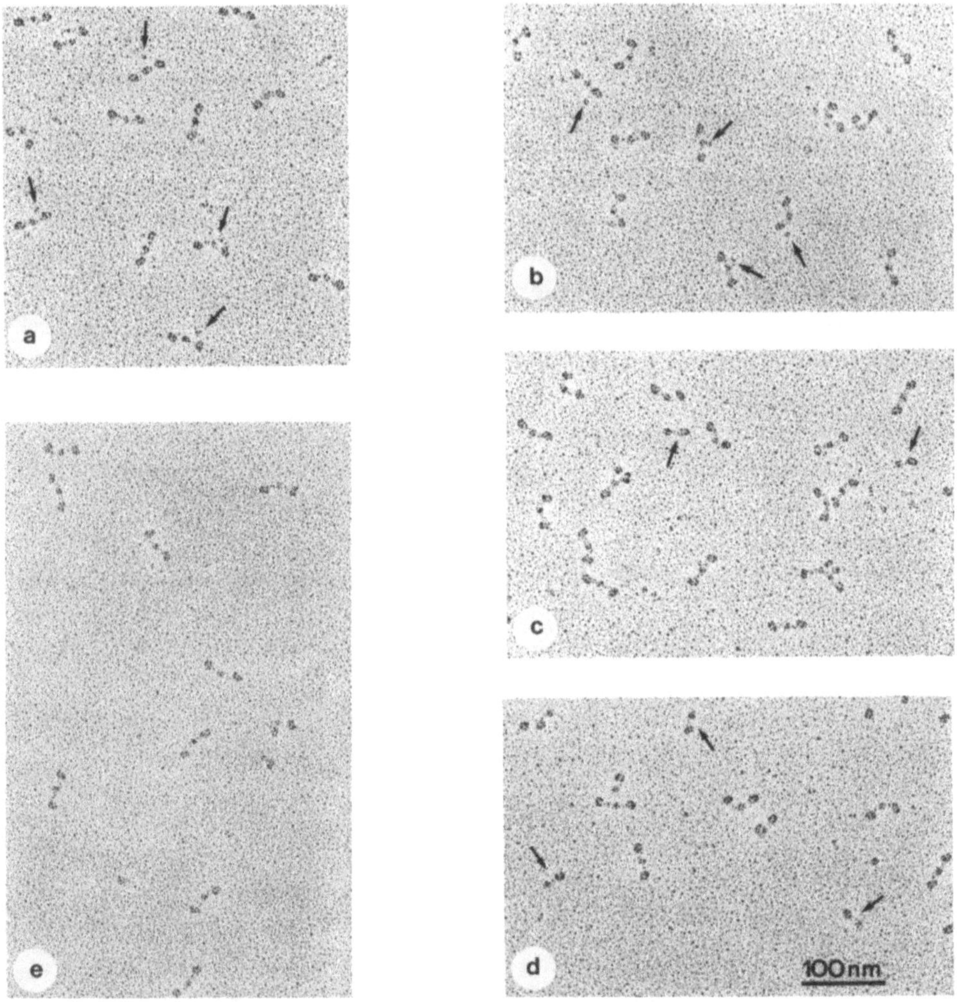

Figure 2. Electron micrographs of rotary shadowed native fibrinogen fraction I-4 (a), unmodified fibrinogen after treatment with 8 M urea (b), fibrinogen after plasmin digestion for 30 minutes (c) and 60 minutes (d), redissolved crystals of PAE modified fibrinogen (e). Arrows indicate satellite nodules (a,b), fragment Y (c,d). Electron optical magnification 50,000.

The α-chain segments connecting the satellite with the outer nodules could envelop the molecular scaffold like a porous sheath. Such a loosely arranged structure could retain the enclosed solvent during shock freezing. This possibly explains the voluminous "saussage-like" appearance of freeze etched fibrinogen molecules observed by Bachmann (12).

Considering the chemical and electron microscopical evidence, X-like fragments still containing the trinodular structure of the native molecule but deprived of its unordered appendix, seem to be most suitable for crystallization. We obtained spherulites under similar crystallization conditions (dialysis against aqueous solutions of low ionic strength) from fibrinogen digested with a crude Pseudomonas aeruginosa exoprotease (PAE), with bovine α-chymotrypsin and curiously enough with a commercially available neuraminidase of Chlostridium perfringens containing a proteolytic contaminant in minor amounts. As shown by sodium dodecylsulfate (SDS) polyacrylamide-gelelectrophoresis (PAGE), all these spherulites (Fig. 5A) consist of a homogeneous 245 kD fragment, apparently identical in size to a late plasminolysis fragment X. This 245 kD fragment is composed of an original 48 kD γ-chain, a modified 50 kD β-chain and smaller fragments probably derived from the α-chain. Spherulites from PAE-modified fibrinogen (Fig.3) displayed a strong radial birefringence, indicating a considerable degree of radial crystalline order. They are clearly composed of platelike mini-crystals, which sometimes grow and extend out of the spherulites. In rare cases homogeneously refracting large crystals (maximal length 0.7 mm) were obtained from PAE-digests. They are rounded off prisms with elliptical cross sections (Fig. 4 A).Most of them have

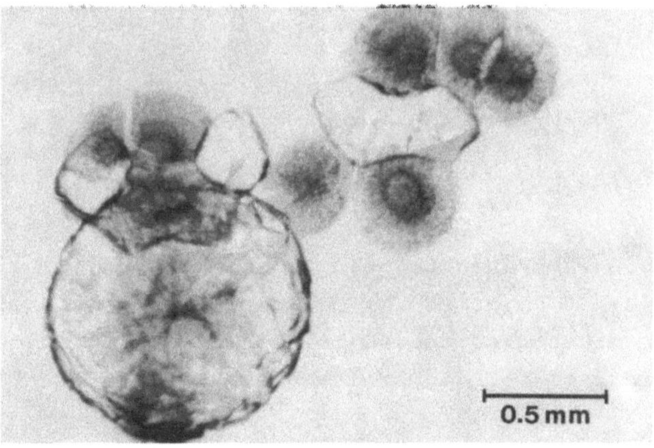

Figure 3. Spherulites of PAE modified fibrinogen

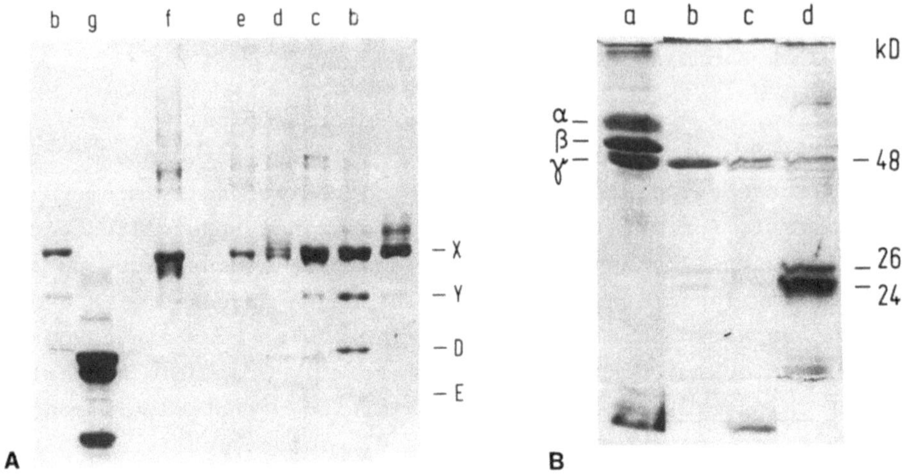

Figure 4. Single crystals from PAE modified human fibrinogen

no smooth surface, but show kinks (Fig. 4B) which not seldom encircle the whole surface. Upon shock treatment the crystals often break along plans parallel to the elliptical faces.
Rotary shadowed samples of the crystalline particles (Fig.2e) are

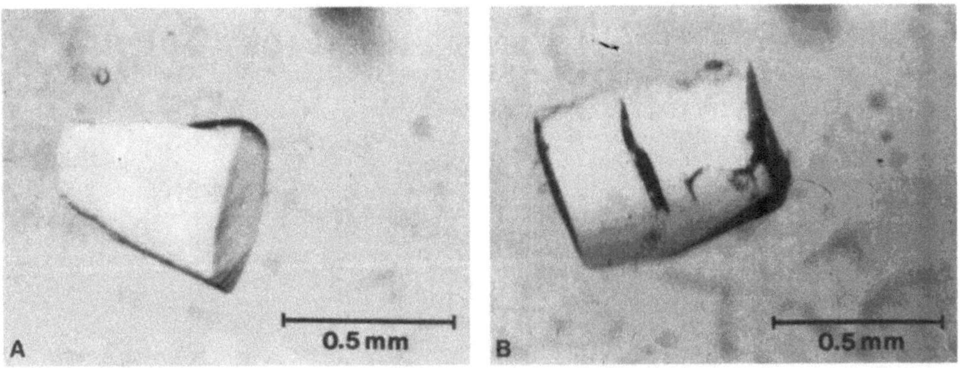

Figure 5A. SDS-PAGE (non-reducing conditions, 3-10% gradient gel). 19 minutes (a), 60 minutes (b) plasmin digest; spherulites from chymotrypsin digest (c); neuraminidase digest (d) and PAE digest (e); crystals from PAE digest (f) and the supernatant of these crystals (g).
Figure 5B. SDS-PAGE (reducing conditions, 15% gel). Unmodified fibrinogen (a); crystals from PAE-digest at high (b) and low (c, d) load; Ccomassie staining (a,b,c), subsequent silver staining (d).

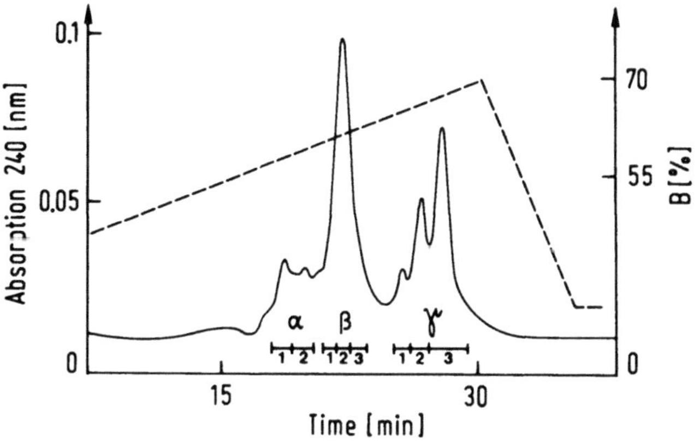

Figure 6. HPLC-chromatography of crystals of PAE-modified fibrinogen after reduction and aminoethylation; gradient: 40 to 70% B (70% acetonitrile in 0.1% trifluoracetic acid).

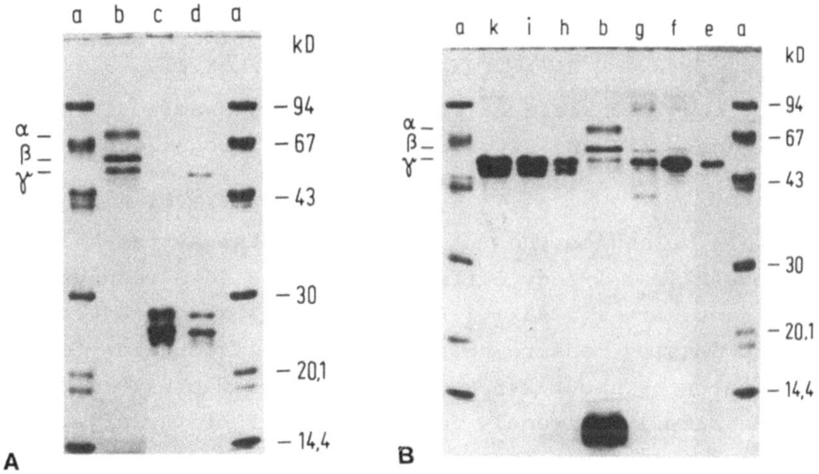

Figure 7. SDS-PAGE (15% gel, reducing conditions) of the fractions obtained by HPLC-chromatography (Fig. 6). Reference proteins (a), native fibrinogen (b), fractions α_1 (c), α_2 (d), β_1 (e), β_2 (f), β_3 (g), γ_1 (h), γ_2 (i), γ_3 (k).

virtually identical to fragment X (Fig. 2c,d). With the exception of the satellite nodules observed in unmodified preparations (Fig. 2a), crystalline particles and fragment X exhibit the same trinodular scaffold, the same overall length and the same dimensions of the constituing globules as the unmodified molecule (Table 1).

According to discelectrophoresis the crystals indeed do contain an X-like fibrinogen derivative of about 245 kD (Fig. 5A). Under reducing conditions (Fig. 5B) two very close bands of molecular weight 48 kD (lane b,c) and two faster migrating bands of apparent molecular weight 24 kD and 26 kD (lane d) are observed. These bands were identified by HPLC-chromatography. The elution profile of reduced and aminoethylated crystalline material (Fig. 6) shows only a shoulder in α-position and a triple peak in γ-position, but an equivalent peak at the position where normally the β-chain elutes. This assignment according to the elution profile of unmodified fibrinogen is supported by SDS-PAGE of the various peak fractions (Fig. 7). We therefore conclude, that the crystals contain a homogeneously modified fibrinogen of almost 245 kD. It consists 1) of a 24 kD or 26 kD remnant α-chain (Fig. 7, lane b,c), which has probably retained its amino-terminal fibrinopeptide A (because partial clottability up to 45 % remains); 2) of a 48 kD β-chain, which has lost about 60 residues probably from its amino-terminus (Fig. 7B lane e,f); and 3) of a slightly heterogeneous γ-chain of 46 to 48 kD (Fig. 7B lane h,i,k).

The crystals belong to the orthorhombic crystal system and are of space group $P2_12_12_1$. They diffract to beyond 10 Å resolution. The cell constants are $\underline{a}$ = 95 ± 1 Å, $\underline{b}$ = 111 ± 1 Å, $\underline{c}$ = 440 ± 4 Å. According to density measurements the unit cell contains four modified molecules of about 245 kD. Due to a value of 4.9 $Å^3$/D the packing density is extremely low, about 75 % of the crystal volume are occupied by solvent and only 25 % by the protein moiety. This rather loose packing may explain the fragility and the limited crystalline order of these crystals.
From these data together with those obtained from electron micrographs of single molecules the presented packing model (Fig. 8) for the crystals was derived. Four almost symmetrical fibrinogen

particles are packed into one unit cell. The length of the fragments is restricted by the unit cell to 440 Å. Special features of the intensity pattern indicate that the molecules are aligned along the c axis and that they are regularly displaced by one fourth along the b and along the c axis of the crystal (Fig. 8A). The symmetry properties of the crystal require special positions of the molecular centers along the b and the c axes (Fig.8 A,B).

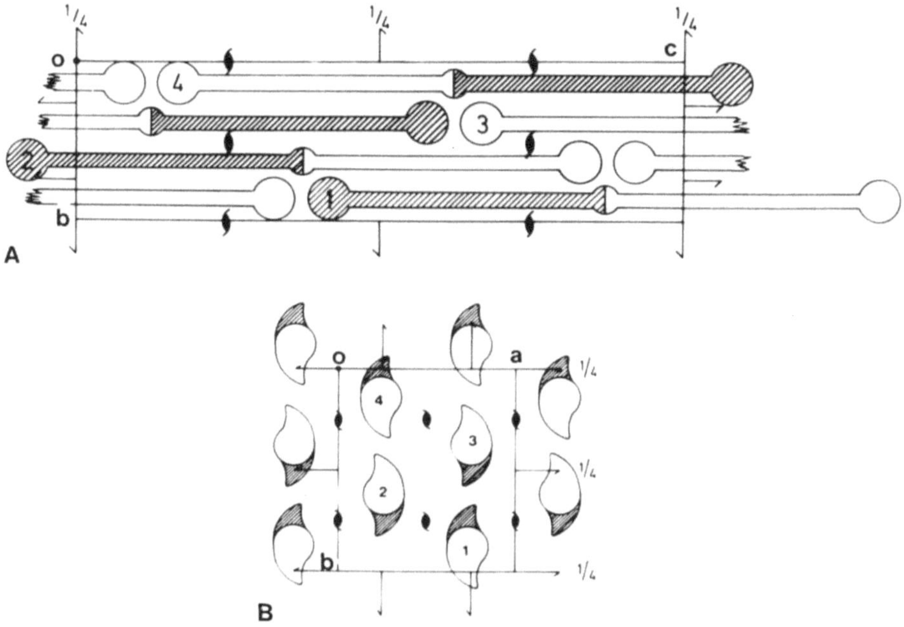

Figure 8. Packing of the fibrinogen molecules in the crystal.
A: projection on the b-c plane; B: projection on the a-b plane.

A two-fold rotation axis relates both halves of the molecules (the hatched and the non-hatched parts of the particles in Fig. 8A). This twofold rotation axis must intersect the disulfide bridge connecting the α-chains of both halves of the molecule and penetrate perpendicularly the plane defined by the two disulfide bridges connecting the γ-chains of both molecular halves. The intensity pattern puts no constraint on the particle placement along the a axis. Several lines of evidence suggest a pseudohexagonal arrangement as shown in Fig. 8B. The center to center distances between nearest neighbours are quite uniform and allow for a lateral packing of the large D-units. Furthermore this packing arrangement could explain the pronounced fragility of the crystals along the b-c plain.

Besides collecting a complete 10 Å intensity data set, we are currently searching for heavy atom derivatives of the crystals. We do hope that a reasonable model with enough details can be provided to improve our knowledge about the undisturbed molecular shape and the domain organization in native fibrinogen.

Acknowledgement

We are obliged to Mrs. H. Wiedemann for the preparation of the rotary shadowed samples and the electron micrographs. The skillful assistance of Mrs. I. Mayr is gratefully acknowledged. The financial support of the Deutsche Forschungsgemeinschaft, SFB 51 (grants B 10, B 22) and the SFB 207 (grants LP A1, LP C7) is greatly appreciated.

References

1. Köppel, G. 1966. Nature 212, 1608-1609.

2. Marguerie, G., H.B. Stuhrmann. 1976. J.Mol.Biol. 102, 143-156.

3. Lederer, K. 1979. Thrombosis Haemostasis (Stuttgart) 41, 641-647.

4. Hall, C.E., H.S. Slayter. 1959. J.Biophys.Biochem.Cytol. 5, 11-17.

5. Doolittle, R.F. 1977. Horizons Biochem.Biophys. 3, 164-191.

6. Cohen, C., N.M. Tooney. 1974. Nature 251, 659-660.

7. Weisel, J.W., G.N. Phillips Jr., C. Cohen. 1981. Nature 289, 263-267.

8. Hewat, E.A., L. Tranqui, R.H. Wade. 1982. J.Mol.Biol. 161, 459-477.

9. Gollwitzer, R., W. Bode, H.J. Schramm, D. Typke, R. Guckenberger. 1980. In: Protides of Biological Fluids, Vol.28 (H. Peeters,ed.) Pergamon Press, Oxford New York. pp. 307-310.

10. Gollwitzer, R., W. Bode. 1980. Haematologica 65, 528-534.

11. Gollwitzer, R., W. Bode, H.J. Schramm, D. Typke, R. Guckenberger. 1983. Annals New York Acad. Sci. 408, 214-225.

12. Bachmann, L., W.W. Schmitt-Fumian, R. Hammel, K. Lederer. 1975. Makromolek.Chem. 176, 2603-2618.

THE C-TERMINAL POLYMERISATION DOMAIN OF FIBRINOGEN

Christopher Southan, Elizabeth Thompson and David A. Lane.

Department of Haematology, Charing Cross and Westminster Medical School, Hammersmith, London W6 8RP, UK.

Introduction

The C-terminal region of the γ chain is essential for many functional interactions of fibrinogen and fibrin. This part of the γ chain is known to be conserved in the fragment D prepared by limited plasmin digestion, in the presence of calcium, known as FgDcate (1). The property of inhibition of fibrin polymerisation by this fragment suggests that it contains a functional fibrinogen C-terminal polymerisation domain (2). This property is lost when FgDcate is further digested in the absence of calcium to a fragment in which a C-terminal section has been cleaved from the γ chain, FgDegta (1). The present work had two principal objectives. Firstly, to isolate and characterise the peptides cleaved from FgDcate by plasmin in the presence of EDTA and secondly, to determine the relationship between the cleavage of these peptides and the fibrinogen C-terminal polymerisation domain.

Methods

For our experiments the FgDcate/FgE complex was prepared from commercial fibrinogen (KabiVitrum AB) and then purified by gel filtration. Further plasmin cleavage in the presence of EDTA was studied by three techniques. SDS-PAGE, run under reducing conditions, was used to monitor the FgD γ chain cleavage into shorter polypeptide chains. The ability of FgDcate to inhibit the polymerisation of pre-formed fibrin was used as an assay for the functional integrity of the C-terminal polymerisation domain on FgD (2). The released peptides were analysed by HPLC, using reverse-phase wide-pore column material. The peptides were then purified, identified by protein chemical techniques and tested for their ability to inhibit fibrin polymerisation. A full description of the experimental details of this work is given in reference (12).

Fibrinogen - Fibrin Formation and Fibrinolysis, Vol. 4
© 1986 Walter de Gruyter & Co., Berlin · New York - Printed in Germany.

Results

SDS-PAGE Analysis: These results (Fig.1) support the work of Niewenhuizen et al. (1) in showing that the DY1 chain is progressively cleaved into two shorter forms. DY2 band predominates over the first hour of digestion and presumably corresponds to the Y chain remenants of FgDint which retains the calcium binding site present in FgDcate. In 4.5 hours the transition to FgDedta is complete and this contains only the shorter Y chain remenant DY3.

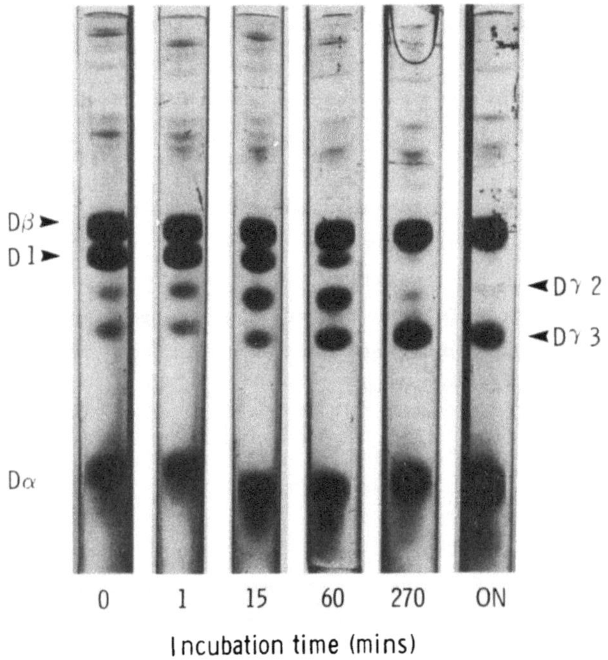

Fig.1:SDS-PAGE of the FgDcate/FgE digest. The bands in these gel sections are those of polypeptides derived from FgD. The general pattern of bands is similar to that reported by Niewenhuizen et al.(1), who also made the following Mr assignments; Dβ 43K, DY1 38K, DY2 29K, DY3 25K and Dα12K. The figures below each gel refer to the time points of digestion. (ON=overnight)

Polymerisation Inhibition: For this assay the complete digestion mixture was added to pre-formed fibrin without the prior removal of cleavage products. Soluble fibrin in 0.02 M acetic acid was mixed with a small aliquot of digest mixture. Polymerisation was initiated by diluting into a cuvette containing phosphate buffer at pH 6.8 (3). The intial conditions were adjusted to give extensive inhibition of fibrin with a molar ratio of fibrin:FgDcate of 3:1. The results are given in Table 1.

Table 1: Inhibition of fibrin polymerisation by FgDcate/FgE digest. The reference for zero inhibition was taken as the absorbance at 350 nm after 20 mins polymerisation of fibrin alone. The percentage inhibition was calculated from a fibrin polymerisation curve which had aliqoits of FgDcate/FgE added after different digest times.

DIGESTION TIME		POLYMERISATION INHIBITION
0 (control)	FgDcate	89 %
1 min		66 %
15 min	||	52 %
60 min	\/	22 %
4.5 hrs	FgDegta	9 %

These results show a progressive loss of polymerisation inhibition activity during progressive digestion and this seems to parallel the γ chain shortening shown in Fig. 1. At 4.5 hours the inhibitory activity of the completed digest could not be restored to the initial levels even by adding a 120 fold excess of reaction mixture.

HPLC Analysis. The chromatograms in Fig. 2 are from FgDcate/FgE digest after complete conversion of FgDcate to FgDegta. The properties of the wide-pore reverse-phase material facilitated direct analysis by HPLC without any pre-treatment to remove high molecular weight material. Over a number of experiments we consistantly observed three major peptide peaks designated as P1 P2 and P3 in Fig. 2, which were cleaved from FgDcate/FgE. Additional experiments using ultrafiltration and heat precipitation failed to detect significant amounts of any other cleavage products separable from the FgD/FgE material.

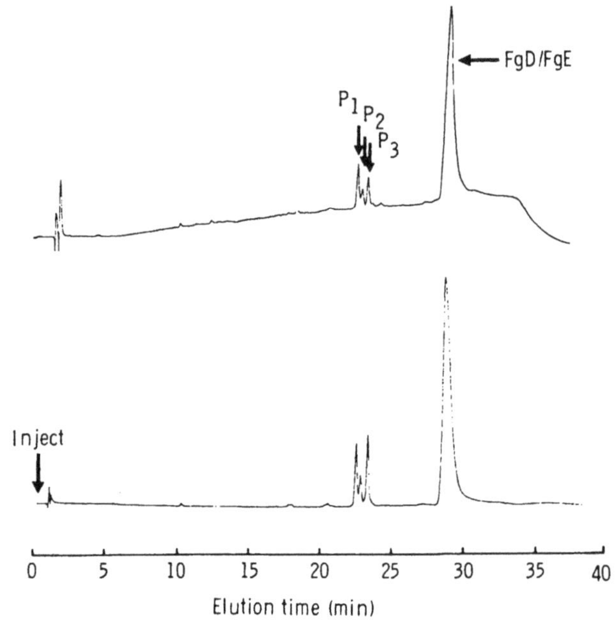

Figure 2: HPLC analysis of FgDcate/FgE digest. 4ul of 5 hour digest (23 mg/ml), after 0.22 um filtration, were injected onto the 0.46 X 25 cm Vydac column. Solvent A was 0.1% TFA/H_2O, and B, 0.1% TFA/CH_3CN. The elution gradient was 0% to 50% B in 30 minutes. The upper profile was recorded at 206 nm, the lower at 280 nm

By including free tryptophan as an internal standard for peak quantification we were able to use this technique to measure the apearance of the three peptides during digestion. The release pattern closely paralled both the γ chain shortening and the loss of polymerisation inhibition activity. There was an indication that P2 had the slowest cleavage rate in the early phase of digestion. Extending the digestion overnight produced a large number of additional peaks and the amount of P1 was reduced by further proteolysis.

Peptide purification. The majority of the high molecular weight material was removed by acid precipitation without affecting peptide recovery for subsequent purification. An isocratic separation, Fig. 3, was developed for the isolation of P1, P2 and P3 directly from the digest supernatant after acid precipitation and filtration.

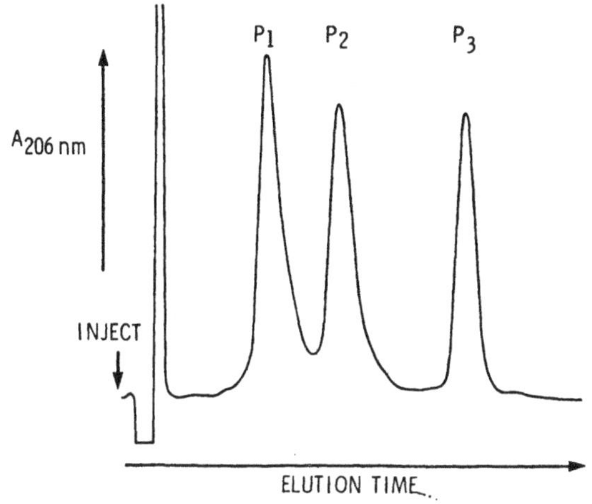

Figure 3: Preparative HPLC for the isolation of P1, P2 and P3: Samples were eluted with the same solvents as Fig. 2 under isocratic conditions at 27% B. The central sections of each peak were collected and freeze-dried.

To check the homogeneity of the purified peptides we employed different HPLC conditions to improve on the peak separation shown in Fig. 2. We were thus able to obtain a complete separation of all three peptides, shown in Fig. 4, and establish the purity of the preparative fractions. Analysis by size-exclusion HPLC further confirmed that each peptide was a distinct molecular size (not shown)

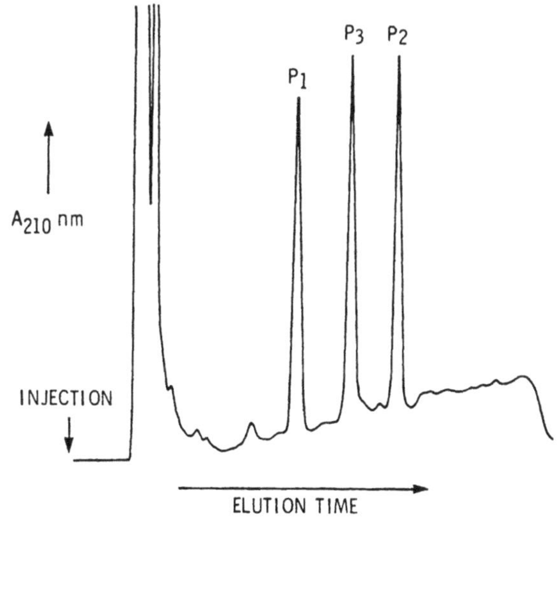

Figure 4: Analytical HPLC of P1,P2, and P3.
Solvent A was 0.025 M ammonium acetate at pH 6.0 which contained 50% acetonitrile in solvent B. The gradient was 45 to 70% B in 15 min at a flow rate of 1.5 ml/min.

Structural investigations of P1,P2 and P3. We used the manual DABITC/Edman sequencing technique (4) to establish that these 3 peptides were pure cleavage products with N-terminals Thr-Arg, Phe-Phe- and Ala-Ser- for P1,P2 and P3, respectively. The same determination for the peak mixture from a complete digest gave all three N-terminals and the indication that they were released in stoichiometricaly similar amounts.

To determine the exact size of these peptides a fast atom bombardment analysis (FAB-mapping) (5) was performed which gave molecular weights of 3698 for P1 and 1893 for P3, accurate to one mass unit. Because of the high molecular weight further FAB mapping was undertaken following chymotryptic digestion of P2. In conjunction with the N-terminal sequences and amino acid analyses these results identified P1 as γ 374 - 405, P2 as γ 303-356 and P3 as 357 - 373. Figure 5 shows the alignment between the known γ chain sequence and the peptides we have isolated We found no evidence of any peptides arising from cleavages at γ 321 or 338 which are presumably protected by the disulphide loop between two nearby cysteine residues.

Polymerisation Inhibition of Peptides. HPLC purified P1 P2 & P3 were added separately and in combination in a 200 fold molar exess to polymerising fibrin to ascertain whether they could directly inhibit polymerisation. We were consistantly unable to demonstrate such inhibitory activity with any of these peptides.

```
                  320        ............340
                   |        :            :|
FFTSHNGMQFSTWDNDNDKFEGNCAEQDGSGWWMNKCHAGHLNGVYYQGGTYSK
|--------(P2,303-356)--------------------------------|


  360                 380                   400      411
   |                   |                     |        |
ASTPNGYDNGIIWATWKTRWYSMKKTTMKIIPFNRLTIGEGQQHHLGGAKQAGDV
|--(P3,357-373)-||------(P1,374-405)------------|
```

Figure 5: The C-terminal section of the γ Chain.The sequence, in single-letter code for amino acids, was taken from Henschen et al (6). Vertical lines mark those residues at the N-terminal or C-terminal. The peptides indicated directly beneath the sequence as P1, P2 and P3, were isolated and identified in this study.

Discussion

This work establishes that the conversion of FgDcate to FgDegta arises from the cleavage of γ chain peptides on the C-terminal side of γ 303. It also seems likely that the fragment FgDint, which retains a calcium binding site (1), arises from the lysine cleavage either at γ 356 or 373. The sequences of the peptides isolated in our study overlap with those of γ 374-411 (7) and γ 396-411 (8) that have been claimed to bind to fibrin and be potent inhibitors of polymerisation. However, we find it difficult to reconcile these findings of inhibitory peptides isolated from plasmin digests of FgDcate with our results which demonstrate a progressive and extensive loss of polymerisation inhibitory activity under conditions where the native peptides are present in maximal amounts in the digest mixture.

Other recent studies also indicate significant structural contributions to this polymerisation domain from residues on the N-terminal side of γ 374. Two variants with the substitutions γ 275 Arg->His (9) and γ 330 Asp->Val (10) have been shown to cause defective polymerisation. Sequence comparisons with lamprey fibrinogen indicate highly conserved regions between γ 318-352 and 363-385 (11). We conclude, therefore, that the polymerisaton domain of fibrinogen may be a more extended region than previously supposed and includes the sequence γ 303-405 when this is contiguous with the remainder of the γ chain.

The authors would like to thank Dr Maria Panico, Professor Howard Morris, and Tony Etienne, the Biochemistry Department of Imperial College, London, for the FAB-mapping and amino acid analysis. This work was supported by a grant from the Wellcome Trust to D.A. Lane.

References

1. Nieuwenhuizen, W., Voskluilen, M., Vermond, A., Haverkate, F. and Hermans, J. 1982. Biochim. Biophys.Acta. 707, 190-192.

2. Williams, J.E., Hantgen, R.R., Hermans, J. & McDonaugh, J. (1981). Biochem. J. 197, 661-668.

3. Belitser, V.A., Varetskaja, T.V. and Malneva, G.V. 1968. Biochim. Biophys. Acta. 154, 367-375.

4. Chang, J.Y., Brauer, D. and Wittman-Liebold, B. 1978. FEBS Lett. 93, 205-213.

5. Morris, H.R., Panico, M. and Taylor, G.W. 1983. Biochem. Biophys. Res. Commun. 117, 299-305.

7. Olexa, S.A. and Budzynski, A.Z. 1981 J. Biol. Chem. 256, 3544-3549.

8. Horwitz, B.H., Varadi, A. and Scheraga, H.A. 1984. Proc. Natl. Acad. Sci. 81, 5980-5984.

9 Kehl, M., Henschen, A., Tavory, S., Rimon, A., Soria, J. and Soria, C. 1984. VIII International Congress on Thrombosis, Istanbul, Abstract No. 82.

10. Reber, P., Furlan, M., Rupp, C., Kehl, M., Lottspeich, F., Henschen, A., Mannuci, P.M. and Beck, E.A. 1985. Proc. 17th Annual Meeting of USEGB, Geneva, Experimentia 41, in press.

11. Strong, D.D., Moore, M., Cottrell, B.A., Bohonus, V.L., Evans, B., Riley, M. and Doolittle, R.F. 1985. Biochemistry, 24, 92-101.

12. Southan, C., Thompson, L., Panico, M, Etienne, T., Morris, H.M., and Lane, D.A. 1985. J. Biol. Chem, in press.

γ- CHAIN CROSSLINKING OF FIBRIN AT DD-TRANS CONTACT

E. Selmayr, W. Thiel, G. Müller-Berghaus

Clinical Research Unit for Blood Coagulation and Thrombosis of the Max-Planck-Gesellschaft at the Justus-Liebig- Universität, Giessen, West-Germany

Introduction

The crosslinking of the γ-chains of fibrin is believed to occur at the so-called DD-long contact of two adjacent fibrin molecules. This model was deduced from electron micrographs of crosslinked fibrinogen dimers (1). Since fibrinogen has no polymerisation sites exposed on its E-domain, the aim of the present investigation was the generation of fibrin-fibrinogen dimers to ascertain the formation of half-staggered overlapping molecules. If crosslinking occurs in a fibrin-fibrinogen dimer, the concept of the crosslinking at DD-long contact is unlikely.

Materials and Methods

Human fibrinogen was purified from freshly drawn ACD blood by glycine and ethanol precipication (2).

Labelling of fibrinogen: Human fibrinogen was labelled with 125-I by the iodine monochloride method (3).

Prearation of desAA-fibrin Sepharose: Fibrinogen was coupled to CNBr-activated Sepharose 4B (Pharmacia, Stockholm, Sweden) according to the manufacturer's instructions, except that the coupling buffer had a pH of 8.0. The amount of coupled fibrinogen was 8 mg/ml gel. Fibrinogen-Sepahrose was incubated with batroxobin for 3 hours. Batroxobin was removed from gel by washing with tris buffer and 3 M urea at pH 7.4.

Activation of FXIII: FXIII in tris buffer was activated with bovine thrombin for 30 minutes at room temperatur. Thereafter, thrombin activity was quenched with hirudin.

Fibrinogen - Fibrin Formation and Fibrinolysis, Vol. 4
© 1986 Walter de Gruyter & Co., Berlin · New York - Printed in Germany.

Reaction mixtures

1. The required volume of the desAA-fibrin Sepharose gel in tris buffer was mixed with anti-batroxobin, 125-I-Fibrinogen, calcium (final concentration: 2.5 mmol) and preactivated FXIII (final concentration: 2 U/ml). A series of four experiments were performed: 125-I-Fibrinogen (final concentration: 1,2,4 or 5 mg/ml) was mixed with des AA-fibrin Sepharose of different concentrations giving fibrin:fibrinogen ratios of 1:1, 1:2, 1:5, 1:10 and 1:20. After incubation for 2 h at 37°C, non-crosslinked fibrinogen was removed by washing the gel two times for 30 minutes with 2 ml 6 M guanidinium chloride, pH 4.1 and consecutive centrifugation. Radioactivities of gel and supernatant were measured in a well-type scintillation counter.
2. Fibrinogen (final concentration: 2 mg/ml) was mixed with either immobilized fibrinogen or immobilized desAA-fibrin as described above but the incubation time was 1 h at 37°C.
3. Control experiments were carried out by a). Incubation of fibrinogen with immobilized fibrinogen or immobilized fibrin in the absence of FXIIIa, b). Incubation of fibrinogen with Sepharose 4B in the presence of FXIIIa.

Results

Under all different experimental conditions, 125-I-fibrinogen was crosslinked to immobilized desAA-fibrin by FXIIIa. In comparison to the crosslinking of fibrinogen to desAA-fibrin Sepharose, fibrinogen was crosslinked to fibrinogen-Sepharose to a much smaller extent (Tab. 1). If fibrinogen was incubated with immobilized fibrinogen or immoblilized fibrin (ratio 1:1) in the absence of FXIIIa only a small amount of the radio-labelled fibrinogen was bound to the gel (Tab. 1). After incubation of fibrinogen with Sepahrose 4B in the presence of FXIIIa, the bound fibrinogen amounted to 1.9% $\pm$ 0.3. In Figure 1 we have calculated how many molecules of fibrinogen were covalently bound to one molecule of immobilized fibrin indicating the formation of crosslinked fibrin-fibrinogen dimers.

Table 1: Crosslinking of ^{125}I-Fibrinogen to immobilized desAA-Fibrin and immobilized Fibrinogen (ratio 1:1) (From: Selmayr, E. et al. (4)).

Presence or absence of Factor XIIIa	^{125}I-Fibrinogen* bound to desAA-Fibrin Sepharose	Fibrinogen-Sepharose	Sepharose
+	21.92 ± 0.49	5.69 ± 0.63	1.93 ± 0.18
-	4.97 ± 0.34	1.93 ± 0.18	

* % of radioactivity applied in the reaction mixtures

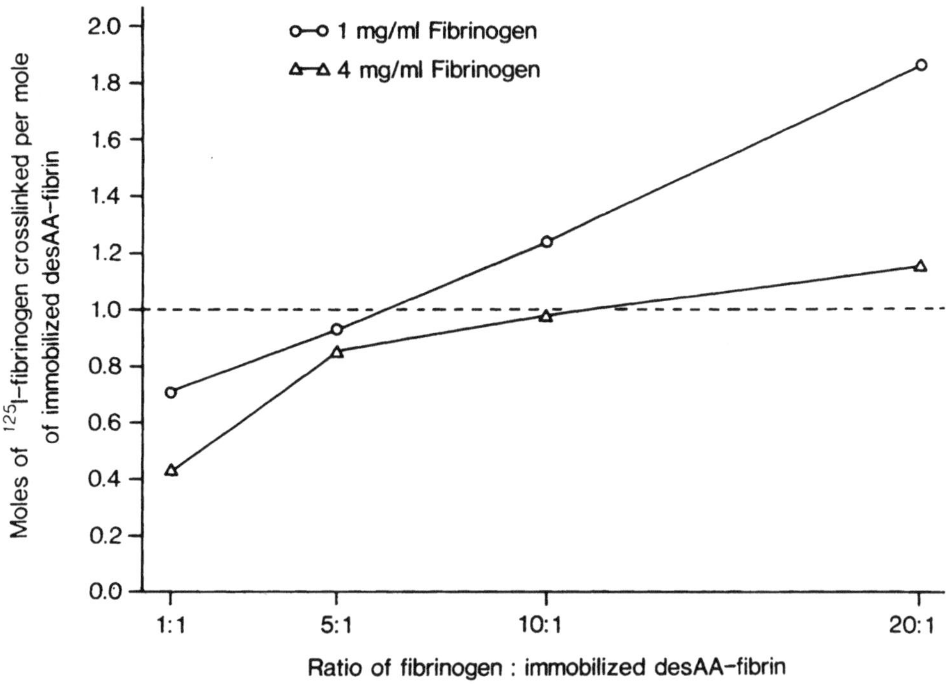

Fig 1: Crosslinked fibrin-fibrinogen dimers. 125-I-fibrinogen/desAA-fibrin Sepharose mixtures were incubated with FXIIIa for 2 h at 37°C. Fibrinogen concentrations were 1 mg/ml and 4 mg/ml and the ratios of fibrinogen to immobilized fibrin differed from 1:1 to 20:1. The broken line represents the crosslinking of one molecule fibrinogen to one molecule immobilized fibrin.

Discussion

The demonstration of a crosslinked fibrin-fibrinogen dimer indicates the half staggered overlap as a prerequisite for crosslinking. In this molecular alignment, only one possibility for the formation of a crosslinking bridge exists, namely between the D-domains of the two overlapping molecules. From these experiments and the findings of Horwitz et al. (5) and Budzynski et al. (6) we present a model which describes the polymerisation and crosslinking of fibrin molecules (Fig. 2). In this model the γ-chains of the polymerised fibrin molecules are retroflected and recurrent from the D- domain in direction to the E-domain. Since the axis of the two crosslinked D-domains runs tranversal we propose the term DD-trans contact for this molecular alignment in fibrin crosslinking.

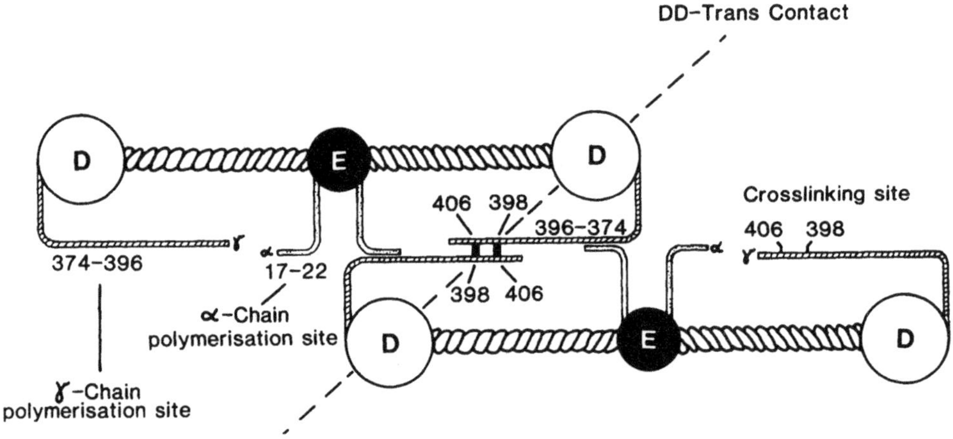

Fig. 2: DD-trans contact in fibrin polymerisation and crosslinking. Fibrin polymerisation starts with the exposure of the N-terminal α-chain polymerisation sites after FPA-release on the E-domain of fibrinogen. The N-terminal α-chain polymerisation site binds to the C-terminal γ-chain polymerisation site of a second fibrin molecule. Since two of this α-γ contacts exist, this represents the mechanism how the γ-chains are directed into an antiparallel position which is necessary for the consecutive crosslinking reaction by FXIIIa. After the alignment of the γ-chains, crosslinking by FXIIIa is possible between two overlapping fibrin molecules at position 398/406. (From: Selmayr, E. & Müller-Berghaus, G. (7)).

Acknowlegement

This study was supported by the Stiftung Volkswagenwerk, Hannover, and by grants (Mu 279) of the Deutsche Forschungsgemeinschaft, Bonn-Bad Godesberg. The authors thank Prof. Dr. E. Sattler for the hospitality at the Zentralabteilung des Strahlenzentrums.

References

1. Erickson, H.P., W.E. Fowler. 1983. Ann.N.Y.Acad.Sci. 408, 146-163.

2. Blombäck, B., M. Blombäck. 1956. Ark.Kemi 10, 415-443.

3. McFarlane, A.S. 1958. Nature 182, 53.

4. Selmayr, E., W. Thiel, G. Müller-Berghaus. 1985. Thromb.Res. (In press).

5. Horwitz, B.H., V. Andrås, H.A. Scheraga. 1984. Proc.Natl. Acad.Sci.USA 81, 5980-5984.

6. Budzynski, A.Z., S.A. Olexa, B.V. Pandya. 1983. Ann.N.Y. Acad.Sci. 408, 301-313.

7. Selmayr, E., G. Müller-Berghaus. (Submitted for publication).

SOLUBLE FIBRIN CONTAINS FIBRIN POLYMERS OF DIFFERENT MOLECULAR WEIGHT. ULTRACENTRIFUGATION STUDIES AT 37°C

K.T. Preissner, J. Rötker, G. Müller-Berghaus
Clinical Research Unit for Blood Coagulation and Thrombosis of the Max-Planck-Gesellschaft at the Justus-Liebig-University, Giessen (F.R.G.)

Introduction

Inhibition of fibrin polymerization occurs through the action of fibrin(ogen) degradation products (1-4) or small peptides, representing the N-terminal sequence of the α- or ß-chain of fibrin (5,6). Fibrinogen has also been described to suppress fibrin polymerization <u>in vitro</u> or <u>in vivo</u> (7-11), thereby enabling the nascent fibrin to circulate in a soluble form. The reversible nature of the fibrin-fibrinogen interaction, which was studied under nearly physiological conditions at 37°C has been documented in former ultracentrifugation studies from our laboratory (12). In the course of these studies, it was noticed that the concentration of fibrin influenced the degree of fibrin polymerization in the presence of fibrinogen.

Experimental

Human fibrinogen was isolated by a modified glycine precipitation procedure (13,14). DesAA-fibrin and desAABB-fibrin were prepared as described (12). Radiolabelling was carried out using the iodine monochloride method (15). Mixtures of fibrin and fibrinogen in various molar ratios were incubated in Tris-buffer, pH 7.4, containing 2.7 M urea, the fibrinogen concentration always amounted to 2 mg/ml. After removal of urea by extensive dialysis, sample mixtures were incubated at 37°C for 1 hr before ultracentrifugation. Ultracentrifugation of fibrin-fibrinogen mixtures was carried out at 37°C for 3.5 hr or 6 hr, respectively, in a SW 41 rotor (Beckman) at 40,000 rpm either with 5-20% (w/v) or

Fibrinogen - Fibrin Formation and Fibrinolysis, Vol. 4
© 1986 Walter de Gruyter & Co., Berlin · New York - Printed in Germany.

5-30% (w/v) linear sucrose density gradients which contained fibrinogen at a uniform concentration of 2 mg/ml. Sedimentation coefficients were approximated (16) by using fibrinogen (8S), thyroglobulin (12.5S, 19.5S) and IgM (19S) as standards and are not corrected for temperature and density of the medium.

Results

Different Polymeric Forms of desAA-Fibrin and desAABB-Fibrin in Fibrin-Fibrinogen Mixtures

If mixtures of fibrin and fibrinogen were centrifuged at 37°C through sucrose density gradients which contained uniformally distributed fibrinogen, calcium ions, and inhibitors to prevent thrombin and Factor XIIIa action, two distinct peaks became separated. Depending on the initial fibrin concentration, the faster migrating fibrin peak was found at various positions within the gradient, whereas the position of radiolabelled fibrinogen re-

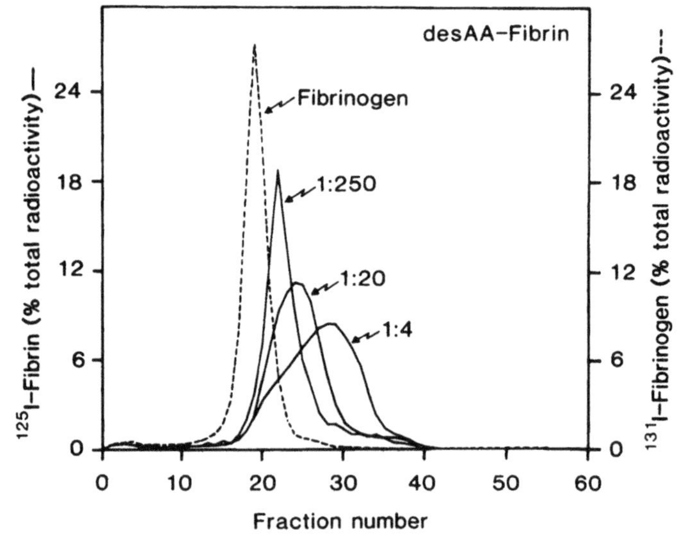

Figure 1: Ultracentrifugation of mixtures of 125I-desAA-fibrin and 131I-fibrinogen in varying molar ratios as indicated through linear 5-30% (w/v) sucrose density gradients containing 2 mg/ml fibrinogen at 37°C for 6 hr. Sedimentation direction is to the right. (From (17)).

mained constant regardless which ratio of fibrin to fibrinogen was employed. This dependence of the size of the polymeric forms of fibrin on their initial concentrations is depicted for desAA-fibrin (Fig. 1) as well as for desAABB-fibrin (Fig. 2) by superimposing the results of three independent ultracentrifugation runs with different initial ratios of fibrin to fibrinogen. The higher the initial fibrin concentration was, the larger became the sedimentation coefficient or the apparent size of the fibrin material. In this respect, at the same fibrin to fibrinogen ratio, desAABB-fibrin always formed higher polymeric forms than desAA-fibrin.

The presence of fibrinogen within the gradients ensured total recovery of the proteins. No co-sedimentation of fibrin with fibrinogen, originated from the sample mixture, was apparent. The approximation of the sedimentation coefficients for the different positions of the polymeric forms of fibrin was accomplished by means of calibration curves which were constructed with three proteins of known sedimentation coefficients. The sucrose gra-

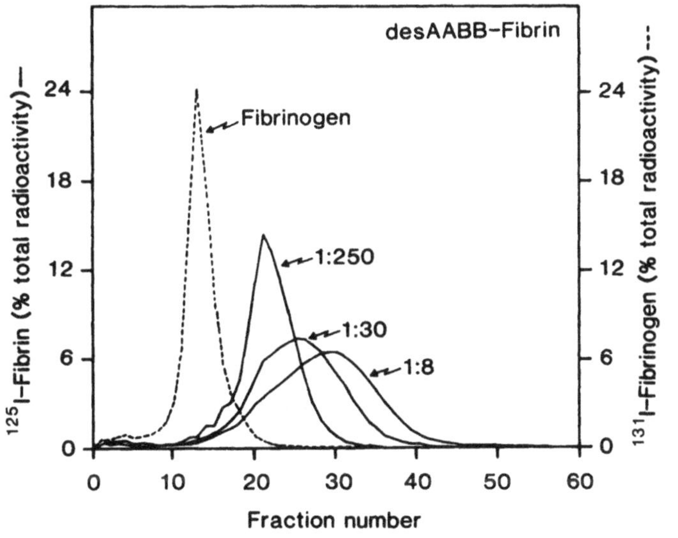

Figure 2: Ultracentrifugation of mixtures of 125I-desAABB-fibrin and 131I-fibrinogen in varying molar ratios as indicated through linear 5-20% (w/v) sucrose density gradients containing 2 mg/ml fibrinogen at 37°C for 3.5 hr. Sedimentation direction is to the right. (From (17)).

Table 1:

Sedimentation Coefficients (S) of Polymeric Forms of Fibrin. Mean values ± SD are given for n experiments.

Sample	Ratio of fibrin to fibrinogen	S	n
DesAA-fibrin/ fibrinogen	1:4	13.3 ± 0.4	3
	1:20	10.4 ± 0.5	9
	1:250	8.9 ± 0.5	9
DesAABB-fibrin/ fibrinogen	1:8	20.6 ± 0.9	4
	1:30	16.9 ± 0.3	4
	1:250	13.5 ± 0.4	4

dients remained linear over the analyzed range after the centrifugation. Table 1 summarizes the sedimentation coefficients of the polymeric forms of fibrin at different fibrin concentrations. The sedimentation coefficients of desAA-fibrin ranged from about 9S to 13S, whereas for des AABB-fibrin values from about 14S to 21S were found. Taking the highest ratio of desAA-fibrin to fibrinogen (1:4) in these mixtures, the material still represented smaller polymeric forms of fibrin than desAABB-fibrin to fibrinogen at its lowest chosen ratio (1:250).

DesAA-fibrin - desAABB-Fibrin Interactions

The interaction between both types of fibrin in the presence of fibrinogen was studied in a similar experimental setting at 37°C in the presence of calcium ions. Equimolar amounts of differently labelled desAA-fibrin and desAABB-fibrin were mixed at three different ratios of total fibrin to fibrinogen with a constant amount of unlabelled fibrinogen. After centrifugation through gradients containing uniformally distributed fibrinogen, a separation of both types of fibrin to remote positions occurs as was found in the former experiments. The same dependence of the size of polymeric forms of both types of fibrin on their initial concentration was observed (Fig. 3). However, co-sedimentation of a fraction of desAA-fibrin with the faster migrating desAABB-fibrin was evident indicating a strong interaction of both types of fibrin. The portion of co-sedimenting desAA-fibrin was also dependent on the initial fibrin concentration and amounted to 12%, 24%, and 29% of total desAA-fibrin, respectively, depending

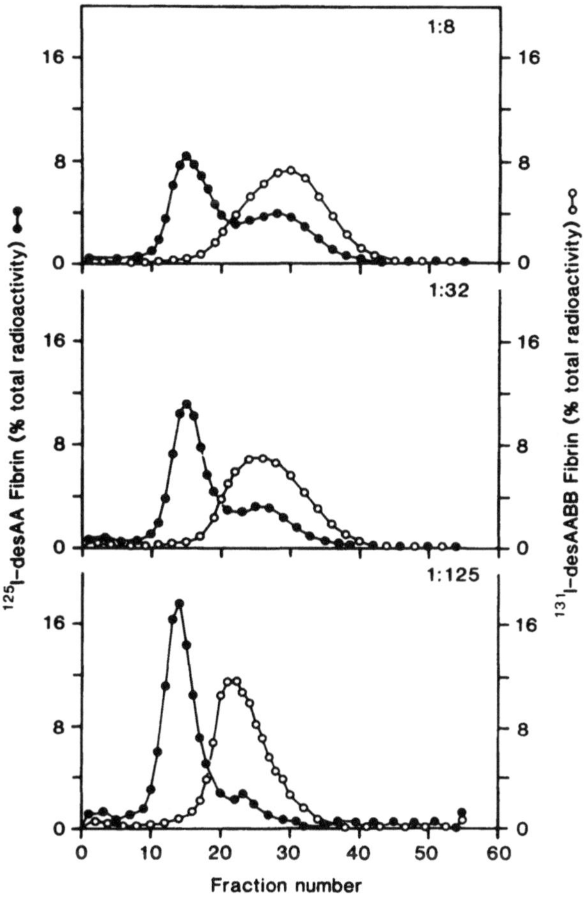

Figure 3: Ultracentrifugation of mixtures of 125I-desAA-fibrin and 131I-desAABB-fibrin together with fibrinogen in varying molar ratios of total fibrin to fibrinogen as indicated through linear 5-30% (w/v) sucrose density gradients containing 2 mg/ml fibrinogen at 37°C for 3.5 hr. Sedimentation direction is to the right.

on the molar ratios of fibrin to fibrinogen of 1:125, 1:32, and 1:8, respectively. In contrast, the presence of 2 mM EDTA in the sample mixtures and the gradients instead of calcium chloride totally abolished the co-sedimentation of both types of fibrin.

Discussion

Numerous studies have provided evidence that fibrinogen or fibrin(ogen) degradation products act as solubilizing agents for soluble fibrin by preventing fibrin polymerization (1-4,10,18,19). During the early phase of the fibrinogen-fibrin conversion, such soluble fibrin becomes also detectable in the circulation (3,8, 11,20,21). The present study continues work that was initiated to define the polymeric forms of fibrin in soluble fibrin in the presence of excess fibrinogen. Depending on the type of fibrin, heterogeneous populations of polymeric forms of fibrin were formed whose sizes were governed by the initial fibrin concentrations. Both types of fibrin exhibited an increase in the size of polymers that was concentration-dependent and more pronounced for desAABB-fibrin. A similar dependence of the yield of cross-linked fibrin-fibrinogen on the fibrin concentration was found by others (22).

Since fibrin with a sedimentation coefficient of about 8S to 9S represents a monomeric form and material with 12S to 13S fibrin dimers (23), it is reasonable to assume that the only product which may be designated as fibrin monomer in these gradients has the characteristics of desAA-fibrin. In contrast, the smallest form of desAABB-fibrin seems to be a dimer. These findings are in agreement with the concept that desAABB-fibrin exhibits a higher tendency for polymer formation than desAA-fibrin (24) due to the expression of additional polymerization sites after the release of fibrinopeptides B (25).

If both types of fibrin coexist during this stage of the clotting process, interactions between desAA-fibrin and desAABB-fibrin might result. In the same ultracentrifugation system, we investigated 1:1 mixtures of both types of fibrin in the presence of excess fibrinogen. The calcium-dependent co-sedimentation of a portion of desAA-fibrin with the faster migrating desAABB-fibrin

suggests a co-polymerization of both types of fibrin. The amount of incorporated desAA-fibrin was dependent on the initial fibrin concentration, whereby the size of the resulting polymer was governed by the polymeric forms of desAABB-fibrin.
In conclusion: Soluble fibrin constitutes a heterogeneous population of different polymeric forms of fibrin in the presence of fibrinogen. The size of these polymers was dependent on the initial fibrin concentration. Under physiological conditions, a cooperative process for the early stage of the fibrin polymerization, involving both types of fibrin, was observed whereby only desAA-fibrin may exist in monomeric form at 37°C.

Acknowledgement

This work was supported by the Stiftung Volkswagenwerk, Hannover.

References

1. Lipinski, B., Z. Wegrzynowicz, A.Z. Budzynski, M. Kopeć, Z.S. Latallo, E. Kowalski. 1967. Thromb. Diath. Haemorrh. 17, 65-77.

2. Marder, V.J., N.R. Shulman, W.R. Carroll. 1969. J. Biol. Chem. 244, 2111-2119.

3. Niewarowski, S., V. Gurewich. 1971. J. Lab. Clin. Med. 77, 665-676.

4. Haverkate, F., G. Timan, W. Nieuwenhuizen. 1979. Eur. J. Clin. Invest. 9, 253-255.

5. Laudano, A.P., R.F. Doolittle. 1978. Proc. Natl. Acad. Sci. USA 78, 3085-3088.

6. Hsieh, K., M.S. Mudd, G.D. Wilner. 1981. J. Med. Chem. 24, 322-327.

7. Shainoff, J.R., I.H. Page. 1962. J. Exp. Med. 116, 687-707.

8. Bang, N.U., M.L. Chang. 1974. Sem. Thrombos. Hemostas. 1, 91-128.

9. Müller-Berghaus, G., I. Mahn, G. Köveker, F.-D. Maul. 1976. Br. J. Haematol. 33, 61-79.

10. Shainoff, J.R., I.H. Page. 1960. Circ. Res. 8, 1010-1022.

11. Kröhnke, I., I. Mahn, W. Krell, G. Müller-Berghaus. 1980. Br. J. Haematol. 45, 131-141.

12. Preissner, K.T., J. Rötker, E. Selmayr, H. Fasold, G. Müller-Berghaus. 1985. Biochim. Biophys. Acta (in press).

13. Blombäck, B., M. Blombäck. 1956. Ark. Kemi 10, 415-443.

14. Mahn, I., G. Müller-Berghaus. 1975. Haemostasis 4, 40-50.

15. McFarlane, A.S. 1958. Nature 182, 53.

16. O'Brien, R.D., C.A. Timpone, R.E. Gibson. 1978. Anal. Biochem. 86, 602-615.

17. Rötker, J., K.T. Preissner, G. Müller-Berghaus. 1985. (submitted)

18. Brosstad, F. 1979. Thromb. Res. 15, 563-568.

19. Alkjaersig, N., A.P. Fletcher. 1983. Biochem. J. 213, 75-83.

20. Godal, H.C.,U. Abildgaard. 1966. Scand. J. Haemat. 3, 342-350.

21. Largo, R., V. Heller, P.W. Straub. 1976. Blood 47, 991-1002.

22. Kanaide, H., J.R. Shainoff. 1976. J. Lab. Clin. Med. 85, 574-579.

23. Smith, G.F. 1980. Biochem. J. 185, 1-11.

24. Nossel, H., K.L. Kaplan. 1979. In: Chemistry and Physiology of the Human Plasma Proteins (D. Bing, ed.) Pergamon Press, New York, pp. 97-110.

25. Olexa, S.A., A.Z. Budzynski. 1980. Proc. Natl. Acad. Sci. USA 77, 1374-1378.

RELATIONSHIP OF FINAL THICKNESS OF FIBRIN FIBERS TO MAXIMAL RATE OF ASSEMBLY AND TO FIBRINOPEPTIDE B RELEASE

H. Pirkle, P. Vukasin, I. Theodor, D. Miyada
Department of Pathology, College of Medicine, University of California, Irvine, CA 92717

Introduction

While Ferry and Morrison put forward the first explicit model for clot formation through longitudinal and lateral growth of fibrin fibers (1), the notion that these two modes of assembly depended, respectively, on the release of fibrinopeptide A (FPA) and fibrinopeptide B (FPB) arose from the light scattering observations of Laurent and Blomback on fibrinogen treated with thrombin or with reptilase (2). Some subsequent studies have supported a role for FPB release in the lateral aggregation of fibrin (3,4), but others have not (5,6).

The present studies focus on the fiber thickness of mature clots formed with and without FPB release, taking into account the effect of other factors which influence fiber thickness. We found that the presence or absence of FPB on fibrin monomers had no effect on the thickness of repolymerized fibers, but that some difference between thrombin and batroxobin in their kinetics of fibrinopeptide release did, under most conditions, produce differences in fiber thickness.

Methods

Fibrinogen was isolated from human plasma by glycine precipitation (7) and freed of factor XIII by chromatography on DEAE-cellulose. Batroxobin was purified from *Bothrops atrox* venom (Sigma) by gel filtration on Sephadex G-200 followed by chromatography with salt gradients on DEAE-cellulose and SP-Sephadex. The product was electrophoretically homogeneous (8) and had a

Fibrinogen - Fibrin Formation and Fibrinolysis, Vol. 4
© 1986 Walter de Gruyter & Co., Berlin · New York - Printed in Germany.

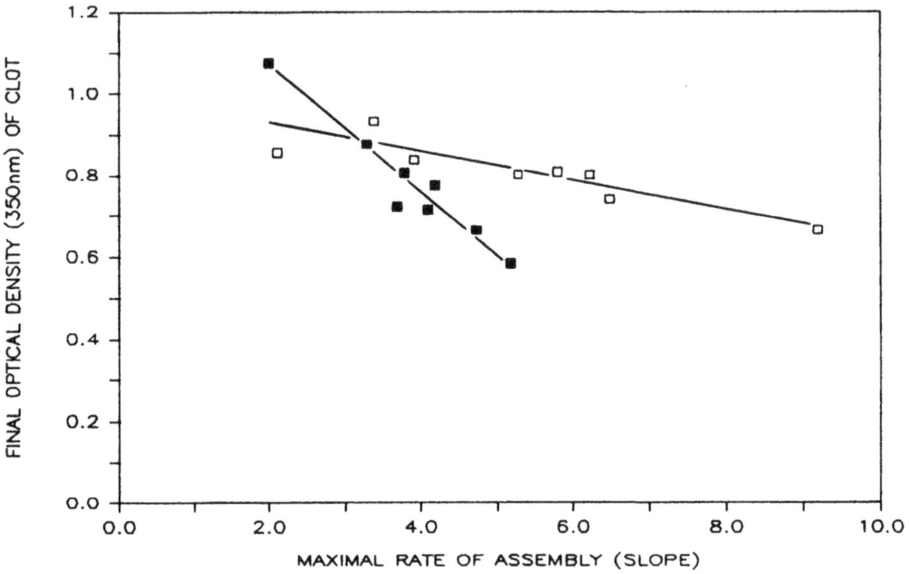

Fig. 1. Final optical density of primary clot as a function of maximal rate of assembly. Batroxobin, closed symbols; thrombin, open symbols. Enzyme concentration, 0.3-1.0 NIH units or equivalents/ml. Fibrinogen concentration, 0.27 mg/ml.

specific activity of 1200 thrombin equivalent units/mg, estimating activity from the crossing point of the batroxobin and thrombin dilution curves. Highly purified human thrombin (3200 NIH units/mg) was kindly supplied by J. W. Fenton, II. Optical density of clotting mixtures in polystyrene cuvettes was monitored in a recording spectrophotometer at 350 nm with the temperature controlled at 24° C. Maximal rate of assembly of the clot was taken as the slope of the manually placed tangent to the point of inflection of the sigmoidal optical density curve. Final optical density was the value beyond which the curve showed no further change. Fibrinopeptide release was determined by HPLC of the clot supernatants (9). Fibrin monomers were prepared by winding the clot onto a glass rod and immersing it in 0.02 M acetic acid. Monomers were repolymerized by adding 0.4 ml to 2 ml of 0.06 M of phosphate buffer of the desired pH, adjusted to the desired ionic strength with NaCl. In some experiments, the

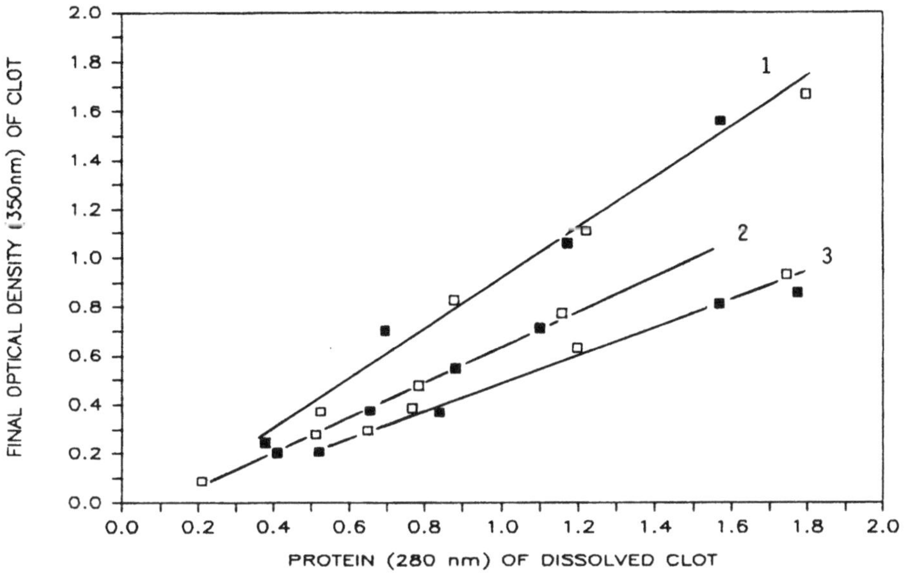

Fig. 2. Final optical density of repolymerized monomer clots, varying in protein content. Batroxobin monomers, closed symbols; thrombin monomers, open symbols. Curve 1: pH 6.8, ionic strength = 0.165. Curve 2: pH 6.8, ionic strength = 0.250. Curve 3: pH 7.2, ionic strength = 0.192.

repolymerization mixture was 0.5 mM in $CaCl_2$. The protein content of the repolymerized clots was determined by absorbance at 282 nm in in alkaline urea solution (10). Both HPLC of clot supernatants and polyacrylamide gel electrophoresis of reduced fibrin chains of mature clots showed complete release of FPA and FPB by thrombin and complete release of FPA only by batroxobin.

Results

Fig. 1 shows that the final optical density of both thrombin and batroxobin clots was an inverse linear function of maximal rate of assembly, varied by varying enzyme concentration. Batroxobin clots showed a stronger dependence of optical density on rate of assembly than did thrombin clots.

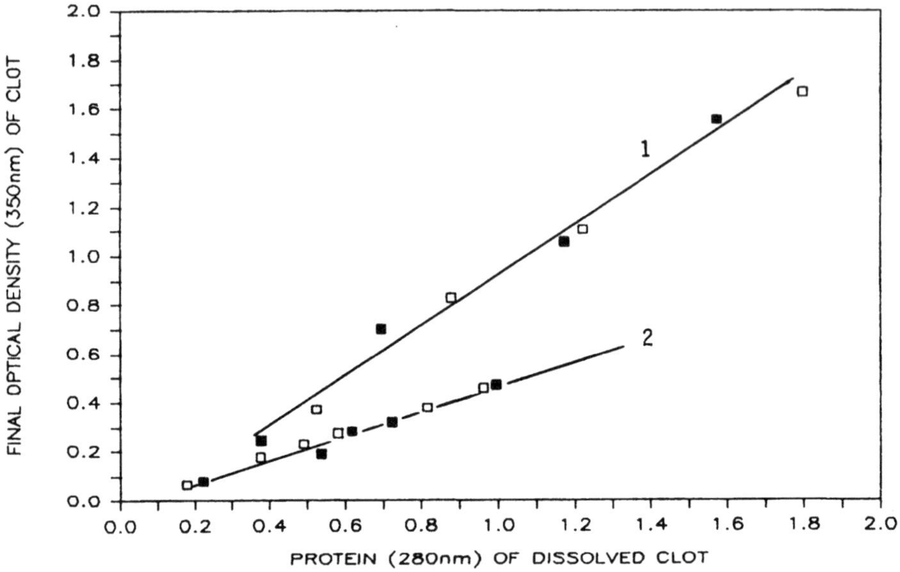

Fig. 3. Final optical density of repolymerized monomer clots, varying in protein content, without calcium (curve 1) and with 0.5 mM calcium (curve 2). Batroxobin monomers, closed symbols; thrombin monomers, open symbols. pH 6.8, ionic strength = 0.165.

To see whether the difference in optical density between thrombin clots and batroxobin clots depended on their different FPB content, we compared repolymerization of the monomers prepared from the two kinds of clots as shown in Fig. 2. Clot turbidity was varied by varying monomer concentration to see if thrombin monomers and batroxobin monomers in the same amount would produce clots with the same turbidity. As seen in Fig. 2, thrombin clots and batroxobin clots with the same protein content had the same optical density, even when optical density was altered by changes in pH, ionic strength, and (Fig. 3) calcium.

Discussion

The effect of rate of clotting on clot turbidity and fiber thickness is well known qualitatively (1,11), but has not previously been expressed in the simple quantitative relationship given here. This relationship allowed us to compare the turbidity of clots standardized to the same maximal rate of assembly and to find that retention of FPB does not necessarily give a less turbid clot, as is commonly thought. On the contrary, we found that, depending on maximal rate of assembly, batroxobin clots which had demonstrably released no FPB were less, equally, or more turbid than thrombin clots that had released all their FPB. This finding may explain some discrepant results of others (3-6).

The basis for the difference between thrombin and batroxobin with respect to turbidity of their primary clots is not clear. However, it is clear from the repolymerization results that this difference does not depend on the FPB content of the fibrin. The difference between the two kinds of primary clots must depend, then, on the presence of the enzymes in the clotting mixture and, presumably, on differences between the ongoing actions that they catalyze. Thus, detailed studies on the kinetics of fibrinopeptide release may hold the answer.

The identity in optical density for repolymerized batroxobin and thrombin clots which we found is in puzzling contrast to the results of Spellman _et al_. (3), who reported that repolymerized ancrod clots were less turbid than thrombin clots under all of a variety of conditions. One possible basis for the contrasting results may be the different venom enzymes used, since ancrod and batroxobin have been shown to have different secondary proteolytic characteristics (12). Another possible factor may be the multiple preparative repolymerizations used by Spellman _et al_., a procedure which we have found to differentially denature desAA monomers or to select species which give less turbid clots.

Here we interpret optical density as reflecting relative mean fiber thickness (13,14) but with the reservation that branching may contribute (15), although not necessarily independently.

Conclusion

In the presence of thrombin or batroxobin, clot opacity (and, presumably, mean fiber thickness) is an inverse linear function of maximal rate of assembly of the clot.

The relationship between opacity of batroxobin and thrombin clots varies according to maximal rate of assembly.

Differences in opacity between batroxobin and thrombin clots do not depend on their content of FPB.

Acknowledgement

This research was supported by a grant from the American Heart Association, California Affiliate.

References

1. Ferry, J. D. and P. R. Morrison. 1947. Preparation and properties of serum and plasma proteins. VIII. The conversion of human fibrinogen to fibrin under various conditions. J. Am. Chem. Soc. 69, 388-400.

2. Laurent, T. C. and B. Blombäck. 1958. On the significance of the release of two different peptides from fibrinogen during clotting. Acta Chem. Scand. 12, 1875-1877.

3. Spellman, G. G., Jr., J. Macoviak and H. R. Gralnick. 1977. Comparison of polymerization of ancrod and thrombin fibrin monomers. Blood 50, 619-624.

4. Shen L. L., J. Hermans, J. McDonagh and R. P. McDonagh. 1977. Role of fibrinopeptide B release: Comparison of fibrins produced by thrombin and ancrod. Am J. Physiol. 232, H629-H633.

5. Brosstad, F., P. Kierulf and H. C. Godal. 1979. The fibrin-solubilizing effect of fibrinogen as studied by light scattering. Thrombos. Res. 14, 705-712.

6. Furlan, M., C. Rupp and E. A. Beck. 1983. Inhibition of fibrin polymerization by fragment D is affected by calcium, Gly-Pro-Arg and Gly-His-Arg. Biochim. Biophys. Acta 742, 25-32.

7. Kazal, L. G., S. Amsel, O. P. Miller and L. M. Tocantins. 1963. The preparation and some properties of fibrinogen precipitated from human plasma by glycine. Proc. Soc. Exp. Biol. Med. 113, 989-994.

8. Laemmli, U. K. 1970. Cleavage of structural proteins during the assembly of the head of bacteriophage T4. Nature 227, 680-685.

9. Kehl, M., F. Lottspeich and A. Henschen. 1981. Analysis of human fibrinopeptides by high-performance liquid chromatography. Hoppe-Seyler's Z. Physiol. Chem. 362, 1661-1664.

10. Blombäck, B. 1958. On the properties of fibrinogen and fibrin. Arkiv Kemi. 12, 99-113.

11. Buchanan, J. M., L. B. Chen, T. Hamazaki, E. Lenk and D. F. Waugh. 1977. In: Chemistry and Biology of Thrombin (R. L. Lundblad, J. W. Fenton, II and K. G. Mann, eds.). Ann Arbor Science Publishers Inc., Ann Arbor, pp. 263-273.

12. Mattock, P. and M. P. Esnouf. 1971. Differences in the subunit structure of human fibrin formed by the action of arvin, reptilase and thrombin. Nature New Biol. 233, 277-279.

13. Hantgan, R., W. Fowler, H. Erickson and J. Hermans. 1980. Fibrin assembly: A comparison of electron microscopic and light scattering results. Thrombos. Haemostas. 44, 119-124.

14. Hermans, J., personal communication.

15. Müller, M. and W. Burchard. 1982. In.: Fibrinogen. Recent Biochemical and Medical Aspects (A. Henschen, H. Graeff and F. Lottspeich, eds.). Walter de Gruyter, Berlin, New York, pp. 29-42.

III. Congenital Variants

FIBRINOGEN NEW YORK 1: THE STRUCTURAL, FUNCTIONAL, AND GENETIC DEFECTS AND AN HYPOTHESIS OF THE ROLE OF FIBRIN IN THE REGULATION OF COAGULATION AND FIBRINOLYSIS

C.Y. Liu, P. Wallen*, and D.A. Handley

Department of Medicine, College of Physicians and Surgeons
Columbia University, New York, New York 10032 and
* Department of Physiological Chemistry, University of Umea.

Introduction

Thrombosis is a frequent pathologic process. Dysfibrinogenemia has been increasingly recognized as a cause of abnormal coagulation tests and, in approximately half the patients, is associated with hemorrhage or thrombosis (1). To-date, five patients have been reported with dysfibrinogenemia associated with recurrent thrombosis (2-6). However, the relationship between the structural abnormalities of the fibrinogen molecule and the clinical manifestations has yet to be established.

Fibrinogen New York 1 (NY-1), a dysfunctional fibrinogen identified in a family with thrombotic tendency, is inherited in a heterozygous, autosomal codominant fashion (6,7). Biochemical studies (7,8) indicated that NY-1 fibrinogen and NY-1a fibrinogen (purified from a brother of the original patient) contain two types of Bβ-chains: a normal and an abnormal chain (Fig. 1). Amino acid sequence analysis (7,9) demonstrated a deletion of 64 residues (from 9 to 72) in the NH_2-terminal region of the abnormal Bβ-chain (Fig. 2), corresponding exactly to exon 2 of the gene.

Plasminogen activation by tissue plasminogen activator (tPA) was shown to be markedly enhanced by normal fibrin. However, the thrombin-nonclottable fibrin derived from NY-1 fibrinogen showed defective potentiation of plasminogen activation by tPA (10). Studies indicated that the binding of tPA and thrombin by NY-1 fibrin were both abnormal. Microscopic studies of the NY-1 fibrin clot showed an abnormal structure with numerous short fibrin aggregates lacking systematically ordered fibrin strands

Fibrinogen - Fibrin Formation and Fibrinolysis, Vol. 4
© 1986 Walter de Gruyter & Co., Berlin · New York - Printed in Germany.

(11). Thus, the deletion of Bβ(9-72) has important structural, functional, and genetic implications. This report presents a summary of the results of these studies.

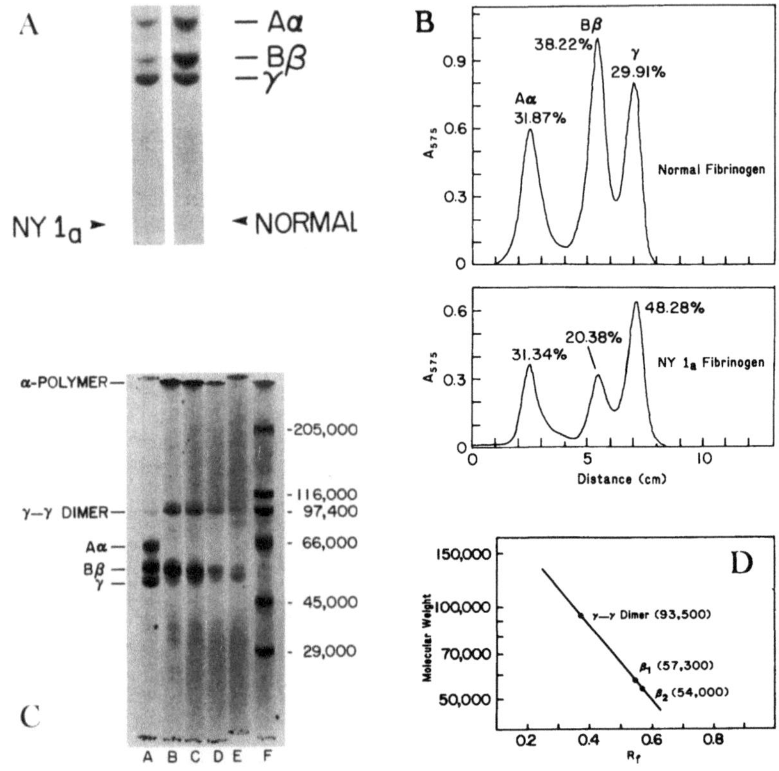

Fig. 1: <u>Identification of the Abnormal Bβ-Chain by SDS-PAGE (7.5%)</u>

A) Gels were run under reducing conditions and stained with Coomassie Blue. B) Densitometric tracings for gels shown in A. C) Fibrin treated with Factor XIIIa and Ca^{+2} (except for samples in gels A and F) was run under reducing conditions, and the gels stained with Coomassie Blue. Gel A, normal fibrinogen (5 mg/ml) in TBS buffer treated with thrombin (2 NIH units/ml); gel B, normal fibrinogen treated with thrombin and Factor XIIIa in the presence of Ca^{+2} (2 mM); gel C, fibrinogen NY-la (clottable and non-clottable treated like gel B; gel D, thrombin-clottable fibrin from fibrinogen NY-la treated like gel B; gel E, thrombin-nonclottable fibrin from fibrinogen NY-la treated like gel B; gel F, standard proteins as molecular weight markers (myosin, 205,000; β-galactosidase, 116,000; phosphorylase b, 97,400; bovine serum albumin, 66,000; ovalbumin, 45,000; carbonic anhydrase, 29,000). D) Determination of the molecular weights of normal (β_1) and abnormal (β_2) Bβ-chains. See ref. 7 for further information.

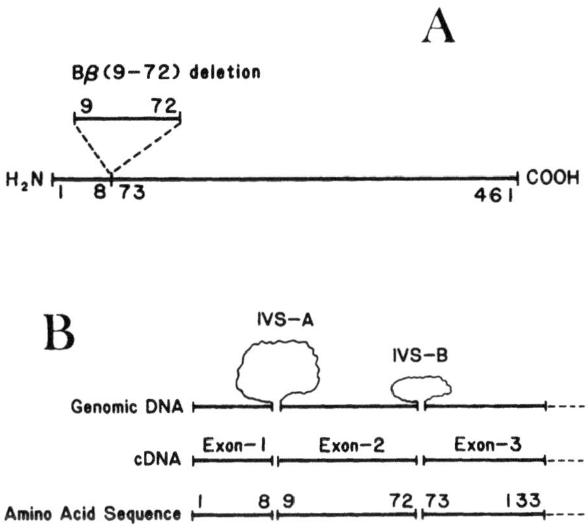

Fig. 2: Amino Acid Sequence Analysis of Bβ-Chain of Fibrinogen NY-1a

A) The abnormal Bβ-chain with a deletion of Bβ(9-72).
B) A portion of the genomic DNA and cDNA structure corresponding to the NH_2-terminal end of the normal Bβ-chain.

The numbers for the Bβ-chain are the amino acid positions corresponding to the respective exons. See ref. 7 for further information.

Experimental Procedures

Materials and Methods were as previously described (7,12,13), with exceptions described in this report.

Results and Discussion

Identification of the Abnormal Bβ-Chain

Treatment of NY-1 and NY-1a fibrinogens with thrombin (2 NIH units/ml) gave rise to a clot that contained the clottable fibrin (presumably normal) and a supernatant that contained the nonclottable fibrin (presumably abnormal) (Table 1). Treatment with higher thrombin concentration (80 NIH units/ml) gave the same results. Although thrombin treatment resulted in quantitative release of fibrinopeptide A (FPA), fibrinopeptide B (FPB) cleavage was approximately half that of normal (Table 2). Thus, this localized the defect to the NH_2-terminus of the Bβ-chain. In the presence of Ca^{2+} the thrombin non-clottable fibrin could clot. The sizes of the three chains of the abnormal fibrinogen were examined by SDS-PAGE (Fig. 1).

Table 1 Percentage of Non-Clottable Fibrinogen

	NY-1	NY-1a	Normal
Clottable	50%	60-65%	98%
Non-Clottable	50%	35-40%	2%

Table 2 Fibrinopeptide Release by Thrombin

	NY-1	NY-1a	Normal
FPA/Fibrinogen (mole/mole)	1.9	1.9	2
FPB/Fibrinogen	0.6-1.0	1.0-1.3	1.9

The Bβ-chain region of NY-1a fibrinogen was less dense than that of normal fibrinogen (Fig. 1A,B), suggesting that the abnormal Bβ-chain had a molecular weight less than that of the normal. Similar results were observed with NY-1 fibrinogen. To confirm this, cross-linked NY-1 fibrin was analyzed by SDS-PAGE (Fig. 1C,D). In addition to the α-polymers, γ, γ-dimers, and the normal Bβ-chain protein bands, there is a band with a slightly lower molecular weight than the normal Bβ-chain (gels C and E). The molecular weight of this defective Bβ-chain (β_2) was estimated to be 54,000 as compared to 57,000 (β_1) for the normal Bβ-chain. These molecular weight differences are consistent with a deletion of about 30 amino acids.

To determine the amino acid sequence of the abnormal Bβ-chain of NY-1a, automated Edman degradation was performed. The results indicated that the abnormal Bβ-chain (7,9) resulted from a deletion of residues Bβ(9-72) (Fig. 2A). The major features and partial sequence of the genomic DNA and cDNA coding for the

Bβ-chain of human fibrinogen have been described (14); seven intervening sequences (IVS) were identified. IVS-A and IVS-B are located between amino acids 8/9 and 72/73, with the sequence 9-72 representing exon-2. Thus, this deletion corresponds exactly to exon-2 of the gene (Fig. 2B). The most likely cause of this deletion is abnormal RNA-splicing (7). The loss of the 3' splice site of IVS-A and the use of the 3' splice site of IVS B would lead to elimination of exon-2 during RNA processing. It is also possible that there are two alternative RNA-splicing pathways for the Bβ-chain of fibrinogen with the abnormal splicing pathway observed in NY-1a less efficiently used in the normal.

The deletion of residues (9-72) is likely to be the only defect in Fibrinogen NY since double mutation in a single gene is very uncommon. The absence of the normal thrombin (14/15) cleavage site (Fig. 2A) explains the decrease FPB recovery following thrombin cleavage (Table 2). Normally Cys-65 of the Bβ-chain forms a disulfide bond with Cys-36 of the Aα-chain. Since this residue is missing, Fibrinogen NY would be expected to have a free SH group at residue 36 of the Aα-chain. Alternatively, a different arrangement of the disulfide bond may result in a conformation change in the NH_2-terminal region. In this way the deletion in the Bβ-chain could lead to a structural change in the Aα-chain. As there is a fibrin polymerization site in the NH_2-terminal region of fibrinogen (15) this may explain why the abnormal fibrin cannot clot in response to thrombin. This deletion represents a new type of genetic and structural defect in the fibrinogen molecule; variants studied in detail to-date have proved to be point mutations only (16).

Functional Defects of the Abnormal Fibrinogen

It is believed that there is a dynamic steady state of coagulation and fibrinolysis in vivo (Fig. 3) as indicated by the observations that: (i) there is a normal FPA level (17) which reflects baseline thrombin or coagulation activity; (ii) there are normal levels of Bβ(1-42) and other fibrinogen degraded products which indicate plasmin or fibrinolytic activity (18,19); and (iii) changes in these levels occur during certain pathological states (19,20,21). Since thrombin can initiate fibrin formation and platelet aggregation, it is inferred (22) that adsorption of thrombin to a fibrin clot serves to regulate the coagulation process (Fig. 4). Thus, thrombin binding by NY fibrin was studied using iodinated thrombin. Trapped thrombin in the fluid within the clot was washed out and the bound thrombin (Fig. 5) was measured as previously described (12). Scatchard analysis of the binding data at the high affinity binding site (Fig. 6) indicate that NY-1 fibrin (mixture of thrombin clottable and non-clottable has comparable binding affinity (K_a = $6x10^5$ M^{-1}) but less binding capacity (50%) than does normal fibrin. Chromatographic studies indicate that only the clottable fibrin could bind thrombin (23). Thus, defective thrombin binding of the non-clottable fibrin was responsible for the decreased thrombin binding capacity. This observation is consistent with the concept that a higher than normal balance level of thrombin in circulation is one possible factor for the thrombotic tendency.

Plasmin activation by tPA has been shown to be markedly enhanced in the presence of fibrin. To study NY fibrin-mediated potentiation of plasminogen activation by tPA, the following experiments were performed (23). The acceleration rate of plasmin formation during plasminogen activation by tPA was measured at A_{405} using the plasmin synthetic substrate S-2251 (11). Using constant amounts of fibrinogen, glu-plasminogen, and synthetic substrate, tPA was added and the acceleration rate determined (Table 3). The addition of thrombin to either normal or abnormal fibrinogen resulted in enhanced plasmin formation.

However, the potentiation by NY-la fibrin is much less than that by normal fibrin (11,23). Although abnormal NY-la fibrinogen can clot in the presence of Ca^{2+}, Ca^{2+} addition does not correct the defective fibrin potentiation. To explore the mechanism for the defective fibrin potentiation, studies of tPA binding by fibrin were performed. These studies indicated that NY-la fibrin had only 40% of the tPA binding capacity of normal fibrin (23).

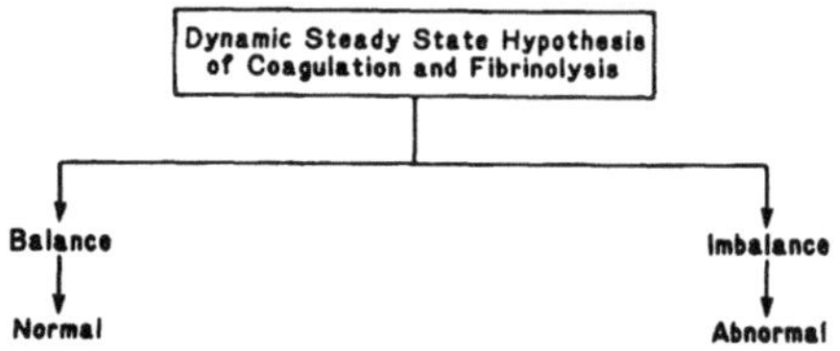

Fig. 3: Dynamic Steady State Hypothesis. Coagulation and fibrinolysis are two normal, dynamic processes and a balance is normally seen between these two processes.

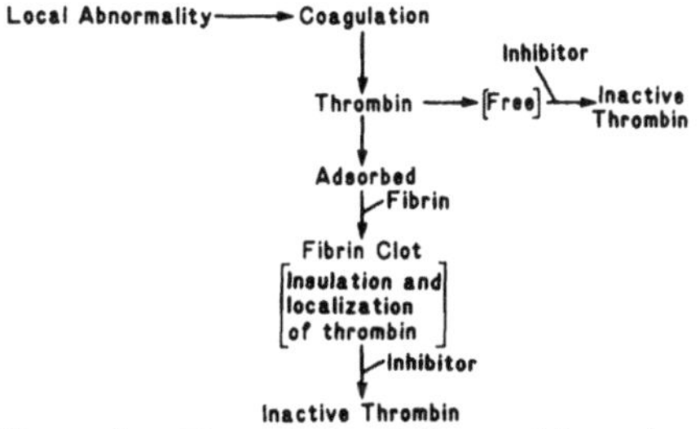

Fig. 4: Thrombin Adsorption by Fibrin. Thrombin bound by fibrin remains active but the adsorption process may physically localize thrombin action.

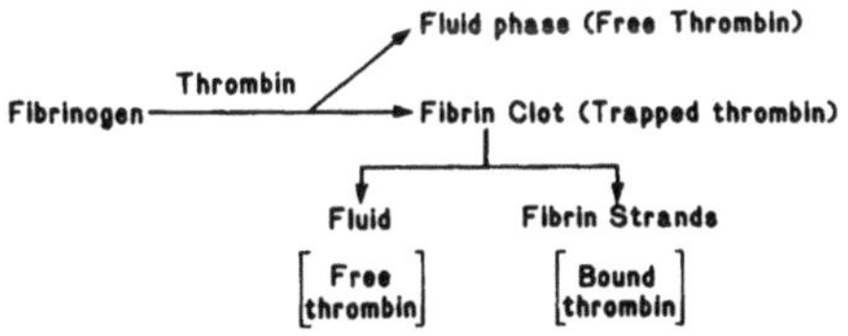

Fig. 5: Mechanism of Thrombin Adsorption by Fibrin in vitro. The fibrin clot consists of fibrin strands and the fluid between the strands. Thrombin adsorbed to the fibrin strands is assumed to be bound while that in the fluid is assumed to be free (12).

Morphological Study of the Fibrin Clots

The structure of the fibrin clot was visualized using polarized dark-field light microscopy (23). Normal fibrin exhibits systematically organized fibrin strands (Fig. 7A). Figure 7B represents a clot containing the mixture of clottable and non-clottable NY-la fibrins. Here numerous short fibrin aggregates were seen lacking systematically ordered fibrin strands. The non-clottable fibrin alone (Fig. 7C) showed only short dispersed aggregates without

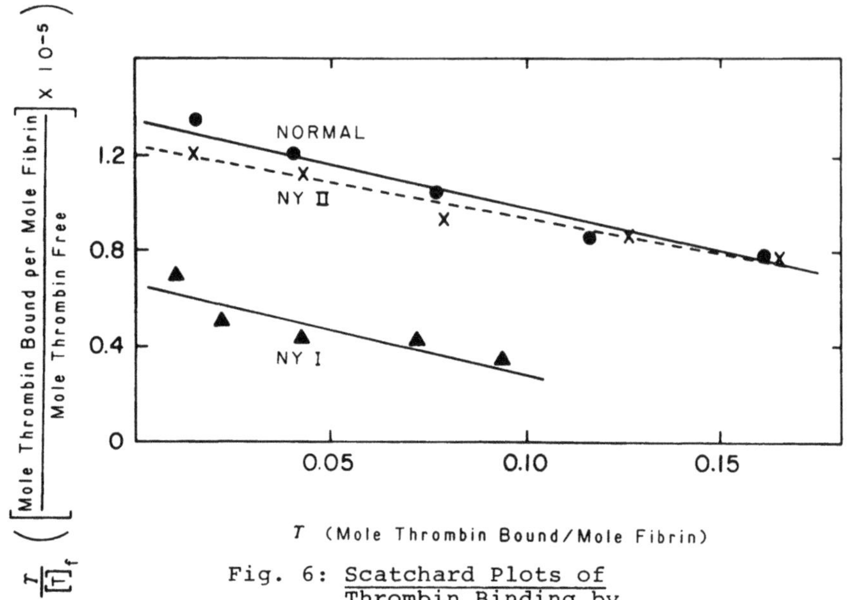

Fig. 6: <u>Scatchard Plots of Thrombin Binding by Fibrin at the High Affinity Binding Site.</u> Fibrinogen New York II (NY-II) is a dysfunctional fibrinogen not associated with a thrombotic tendency. See refs 12 and 23 for procedures and calculations.

long fibrin strands. Electron microscopic studies of the ultra-structure of the fibrin clots confirmed these results (23).

Thus, the Bβ(9-72) region may be a functional domain, or may be related to a functional domain(s), involved in normal fibrin polymerization, thrombin and tPA binding, and fibrin potentiation of plasminogen activation by tPA. The possible inter-relationships between these defects are: (i) the deletion may be directly related to these defects; and (ii) it may be indirectly related to the defective thrombin and tPA binding through defective fibrin polymerization, and the defective tPA-binding by fibrin may be related to the defective fibrin potentiation of plasminogen activation because of the defective formation of a trimolecular complex of fibrin, tPA and plasminogen. This interpretation is consistent with the observation (4) that an abnormal plasminogen-fibrin

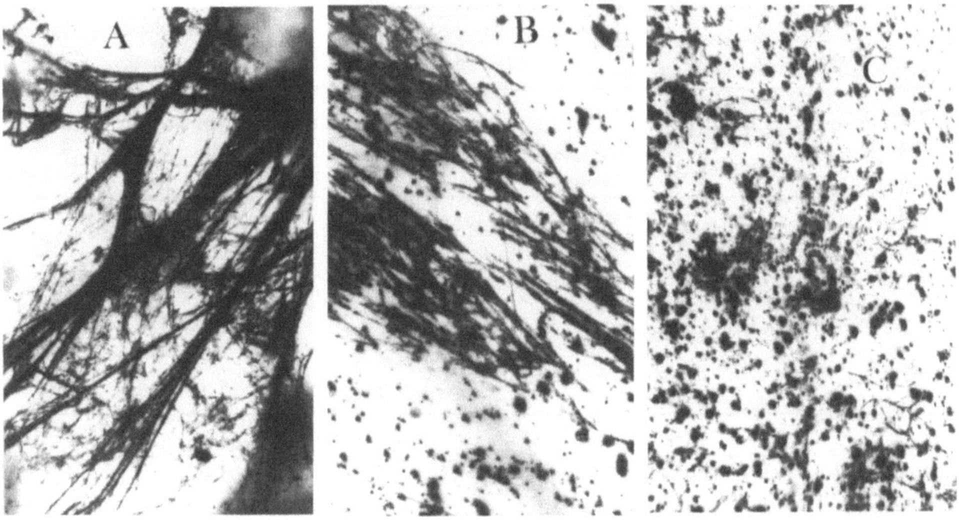

Fig. 7: Structure of Fibrin Clots Viewed by Light Microscopy. Fibrinogen was clotted with thrombin. See refs. 12 and 23 for experimental conditions. A) Normal fibrin clots. B) NY-1 fibrin clots, mixture of clottable and non-clottable. C) NY-1 fibrin clots, non-clottable only. (All pictures X750).

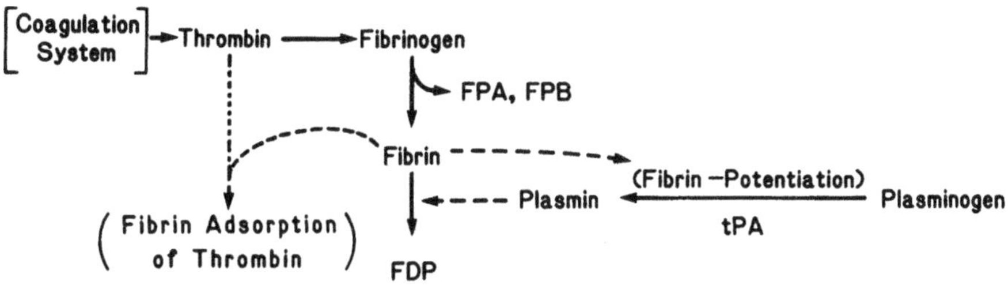

Fig. 8: A Hypothesis - The Role of Fibrin in the Regulation of Coagulation and Fibrinolysis. Fibrin may link the coagulation and fibrinolytic pathways as one dynamic continuous coagulation-fibrinolytic system. Fibrin may also act as a regulator of this dynamic system. It may regulate coagulation by absorbing thrombin and other coagulation factors, while it may serve to regulate fibrinolysis by potentiating tPA-mediated plasminogen activation.

FDP = Fibrin degraded products.

Table 3 Defective Fibrin Potentiation of Plasminogen Activation by tPA

Experimental Condition	Plasmin Formation Rate $(\Delta A_{405}/min^2) \times 10^4$	
Normal Fibrinogen	0.09	
Normal Fibrinogen + Thrombin	1.10	100%
NY-la Fibrinogen + Thrombin	0.73	60%
NY-la Fibrinogen + Ca^{2+} + Thrombin	0.51	42%

binding was associated with thrombotic tendency. Since Fibrinogen NY-1 was found in a family with thrombotic tendency, the deletion of Bβ(9-72) of fibrinogen molecule may not only have important structural, functional, and genetic, but also clinical implications.

The Role of Fibrin in Coagulation and Fibrinolysis

In conclusion, the results of these studies appear to support the following hypothesis regarding the role of fibrin (Fig. 8): (i) fibrin, the final product of coagulation and the initial substrate of plasmin in fibrinolysis, may serve to link these two pathways as one dynamic continuous coagulation-fibrinolytic system; and (ii) fibrin also may be a physiologically important regulator, controlling coagulation by absorbing thrombin and other coagulation factors and regulating fibrinolysis by potentiating tPA-mediated plasminogen activation. Further studies are in progress to evaluate this hypothesis.

Acknowledgements

This work was supported by NHLBI grant HL-15486 and Swedish Medical Research Council grant No. 13X-03906.

References

1. Menache, D. 1973. Thromb. Diath. Haemorrh. 29, 525.

2. Beck, E.A., J.R. Shainoff, A. Vogel, D.P. Jackson. 1971. J. Clin. Invest. 50, 1874.

3. Fuchs, G., R. Egbring, K. Haveman. 1977. Blut 34, 107.

4. Soria, J., C. Soria, J.P. Caen. 1983. Br. J. Haematol. 53, 575.

5. Carrell, N., D.A. Gabriel, P.M. Blatt, M.E. Carr, J. McDonagh. 1983. Blood 62, 439.

6. Al-Mondhiry, H., S.B. Bilezikian, H.L. Nossel. 1975. Blood 45, 607.

7. Liu, C.Y., J.A. Koehn, F.J. Morgan. 1985. J. Biol. Chem. 260, 4390.

8. Liu, C.Y., J.A. Koehn, H.L. Nossel. 1983. Thromb. Haemost. 50, 336.

9. Liu, C.Y., F.J. Morgan. 1984. Circulation 70, 1404.

10. Liu, C.Y., P. Wallen. 1984. Circulation 70, 1462.

11. Liu, C.Y., P. Wallen, D.A. Handley. 1985. Thromb. Haemost. 54, 640.

12. Liu, C.Y., H.L. Nossel, K.L. Kaplan. 1979. J. Biol. Chem. 254, 10421.

13. Liu, C.Y., D.A. Handley, S. Chien. 1985. Anal. Biochem. 147, 49.

14. Chung, D.W., B.G. Que, M.W. Rixon, M. Mace, Jr., E.W. Davie. 1983. Biochem. 22, 3244.

15. Kudryk, B.J., D. Collen, K.R. Woods, B. Blomback. 1974. J. Biol. Chem. 249, 3322.

16. Southan, C., A. Henschen, F. Lottspeich. 1982. In: Fibrinogen (A. Henschen, H. Graeff and F. Lottspeich, eds.) Walter de Gruyter, Berlin, p. 153.

17. Nossel, H.L., I. Yudelman, R.E. Canfield, V.P. Butler, K. Spanondis, G.D. Wilner, G.D. Qureshi. 1974. J. Clin. Invest. 54, 43.

18. Weitz, J., J. Koehn, H.L. Nossel, R.E. Canfield. 1983. Blood 62, 1086.

19. Nossel, H.L., J. Wasser, K.L. Kaplan, K.S. LaGamma, I. Yudelman, R.E. Canfield. 1979. J. Clin. Invest. 64, 1371.

20. Owen, J., D. Kvam, H.L. Nossel, K.L. Kaplan, P. Kernoff. 1983. Blood 61, 476.

21. Borok, Z., J. Weitz, J. Owen, M. Auerbach, H.L. Nossel. 1984. Blood 63, 525.

22. Liu, C.Y. 1981. Ann. N.Y. Acad. Sci. 370, 545.

23. Liu, C.Y., P. Wallen, D.A. Handley. 1985. Manuscript in preparation.

FIBRINOGEN PONTOISE - A GENETICALLY ABNORMAL FIBRINOGEN WITH DEFECTIVE FIBRIN POLYMERISATION BUT NORMAL FIBRINOPEPTIDE RELEASE

H.Kaudewitz, A.Henschen
Max-Planck-Institute for Biochemistry, D-8033 Martinsried München, German Federal Republic

J.Soria, C.Soria
Laboratories de Biochimie et d'Hematologie, Hotel Dieu, Paris, France

Introduction

The detailed understanding of the various properties of fibrin(ogen) is of great clinical importance and biochemical interest. An excellent tool for the investigation of many of the functions of fibrinogen is provided by the genetically abnormal variants. These fibrinogen variants usually differ from the normal molecule in only a single amino acid residue. The functional defect revealed by clinical observations and laboratory tests indicates the importance of the substituted amino acid residue. So far genetically abnormal fibrinogens have been detected in more than 130 families. Proteinchemical analyses of about 25 variants with defective fibrin formation, due to incomplete or slow fibrinopeptide release, showed an amino acid substitution in the neighbourhood of the thrombin cleavage site. Only three cases have been elucidated where the polymerisation defect was unrelated to fibrinopeptide release; here the amino acid substitutions were found to be located in the C-terminal part of the Bβ- or γ-chain. In this report the first

Fibrinogen - Fibrin Formation and Fibrinolysis, Vol. 4
© 1986 Walter de Gruyter & Co., Berlin · New York - Printed in Germany.

proteinchemical analyses of one of these cases, fibrinogen Pontoise, are discribed.
The heterozygously expressed genetically abnormal fibrinogen Pontoise is characterised by a highly prolonged clotting time of 88 sec compared to 20 sec for normal fibrinogen (1). Investigations of the three stages of fibrin formation showed that the aggregation of the fibrin monomers was defective, whereas the release of the fibrinopeptides after treatment with thrombin and the factor XIIIa dependent fibrin stabilisation were normal (2). The SDS gel electrophoresis of fibrinogen Pontoise after plasmin digestion showed the presence of two types of D-fragments, the normal one and a larger one. It was found that the higher molecular weight of the abnormal D-fragment was due to its β-chain component. The difference in size between the abnormal and the normal component corresponded to about 3000 Dalton and was assumed to be caused by a Bβ-chain extension (3).

Results and Discussion

In order to find the predicted extension of the Bβ-chain fibrinogen Pontoise was cleaved in parallel with normal fibrinogen with cyanogen bromide (4) and the fragments separated on a Sephadex G-50 column (Fig.1). Those parts of the two chromatographies in which a difference was observed (pools I and Ia) were subjected to new fractionations by high-performance liquid chromatography (HPLC) on a reversed phase column (Fig.2). The sample from the abnormal fibrinogen was found to contain an additional component. On N-terminal sequence analysis it was identified as a cyanogen bromide fragment of the β-chain with the starting sequence Glu-Asp-Trp-Lys (5,6). The amino acid analysis of the abnormal fragment showed, surprisingly, the presence of glucosamine, whereas the corresponding normal fragment is devoid of carbohydrate. The abnormal and normal fragment

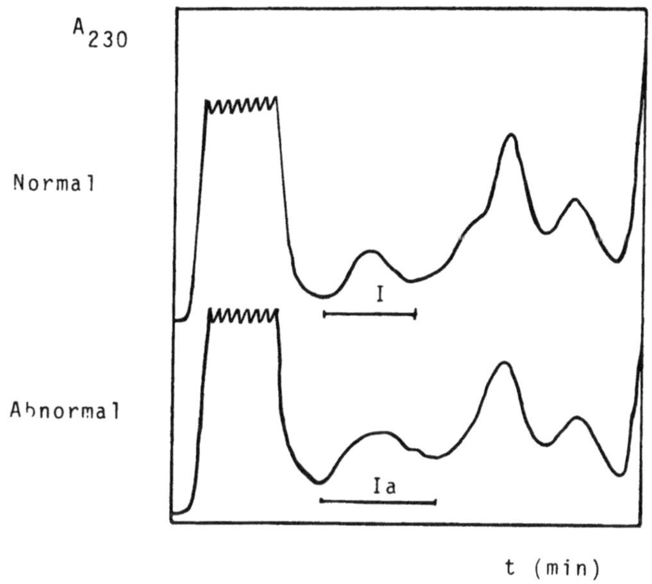

Fig.1: Separation of cyanogen bromide fragments from normal fibrinogen and fibrinogen Pontoise on a Sephadex G-50 column.

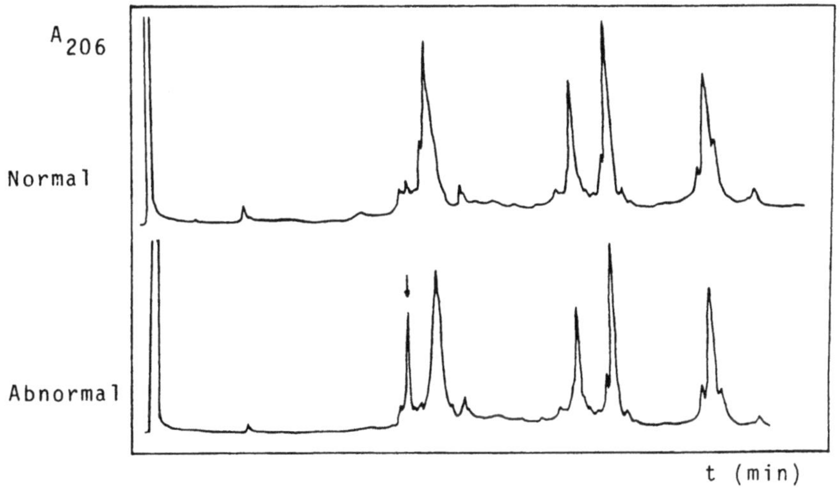

Fig.2: Separation of fraction I and Ia from the Sephadex chromatographies on an HPLC reversed phase column. ↓Extrapeak.

were both digested with trypsin and the cleavage mixtures fractionated on an HPLC reversed phase column (Fig.3). All tryptic fragments were identified by amino acid analysis.

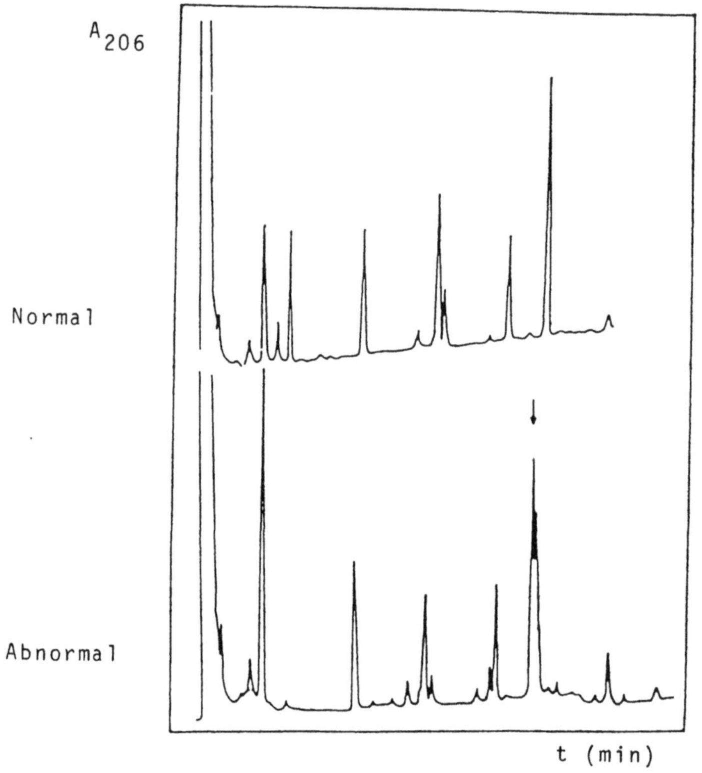

Fig.3: Separation of the tryptic cleavage products from the normal and the abnormal cyanogen bromide fragment on an HPLC reversed phase column. ↓ Extrapeak.

The single tryptic fragment from the abnormal fibrinogen sample, which differed in retention time from the corresponding normal component, was subjected to sequence analysis (Fig.4). It showed an exchange of the alanine residue in position 335 of the Bβ-chain with threonine. However, as the amino acid position penultimate to the substituted one is occupied by an asparagine residue, (position 333) a new sequence coding for N-glycosylation had

Ala-His-Tyr-Gly-Phe-Thr-Val-Gln Asn Glu-Ala-Asn-Lys-

Mutation ↓

Ala-His-Tyr-Gly-Phe-Thr-Val-Gln-Asn-Glu-Thr-Asn-Lys-

Posttranslational ↓

CHO

Ala-His-Tyr-Gly-Phe-Thr-Val-Gln-Asn-Glu-Thr-Asn-Lys-

Fig.4: Amino acid substitution in position 335 and glycosylation in position 333 of the Bβ-chain of fibrinogen Pontoise.

been formed. This asparagine was indeed found to be fully glycosylated. The results explained both the unexpected presence of glucosamine in the amino acid composition and the higher molecular weight due to the additional carbohydrate side chain of the abnormal Bβ-chain. It may be concluded that in the heterozygously expressed fibrinogen Pontoise one half of the Bβ-chain population contains a single carbohydrate side chain and the other half contains two side chains. Even though the additional side chain seems to be relatively far away from the predicted polymerisation site, it strongly interferes with the fibrin monomer polymerisation. Fibrinogen Pontoise is a striking example of how a genetically determined abnormality, caused by a mutation, may induce a non-genetic, posttranslational abnormality (Fig.4).

References

1. Haverkate, F., G. Timan, J. Soria, C. Soria, M.M. Samama. 1978. Thromb. Research 13, 698-692.

2. Soria, J., C. Soria, F. Haverkate, A.M. Guyader, F. Sabater: 1984 XVII Congress Internat. Soc. Hematol., Abstr.

3. Soria, C., J. Soria, M.M. Samama, J.P. Caen: 1984. 7th Meeting Internat. Soc. Haemat. Eur. Afr. Div., Abstr. 134.

4. Lottspeich, F., A. Henschen. 1977. Hoppe-Seylers Z. Physiol. Chem. 358, 1521-1524.

5. Edman, P., A. Henschen. 1975. In: Protein Seqence Determination (S.B. Needleman, ed.) 2nd edn. Springer, Berlin, pp. 232-279.

6. Lottspeich, F. 1985. J. Chromatog. 326, 321-327.

FIBRINOGEN MILANO I: ABNORMAL FIBRIN POLYMERIZATION RELATED TO A CARBOXY-TERMINAL DEFECT OF THE γ-CHAIN (γ-330 ASP $\rightarrow$ VAL)

Peter Reber[1], Miha Furlan[1], Christoph Rupp[1], Maria Kehl[2], Agnes Henschen[2], Piero M. Manucci[3], Eugene A. Beck[1]

[1] Central Hematology Laboratory, Inselspital, CH-3010 Berne, Switzerland

[2] Max-Planck-Institute for Biochemistry, D-8033 Martinsried, Germany

[3] Centro Angelo Bianchi Bonomi, I-20122 Milano, Italy

Introduction

Inherited structural abnormalities may affect functional properties of human fibrinogen. Thus far, exact localization of structural defects was mainly restricted to the amino-terminal part of the fibrinogen $A\alpha$-chain (1). In contrast, abnormal fibrin polymerization in the presence of normal fibrinopeptide release may be caused by defective polymerization sites residing in the carboxy-terminal part of the γ-chain. Abnormal fibrinogens with this type of molecular defect represent ideal models for studies of structural sites responsible for fibrin polymerization.

We report on a new fibrinogen variant which, following thrombin treatment, exhibits normal fibrinopeptide release. However, fibrin polymerization is markedly delayed. The defect responsible for abnormal clot formation was shown to reside in the carboxy-terminus of the fibrinogen γ-chain. According to the accepted nomenclature this new variant was called "fibrinogen Milano I".

Fibrinogen - Fibrin Formation and Fibrinolysis, Vol. 4
© 1986 Walter de Gruyter & Co., Berlin · New York - Printed in Germany.

Materials and Methods

Fibrinogen was isolated from citrated plasma by affinity chromatography on fibrin monomer-Sepharose CL-2B (2). Fibrinopeptide release was studied as previously described (3). Fibrin aggregation was measured by turbidimetry at 350 nm and 37 °C following thrombin treatment (0.5 NIH U/ml, bovine thrombin, Hoffmann-La Roche, Basel, Switzerland) of purified fibrinogen (0.5 mg/ml) in the presence of 0.1 mM Ca^{2+}. Isoelectric focusing was performed in urea-containing gel rods according to Kuyas et al. (4), the pH interval being between 4 and 9. The γ-chain was isolated from both normal fibrinogen and fibrinogen Milano I by HPLC, following reduction and carboxymethylation of half-cystine residues (5). Lyophilized γ-chain was dissolved in 70% formic acid and treated with a 100 to 200 fold molar excess of CNBr over methionine (6). The reaction was stopped with distilled water. Resulting peptides were concentrated on a rotary evaporator and separated on a Vydac TPRP 10 (0.46 x 25 cm) column using 0.1% trifluoroacetic acid in water (solvent A) or acetonitrile (solvent B). Gradients were 10% B for 5 mins, then from 10% to 50% B for 65 mins. Flow rate was 1.5 ml/min.

Results and Discussion

Fibrinogen Milano I was found by a routine test in the plasma of two members of a Northern Italian family (father and daughter) who did not exhibit any signs of an abnormal bleeding tendency. Thrombin and reptilase clotting times were prolonged, as was the rate of fibrin formation in a functional fibrinogen assay. In studies of fibrinopeptide release, relative amounts of fibrinopeptides A and B, cleaved from normal purified fibrinogen under specified experimental conditions, were taken as 100%. Corresponding values following thrombin treatment (0.1 NIH U/ml) of fibrinogen Milano I were 96% for fibrinopeptide A and 107% for fibrinopeptide B. Fifty percent of fibrinopeptides A and B were split off from fibrinogen Milano I at 1.5 and 3.7 min, respectively, while the corresponding time-intervals for normal fibrinogen were 2.8 and 6.9 min.

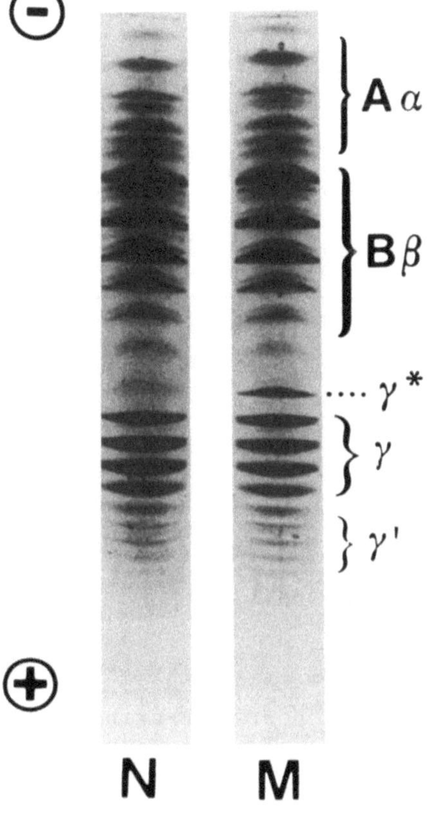

Fig.1: Isoelectric focusing gels of normal fibrinogen (N) and fibrinogen Milano I (M). The abnormally migrating band was marked by an asterisk.

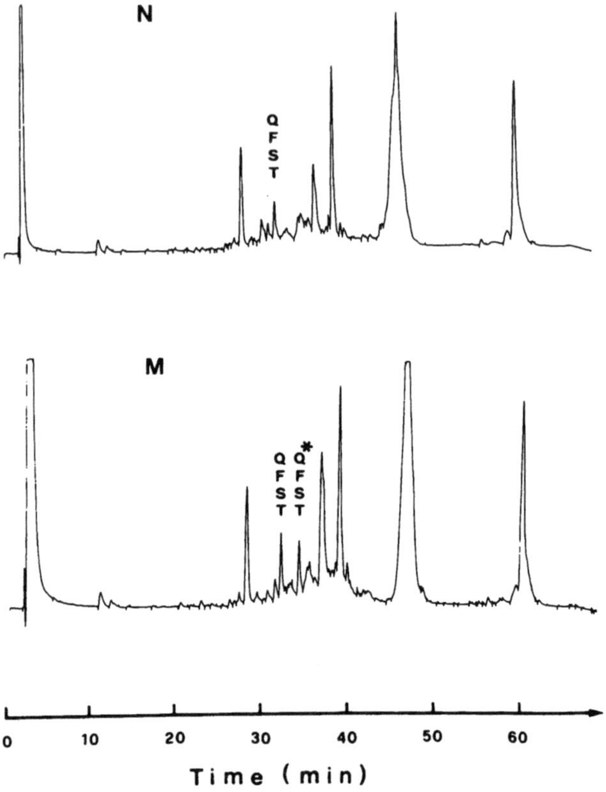

Fig.2: Separation of CNBr fragments derived from isolated normal (top) or abnormal (bottom) γ-chain by HPLC. The abnormal peak, marked by an asterisk, corresponds to CNBr fragment QFST (6) as shown by subsequent amino acid analysis. Q, F, S and T are the first four amino-terminal residues of the peptide.

These results clearly indicate that delayed clotting of fibrinogen Milano I was caused by abnormal fibrin polymerization. In fact, turbidimetric studies, in the presence of 0.1 mM Ca^{2+}, showed a lag time of 110 sec following addition of thrombin to fibrinogen Milano I, with a corresponding value of 13 sec for normal fibrinogen. Interestingly, the subsequent increase in turbidity was comparable for both fibrinogens (0.89 and 0.76 absorbance units per min for abnormal and normal fibrinogen, respectively).

Isoelectric focusing (Fig.1) revealed an abnormal γ-chain with cathodic shift in fibrinogen Milano I, suggesting replacement of either an acidic amino acid by a neutral residue or of a neutral amino acid by a basic one, possibly close to a polymerization site of the fibrinogen γ-chain.

In an attempt to characterize the molecular defect of fibrinogen Milano I, its γ-chain was first purified by reversed phase HPLC and then subjected to cyanogen bromide treatment. HPLC patterns, using a shallow gradient, were different regarding a single peptide, derived from fibrinogen Milano I, emerging at 34.5 min (Fig.2). Both amino acid analysis and sequencing indicated that the abnormality of fibrinogen Milano I resides within the carboxy-terminal part of the γ-chain, asparagine in position 330 being replaced by valine. Comparison of the sequences of human, rat (7) and lamprey (8) fibrinogen suggests that the exchange in fibrinogen Milano I took place in a very conservative area of the molecule, which points to the structural importance of this region.

Acknowledgements

The authors wish to thank Dr F. Lottspeich and Dr D. Georgopoulos (Max-Planck-Institute for Biochemistry, D-8033 Martinsried/Munich, Germany) for performing sequence and amino acid analyses. We would also like to acknowledge the valuable technical assistance of Ms. B. Isenschmid and Mr. R. Sievi. We are greatful to the Swiss National Foudation for supporting this study.

References

1. Henschen, A., Kehl, M., Southan, C.: In Variants of Human Fibrinogen (eds. Beck, E.A., Furlan, M.), Hans Huber, Bern, 273-320 (1984).

2. Furlan, M., Rupp, C., Beck, E.A. and Svendsen, L.: Thromb. Haemostas. 47, 118-121 (1982).

3. Kehl, M., Lottspeich, F., Henschen, A.: Hoppe-Seyler's. Z. Physiol. Chem. 362, 1661-1664 (1981).

4. Kuyas, C., Haeberli, A., Straub, P.W.: J. Biol. Chem. 257, 1107-1109 (1982).

5. Kehl, M., Lottspeich, F., Henschen, A.: Hoppe-Seyler's Z. Physiol. Chem. 363, 1501-1505 (1982).

6. Kehl, M., Lottspeich, F., Henschen, A: In Practical Aspects of Modern HPLC (ed. Molnar, I.), Walter de Gruyter, Berlin, 137-159 (1982).

7. Crabtree, G. R., Kant, J. A.: Cell, 31, 159-166 (1982).

8. Strong, D.D., Moore, M., Cottrell, B.A., Bohonus, V.L., Pontes, M., Evans, B., Riley, M., Doolittle, R.F.: Biochemistry 24, 92-101(1985).

FIBRINOGEN "BERGAMO I" (Aα 16 Arg ⟶ Cys): ALTERNATIVE METHODS FOR STRUCTURE ELUCIDATION

Peter Reber, Miha Furlan and Eugene A. Beck
Central Hematology Laboratory, Inselspital, CH-3010 Berne, Switzerland

Introduction

Among inherited structural defects of human fibrinogen residing in the amino terminal part of the Aα-chain, the substitution of arginine in position 16 by cysteine is remarkable in that it prevents cleavage of the adjacent peptide bond by thrombin and, consequently, release of fibrinopeptide A. This defect has been found thus far in fibrinogens Amsterdam I, Frankfurt II and III, London III, Marseille I, Stony Brook, Schwarzach and Zurich I (1). The structural defect has at first been revealed by sequence analysis of isolated Aα-chain (2). Henschen et al. (3) developed an alternative approach in studies of fibrinogen Schwarzach whereby the abnormal fibrinogen was modified by mercaptolysis and S-aminoethylation; S-aminoethylcysteine in position 16 of the Aα-chain thus acquired properties of a lysine analogue, and a fibrinopeptide A containing modified cysteine was cleaved off by thrombin.

Another fibrinogen variant of this type, fibrinogen Bergamo I (4), has recently been found in two members of a Northern Italian

Fibrinogen - Fibrin Formation and Fibrinolysis, Vol. 4
© 1986 Walter de Gruyter & Co., Berlin · New York - Printed in Germany.

family (father and son). In addition to S-aminoethylation, we used methylation and carboxamidomethylation in order to modify substrate properties of the abnormal fibrinogen. The proposed additional modifications are helpful for separating abnormal fibrinopeptide A from its normal counterpart by HPLC.

Materials and Methods

Purification of fibrinogen: Both normal and abnormal fibrinogen were isolated from citrated plasma by affinity chromatography on fibrin monomer-Sepharose CL-2B (5). No attempt was made to separate normal from abnormal fibrinogen. In this article, the terms "abnormal fibrinogen" or "fibrinogen Bergamo I" refer to this mixture originating from a heterozygous carrier of the variant.

Thrombin and reptilase times were performed with solutions of purified fibrinogen (2 mg/ml) in 0.1 M NaCl/0.05 M triethanolamine/1 mM $CaCl_2$, pH 7.4.

Polymerization studies: Ca^{2+} or EDTA, at final concentrations of 1 mM, were added to solutions of purified fibrinogen (0.5 mg/ml) in 0.1 M NaCl/0.05 M triethanolamine (pH 7.4), and the turbidity increase was measured at 350 nm in a thermostated (37°C) photometer following addition of thrombin (0.5 NIH U/ml final concentration).

Measurement of fibrinopeptide release: Purified normal or abnormal fibrinogen in ammonium acetate buffer was treated with bovine thrombin (5 mg/ml and 0.04 NIH U/ml, respectively). Fibrinopeptide analysis was performed by HPLC following boiling of samples as previously described (6).

Two-dimensional electrophoresis: Isoelectric focusing of fibrinogen and fibrin samples was carried out between pH 4 and pH 9 as described by Kuyas et al (7). In the second dimension, an 8% Laemmli polyacrylamide gel system was used (8).

Chemical modifications of fibrinogen: Lyophilized fibrinogen was dissolved in 6M guanidinium hydrochloride, pH 5, and reduced by addition of 2-mercaptoethanol (16 h, 40 °C.) according to Henschen and Edman (9). Cysteine residues were modified by S-aminoethylation (3) or S-methylation (10). Iodoacetamide was employed for S-carboxamidomethylation under otherwise identical conditions as described for carboxymethylation (9).

Results and Discussion

Functional studies of purified normal and variant fibrinogen yielded the following results: thrombin and reptilase times of fibrinogen Bergamo I were 37.0 s and 51.2 s, respectively, whereas the corresponding normal values were 10.4 s and 10.6 s. The slope of the fibrin polymerization curve was remarkably depressed (0.06 absorbance units/min), and the lag-time strongly prolonged (246 s); the respective normal values were 0.45 absorbance units/min and 30 s. Only 57 % fibrinopeptide A and 83 % fibrinopeptide B were released from fibrinogen Bergamo I during 24 h by a thrombin concentration (0.04 NIH U/ml) that completely cleaved both fibrinopeptides from normal fibrinogen within the same incubation interval.

Two-dimensional electrophoresis revealed no significant difference between constituent polypeptide chains of normal and variant fibrinogen (Fig.1). Release of the negatively charged fibrinopeptides

A and B caused an increase in isoelectric points of both α - and β -chain. As a consequence, reduced α - and β -chains of fibrin showed an anodic shift in isoelectric focusing, while the position of the γ-chain remained unchanged. Two-dimensional electrophoresis of fibrinogen Bergamo I showed that only about one half of the α -chain-related material was shifted towards the anode following extensive thrombin treatment, thus confirming the defective fibrinopeptide release in the abnormal variant. The described two-dimensional electrophoretic method can be used as a simple screening procedure for abnormal fibrinogens carrying a functional defect in the amino terminal domain, if the HPLC approach is not feasible.

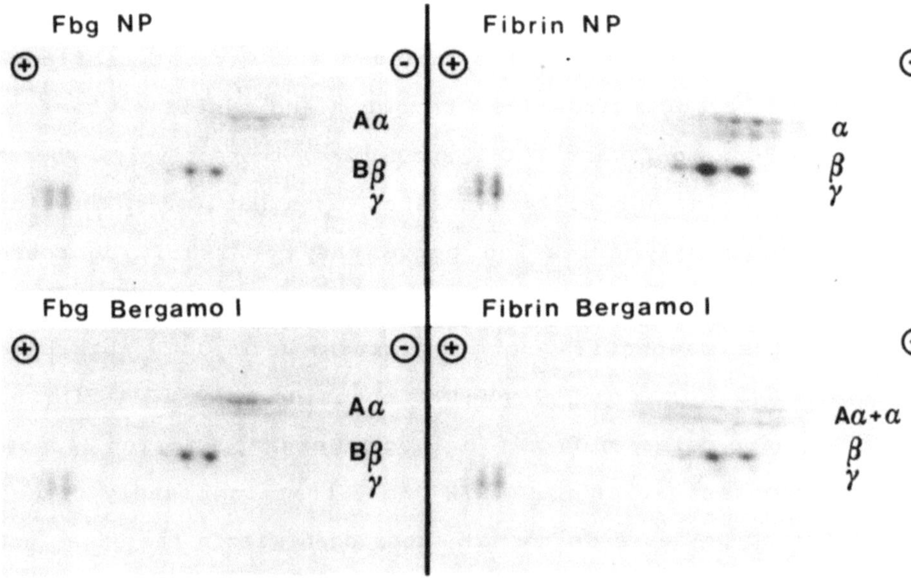

Fig. 1: Two-dimensional electrophoresis of reduced fibrinogen and fibrin: Top gels; normal fibrinogen (left) and fibrin (right); bottom gels; variant fibrinogen (left) and fibrin (right).

To render the Cys-Gly bond (A α 16-17) in a fibrinogen variant susceptible to thrombin, ethylation of the cysteine residue has been proposed by Henschen et al. (3). Using this method, we were able to isolate an abnormal fibrinopeptide A (A*, Fig. 2-2) containing no arginine but rather 0.6 mole aminoethylcysteine per mole peptide. Thus, we confirmed the molecular defect in fibrinogen Bergamo I as the substitution Aα 16 Arg by Cys. The alternative procedures for chemically modifying the abnormal fibrinogen were studied because, following aminoethylation, the abnormal fibrinopeptide A (A* in Fig. 2-2) migrated very closely to its normal counterpart. The major peak, eluted between fibrinopeptides A and B, presumably resulted from proteolytic degradation of the α-carboxy-terminus by thrombin, as SDS-polyacrylamide gel electrophoresis of the thrombin-treated modified fibrinogen showed extensively degraded α-chain remnants.

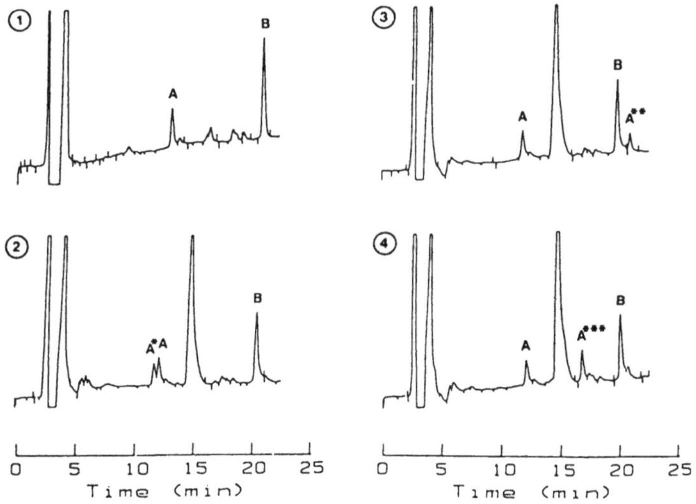

Fig. 2: HPLC-patterns of fibrinopeptides released from fibrinogen Bergamo I by thrombin. Panel 1, unmodified fibrinogen; panel 2, aminoethylated fibrinogen; panel 3, methylated fibrinogen; panel 4, carboxamidomethylated fibrinogen.

Methylated fibrinopeptide A (A^{**} Fig.1-3) and the carboxamidomethylated derivative (A^{***} Fig.1-4) were well separated from normal fibrinopeptide A by HPLC. Their respective amino acid analyses revealed the presence of about 1 mole proline per mole peptide. Furthermore, both the methylated and the carboxamidomethylated derivative contained 1 mole arginine per mole of peptide. These findings are compatible with an elongated fibrinopeptide structure, comprising the sequence Aα 17-19 (Gly-Pro-Arg), adjacent to the modified cysteine residues. We conclude that both methylation and carboxamidomethylation represent methods for improved separation of abnormal fibrinopeptides A containing cysteine instead of arginine in position 16. In contrast to aminoethylation both alternative modifications shift the site of thrombin attack to position 19-20. The proposed procedures may be useful for studies of abnormal fibrinogen variants with absent fibrinopeptide A cleavage by thrombin.

Acknowledgements

This work was supported by the Swiss National Foundation. Dr. D. Georgopoulos (Max-Planck-Institute for Biochemistry, D-8033 Martinsried / Munich, Germany) and Dr. J. Schaller (Institute for Biochemistry, University of Berne, 3012 Berne, Switzerland) are acknowledged for performing the amino acid analyses.

References

1. Henschen, A., Kehl, M., Southan, C.: In Variants of Human Fibrinogen (eds. Beck, E.A., Furlan, M.), Hans Huber, Bern, 273-320 (1984).

2. Southan, C., Henschen, A., Lottspeich, C.: In Fibrinogen, Recent Biochemical and Medical Aspects (eds. Henschen A., Graeff, H., Lottspeich, F.), Walter de Gruyter, Berlin, 153-166 (1982).

3. Henschen, A., Kehl, M., Deutsch, E.: Hoppe-Seyler's Z. Physiol. Chem. 364, 1747-1751 (1983).

4. Reber, P., Furlan, M., Beck, E.A., Finazzi, G., Buelli, M., Barbui, T.: Thromb. Haemostas. (in press).

5. Furlan, M., Rupp, C., Beck, E.A., Svendsen, L.: Thromb. Haemostas. 47, 118-121 (1982).

6. Kehl, M., Lottspeich, F., Henschen, A.: Hoppe-Seyler's Z. Physiol. Chem. 362, 1661-1664 (1981).

7. Kuyas, C., Haeberli, A., Straub, P.W.: J. Biol. Chem. 257, 1107-1109 (1982).

8. Laemmli, U.K.: Nature 227, 680-685 (1970).

9. Henschen, A., Edman, P.: Biochim. Biophys. Acta 263, 351-367 (1972).

10. Henschen, A., Lottspeich, F., Hessel, B.: Hoppe-Seyler's Z. Physiol. Chem. 359, 1607-1610 (1978).

SCREENING SMALL PLASMA SAMPLES BY HPLC FOR ABNORMALITIES OF FIBRINOPEPTIDE RELEASE

Christopher Southan and David A. Lane.

Department of Haematology, Charing Cross and Westminster Medical School, Hammersmith, London W6 8RP, UK.

Introduction

The analysis by HPLC of fibrinopeptides released by thrombin and various snake venom proteases has become an essential step in the characterisation of genetically abnormal fibrinogens (1). A recent review indicates that some kind of fibrinopeptide release defect is associated with the majority of congenital dysfibrinogenaemias so far examined by HPLC (2). Quantitative defects are those that show an alteration in the normal FPA:FPB ratio of 1:1, which persists after extensive thrombin treatment. Heterozygotes cases with 50% non-cleavable FPA, such as fibrinogen London III (3), give ratios of 0.5:1. The majority of cases with this type of FPA release defect have been caused by an Arg->Cys exchange at position Aα 16 which prevents the normal thrombin cleavage (1). Those with 50% non-cleavable FPB, such as New York I (4), give ratios of 1:0.5. HPLC can also detect abnormal fibrinopeptides containing amino acid substitutions. Two types have been reported so far, [His^{16}]FPA and [Val^{12}]FPA, illustrated by cases such as fibrinogens Sydney I (5) and Rouen (6), respectively. Including preliminary reports there are at least 15 cases of [His^{16}]FPA comprising approximately 10% of all congenital dysfibrinogenemias so far reported (2). It seems probable that the standard coagulation testing by which most dysfibrinogenemias are diagnosed, is selective for fibrinopeptide release defects. For laboratories involved in the investigation of such cases it would be particularly convenient if preliminary HPLC analysis of fibrinopeptide release could be performed on plasma samples without the necessity of fibrinogen purification. Another possible application would be the simultaneous measurement of plasma fibrinogen concentrations, especially in cases where hypodysfibrinogenemia is suspected. In this report we describe a method that enables abnormalities in the amount or type of fibrinopeptides released by thrombin to be readily detected using small amounts of plasma.

Methods

Plasma, fresh or re-constituted from freeze-dried samples, was first passed through a 0.45 um membrane filter. An aliquot of 200 ul was then gel-filtered rapidly through a small Sephadex G25 column connected to an HPLC system and eluted with 0.05 M

Fibrinogen - Fibrin Formation and Fibrinolysis, Vol. 4
© 1986 Walter de Gruyter & Co., Berlin · New York - Printed in Germany.

Tris, 0.05 M NaCl, pH 7.0. The collected peak was then treated with thrombin, 50 u/ml, for 10 min at room temperature. The sample was boiled for 3 min followed by centrifugation for 10 min. Supernatants were filtered with 0.22 um membrane filters before examination by HPLC. A refillable guard column was used in conjunction with a Shandon Hypersil 3u ODS 0.46 X 10cm analytical column. The HPLC conditions were those of Kehl et al. (7), except for the use of an extended steeper gradient of 0% to 40% B in 30 min.

Results

A section of a chromatogram obtained from thrombin treated gel-filtered plasma is shown in Fig 1(a). All the normal forms of fibrinopeptide can be identified by their identical elution positions to the control fibrinopeptides from purified fibrinogen.

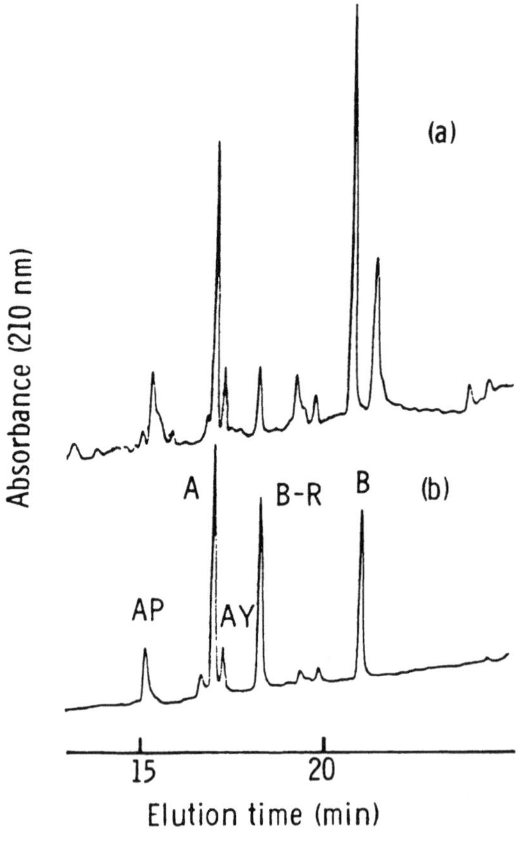

Figure 1: Analysis of Fibrinopeptides. Trace (a) is from an aliquot of gel-filtered plasma treated with thrombin as described. The injection volume was equivalent to approximately 1/5 of the total gel-filtration peak i.e. about 40ul of plasma. The absorbance unit full-scale was 0.08. The control fibrinopeptides in (b) are from 20ul of a 2 hr thrombin clot supernatant from a 10mg/ml fibrinogen solution. The fibrinopeptides are labled according to (7). FPA/FPB peak ratios were 0.92 in (a) and 0.89 in (b).

A control chromatogram from a non-thrombin treated sample showed a very low background of endogenous peptides in this section of the chromatogram except for a peak eluting approximately 1 min after FPB. This was present to a varying extent in all plasma samples but did not interfere with the automatic integration of FPB peak areas. The peak areas or peak heights were used for fibrinopeptide quantitation.

The result for the first case of dysfibrinogenemia we analysed, provisionally designated fibrinogen Ashford, is shown in Fig. 2. Because of a prolonged thrombin time in the patients plasma we performed both a short and an extended thrombin digestion to ensure complete fibrinopeptide release. In this particular case the control fibrinopeptides, shown in Fig. 2(a), were derived from purified fibrinogen Ashford and we were able to confirm identical FPA/FPB ratios from the plasma sample and purified fibrinogen.

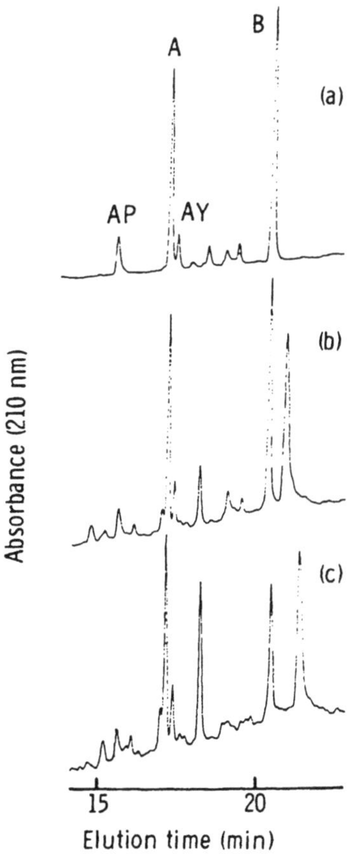

Figure 2: Analysis of fibrinopeptides from fibrinogen Ashford. Trace (a) shows the fibrinopeptides released from purified fibrinogen Ashford. Trace (b) is derived from a gel filtered patient plasma sample treated for 10 min with thrombin and trace (c) after 1 hour thrombin treatment at room temperature. The % proportion of AY/total A is 10.8, 18.6 and 25 % for (a), (b) and (c), respectively

We observed over the extended digestion the expected increased conversion of FPB to the degraded form des Arg B which has been previously shown to be the result of carboxypeptidase activity in plasma (7). We also detected an increase in the AY peak which indicates that some conversion of FPA to AY has occured. A family study has already established the prolonged plasma thrombin time as a congenital abnormality (T. Bowden, personal communication). The demonstration of complete fibrinopeptide release therefore suggests a fibrin polymerisation defect and this was confirmed by subsequent studies on purified fibrinogen Ashford (Southan et al., unpublished observations).

The cases of dysfibrinogenemia refered to next are provisionally designated fibrinogens Sheffield and Paris VI. The analysis by the rapid HPLC technique is shown in Fig. 3

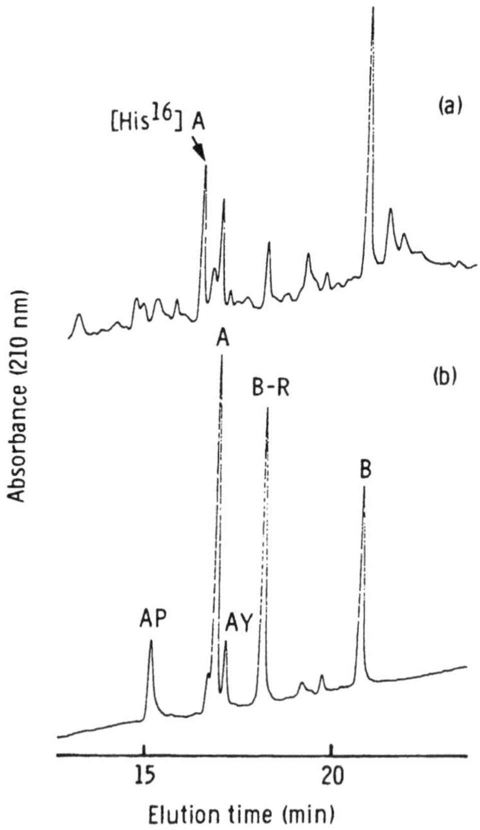

Figure 3: Fibrinopeptide analysis from plasma of fibrinogen Paris (VI). This is shown in trace (a) and control fibrinopeptides from normal fibrinogen in trace (b). The abnormal peak observed in (a) was identifiable as [His^{16}]A on the basis of its 1 min shorter retention time and peak area ratios of abnormalFPA/total FPA of 0.57, essentialy identical to that reported for other cases analysed under the same HPLC conditions (5,8).

Fibrinogen Sheffield (result not shown) exibited essentialy the same pattern of fibrinopeptide release as observed for fibrinogen Paris VI in fig. 3. The apparent splitting of the FPA into two peaks, one of which has both a shorter elusion time and a larger peak area than the normal FPA, can be considered diagnostic for cases of the Aa16 Arg->His substitution.

Amongst the dysfibrinogenemias that we have been screening for fibrinopeptide release defects was a suspected case of hypodysfibrinogenemia. The analysis by this technique is shown below in Fig 4.

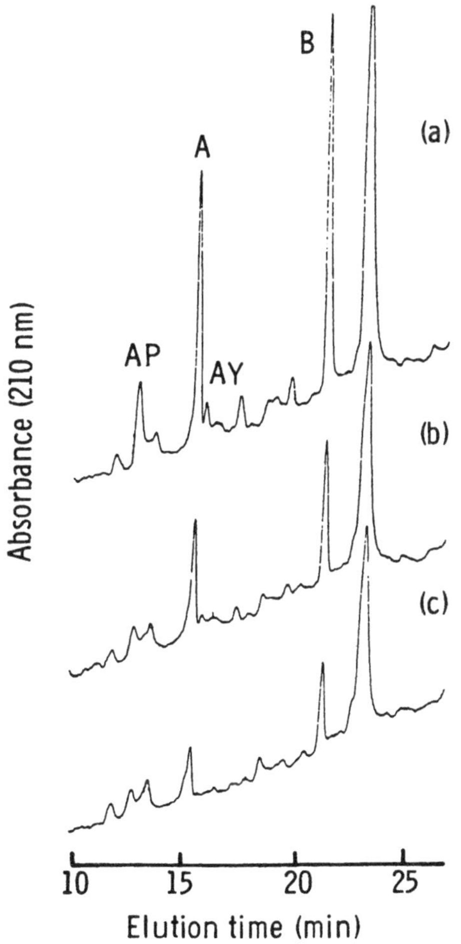

Figure 4: Analysis of family members from a case of suspected hypo-dysfibrinogenemia. For each plasma sample the volumes were kept constant at each stage of preparation. This facilitated quantitation of plasma fibrinogen concentrations dirctly from FPB peak heights. Incubation times with thrombin were shortened to 5 min avoid the conversion of FPB to des-Arg B Trace (a)was obtained from the normal father, trace (b) from the affected mother and trace (c) from the daughter.The FPA:FPB ratio from the mother indicated a normal stoichiometry of fibrinopeptide release.

For this particular family we were able to measure, on the basis of the amount of FPB released, that the mother has a fibrinogen concentration of 36% compared to the normal father (3.1 mg/ml) and the daughter has an even lower level of 22%. The difference between the two affected family members is in reasonable agreement with the same comparative plasma fibrinogen concentrations determined by clot weight of 38% and 11%, (I. Mackie, personal communication). Although these results have established congenital low fibrinogen levels further investigations with purified fibrinogen will be necessary to establish the case as a hypodysfibrinogenemia.

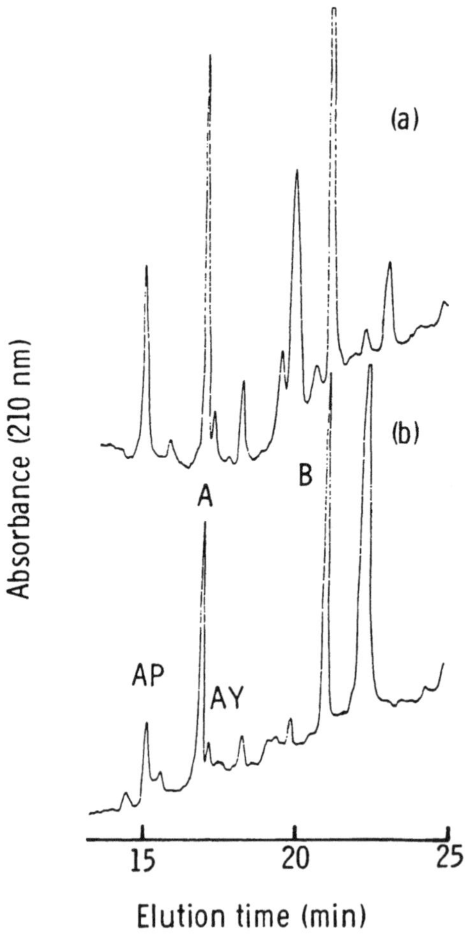

Figure 5: Fibrinopeptide analysis of a post operative plasma sample The patient, trace (a), had had a femoral bypass surgery three days prior to the sample being taken. In the absence of a pre-operative sample a normal individual was used as a control in trace (b). The analysis was performed quantitatively as described in the legend to Fig 4. From peak measurements the fibrinogen level in the patient was 1.7 times that of the control and the % of AP compared to total FPA was 30 % compared with 20% for the normal control.

From the chromatograms in Fig 1 it was possible to quantitate the proportion of phosphorylated FPA (AP) released from normal plasma fibrinogen. The physiological significance of AP levels is not clear at the present time but the very high levels associated with foetal plasma indicate that this may be related to the presence of newly-synthesised fibrinogen in the circulation (9). In a preliminary investigation we examined a post-operative plasma sample where the patient was expected to have very high fibrinogen levels resulting from the acute-phase response (10). The result shown above in Fig.5 must be considered preliminary because a complete series including pre-operative samples was not available . However, there does appear to be an increase in fibrinogen and in the level of AP which may be an index of fibrinogen synthesis in this clinical situation.

Discussion

By using the methods outlined above it is possible to perform a quantitative HPLC analysis on the fibrinopeptides released from plasma samples of 200 ul. Much smaller samples would be well within the sensitivity limits of the instrumentation.The ability to test freeze-dried plasma samples sent by post, or small volumes obtained from a fingerprick, is of particular advantage for a preliminary screening test and is unaffected by the yield and selectivity problems associated with fibrinogen purification from dysfibrinogenemias. In two cases with abnormal fibrinopeptides the molecular defect could be identified from the plasma sample alone although for cases where the fibrinopeptide pattern is normal fibrinogen purification is required to confirm the diagnosis of dysfibrinogenemia.

Although no statistical comparisons have yet been made with standard fibrinogen assays the method is also potentially useful for quantitating plasma fibrinogen levels as the family study of hypofibrinogenemia clearly demonstrated. Although the possible relationship between fibrinogen synthesis and phosphorylation levels is not yet clear, the analysis of small plasma samples will facilitate further investigations of physiological fluctuations in fibrinogen concentrations and AP levels.

This work was supported by a grant to the Wellcome Trust to D.A. Lane. We would like to thank the following people for supplying plasma samples: Tony Bowden and Dr. Wells of the William Harvey Hospital, Ashford, Kent: Dr. Mike Greaves and Peter Cooper of the Royal Hallamshire Hospital, Sheffield: Dr. Anne-Maria Fischer of the Assistance Publique, Paris: Dr. Ian Mackie from the Central Middlesex Hospital, London: Dr. Sheila Ryan from Charing Cross Hospital, London.

References

1. Henschen A., Kehl, M. and Southan, C. 1984. In: variants of human fibrinogen. (Beck E.A. and Furlan M. eds) H. Huber Verlag, Berne, pp 273-320.

2. Lane, D.A. and Southan, C. 1985. In: Haemostasis and Thrombosis, 2nd Edition, (Bloom, A.L. and Thomas, D.P. eds) Chruchill Livingstone, Edinburgh, in press.

3. Southan, C., Lane, D.A. and Henschen, A., 1982. In: Fibrinogen; structure, functional aspects, metabolism. Haverkate, F., Henschen, A., Niewenhuizen, W. & Straub, P.W. eds. Walter de Gruyter, Berlin, New York, pp 167-182.

4. Liu, C.Y. Koehn, J.A. and Morgan, F.J. 1985. J. Biol. Chem. 260, 4390-4396.

5. Southan, C., Lane, D.A., Bode, W. and Henschen, A. 1985. Eur. J. Biochem. 147, 593-600.

6. Kehl, M., Lottspeich, F., Henschen, A. 1982. In: Fibrinogen, structure, functional aspects, metabolism. Haverkate, F., Henschen, A., Niewenhuizen, W. and Straub, P.W. eds, Walter de Gruyter, Berlin, New York, pp 182-193.

7. Kehl, M., Lottspeich, F. and Henschen, A. 1981. Hoppe-Seyler's Z. Physiol. Chem. 362, 1661-1664.

8. Southan, C., Kehl, M., Henschen, A. and Lane, D.A. 1983. Brit. J. Haem. 54, 143-151.

9. Galanakis, D.K., Martinez, J., McDevitt, C.and Miller, F. 1983. Annal. NY Acad. Sci. 408, 640-643.

10. Holm, B. and Godal, H.C. 1984. Thrombosis. Res. 35, 279-290.

IV. Fibrin(ogen) and Fibrinolysis

ON THE ROLE OF FIBRIN IN THE FIBRINOLYTIC SYSTEM

H.R. Lijnen

Center for Thrombosis and Vascular Research, University of Leuven, Campus Gasthuisberg, Herestraat 49, B-3000 Leuven, Belgium

INTRODUCTION

The main role of the fibrinolytic enzyme system in the blood is the removal of fibrin from the vascular bed. The system comprises a proenzyme, plasminogen, which can be activated to the active enzyme plasmin, which will degrade fibrin by several different types of plasminogen activators. These include the activators of the "intrinsic" system, streptokinase, urokinase or pro-urokinase, and tissue-type plasminogen activators. All plasminogen activators studied so far exert their action through hydrolysis of the Arg 560-Val 561 peptide bond in plasminogen. Inhibition of the fibrinolytic system may occur at the level of plasmin or at the level of the activators.

The fibrinolytic system is schematically represented below :

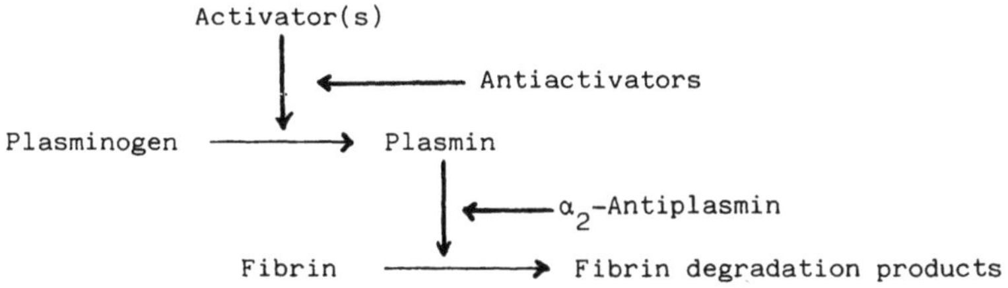

During the last few years, significant progress has been made in our understanding of the molecular mechanisms involved in the regulation of the fibrinolytic enzyme system in vivo (1-3). This has resulted in a better understanding of the role of fibrin. This manuscript will deal with the role of fibrin in fibrinolysis induced by tissue-type plasminogen activator (t-PA) or by pro-urokinase (pro-UK).

Fibrinogen - Fibrin Formation and Fibrinolysis, Vol. 4
© 1986 Walter de Gruyter & Co., Berlin · New York - Printed in Germany.

ACTIVATION OF PLASMINOGEN TO PLASMIN

Human plasminogen is a single chain glycoprotein with a molecular weight of about 92,000, containing about 2 percent carbohydrate. The plasminogen molecule consists of 790 amino acids, it contains 24 disulfide bridges and five homologous triple loop structures or "kringles" (4). Native plasminogen has NH_2-terminal glutamic acid ("Glu-plasminogen") but is easily converted by limited plasmic digestion to modified forms with NH_2-terminal lysine, valine or methionine (5,6), commonly designated "Lys-plasminogen". This conversion occurs by hydrolysis of the Arg 67-Met 68, Lys 76-Lys 77 or Lys 77-Val 78 peptide bonds.

Lys-plasminogen forms are converted to plasmin by cleavage of a single Arg-Val bond (7), corresponding to the Arg 560-Val 561 bond. The two-chain plasmin molecule is composed of a heavy chain or A-chain, originating from the NH_2-terminal part of plasminogen and a light chain or B-chain constituting the COOH-terminal part (7). The B-chain was found to contain an active site similar to that of trypsin, composed of His 602, Asp 645 and Ser 740 (4).

The plasminogen molecule contains structures, called lysine-binding sites which interact specifically with certain amino acids such as lysine, 6-aminohexanoic acid and trans-4-aminomethylcyclohexane-1-carboxylic acid (tranexamic acid) (8-10). Plasminogen contains one binding site with high affinity for 6-aminohexanoic acid (K_d = 9 µM), and about four with low affinity (K_d = 5 mM) (11). These lysine-binding sites are located in the plasmin A-chain (9). The high affinity lysine-binding site has been shown to be comprised within the first kringle structure of plasminogen (12).

These lysine-binding sites in plasminogen mediate its interaction with fibrin (10,13) and its interaction with α_2-antiplasmin (14-17) and with histidine-rich glycoprotein (18). On the basis of these interactions it was suggested that the lysine-binding sites play a crucial role in the regulation of fibrinolysis (1,19).

Tissue-type plasminogen activator

The first satisfactory purification of human t-PA has been obtained from uterine tissues (20). Using an antiserum raised with this preparation, it has been shown that the blood, vascular and tissue plasminogen activator are identical, but different from urokinase. t-PA has been purified from the culture fluid of a stable human melanoma cell line (21). Sufficient amounts were obtained to study its biochemical and biological properties (22).

Recently, the gene of human t-PA has been cloned and expressed (23). Human t-PA, obtained by expression of recombinant DNA coding for its entire sequence in eukaryotic cells, was shown to be indistinguishable from the natural activator isolated from human melanoma cell cultures, with respect to biochemical properties, turnover in vivo and specific thrombolytic effect (24,25).

Native t-PA is a serine protease with a molecular weight of about 70,000, composed of one polypeptide chain containing 527 amino acids. Upon limited plasmic action the molecule is converted to a two-chain activator linked by one disulfide bond (21,26). This occurs by cleavage of the Arg 275-Ile 276 peptide bond yielding a heavy chain derived from the NH_2-terminal part of the molecule and a light chain comprising the COOH-terminal region. The catalytic site located in the light chain of t-PA is composed of His 322, Asp 371 and Ser 478. The amino acid sequences surrounding these residues are highly homologous to corresponding parts of other serine proteases (23).

The heavy chain contains two regions of 82 amino acids each (residues 92-173 and 180-261) which share a high degree of homology with the five kringles of plasminogen and with similar kringles in prothrombin and urokinase. Comparison of the primary structures of high-$\underline{M}_r$ urokinase and t-PA has revealed a high degree of homology between the two proteins, except that t-PA contains a 43 residue long aminoterminal region, which has no counterpart in urokinase; this segment was shown to be homologous with the finger-domains responsible for the fibrin-affinity of fibronectin. Limited proteolysis of this region leads to a loss of the fibrin-affinity of the enzyme (27).

The mechanism of the release of t-PA remains unknown. Cash (28) has speculated that t-PA release may be under neurohumoral control and that a plasminogen activator releasing hormone would constitute the major pathway for its release from the endothelial cells. This hormone could, however, not be identified in bovine pituitary or hypothalamic extracts (29). From infusion experiments of bovine protein C in dogs, Comp and Esmon have concluded that activated protein C might be involved in the release of t-PA in vivo (30). This could, however, not be confirmed in squirrel monkeys using human protein C (31).

The mechanisms involved in the removal of t-PA from the blood are multiple and poorly understood. One main mechanism is through clearance by the liver, which results in a t½ of a few min (32). ^{125}I-labeled t-PA was found to disappear from the plasma of human volunteers with a half-life of 3-4 min (33).

t-PA occurs in plasma as a free active form and as complexes with α_2-antiplasmin and α_1-antitrypsin (34). In several pathological conditions (liver disease, pancreatitis, myocardial infarction or venous thrombosis) the patients may present with a (transient) fast inhibitory activity for t-PA in plasma (35). Assuming formation of a 1:1 stoichiometric complex of t-PA with this inhibitor, the second order rate constant has been estimated at 10^7 $M^{-1}s^{-1}$

(36). A positive correlation was found between inhibition of t-PA and of urokinase (35). Several laboratories have recently obtained evidence for the existence of this rapidly acting inhibitor of t-PA at low concentrations in plasma of healthy individuals, or at higher levels in pathological plasma samples (35-40). It has been suggested that this fast-acting t-PA inhibitor is neutralized by activated protein C, which might explain the apparent pro-fibrinolytic activity of protein C (41).

Several groups have studied the kinetics of the activation of plasminogen by tissue-type plasminogen activator in the presence or the absence of fibrin. The activation obeys Michaelis-Menten kinetics with more favourable kinetic constants in the presence of fibrin than in its absence (42-44). The plasminogen activating properties of one- and two-chain forms of t-PA were found to be very similar (45). Hoylaerts et al. (42) found a marked decrease of K_m (from 65 to 0.16 μM) while the catalytic rate constant did not change significantly (k_{cat} from 0.06 to 0.1 per s) in the presence of fibrin. These kinetic data support a mechanism in which t-PA and plasminogen adsorb to a fibrin clot in a sequential and ordered way yielding a ternary complex.

Fibrin essentially increases the local plasminogen concentration by creating an additional interaction between t-PA and its substrate. In the presence of fibrin the affinity of t-PA for plasminogen is high, indicating that efficient activation can occur. Plasmin formed on the fibrin surface has both its lysine-binding sites and active site occupied and is therefore only slowly inactivated by α_2-antiplasmin. Efficient fibrinolysis in vivo, however, seems to require a continuous replacement at the fibrin surface of inactivated plasmin molecules by plasminogen molecules. In this respect, the finding that binding of plasminogen to fibrin is enhanced by the presence of t-PA (46) might be relevant. In plasma no efficient plasminogen activation by t-PA occurs and

α_2-antiplasmin rapidly binds free plasmin thereby protecting fibrinogen. These interactions thus indicate that the fibrinolytic process is triggered by and confined to fibrin.

Over the last few years the potential of t-PA as a thrombolytic agent has been intensively investigated in several animal models and in humans (for references see 47).

PRO-UROKINASE

Evidence that urokinase is secreted in an inactive form (pro-urokinase) which can be activated by plasmin, was already provided in 1973 (48), but the mechanism of activation remained unknown. Nolan et al. (49) identified a plasminogen activator in human embryonic kidney cell cultures which reacted with anti-urokinase antibodies, was separated from active urokinase by chromatography on benzamidine-Sepharose and was activated by trypsin. They concluded that they had identified a pro-activator form of urokinase. Recently, several groups have apparently independently isolated a single chain form of urokinase (50-54), but differences in kinetic properties were reported. Sumi et al. (55) found no significant difference in enzymatic properties between the single chain and two-chain forms. The other groups, however, found that single chain urokinase is a proenzyme which, following limited digestion with plasmin, is converted to fully active two-chain urokinase. Sumi et al. (55), Husain et al. (52) and Gurewich et al. (56) have reported that the single chain urokinase has a higher specific thrombolytic activity and/or a better selectivity for fibrin than two-chain urokinase. The gene of human urokinase was recently cloned and expressed in E. coli (57). The purified translation product normally consists of active two-chain urokinase but may be obtained as a single chain form if proteolytic degradation is carefully avoided during purification.

In vitro, the recombinant pro-urokinase is a true proenzyme, inactive in plasma but slowly activated in the presence of a fibrin clot (58). The recombinant pro-urokinase was found to have higher specific thrombolytic activity and a better thrombus-selectivity than natural and recombinant two-chain urokinase in rabbits with experimental jugular vein thrombosis (59).

Detailed mechanistic and kinetic studies (60-62) on the activation of plasminogen by (recombinant) pro-urokinase (Rec-pro-UK) yielded the following findings :

1) Activation of plasminogen by both Rec-UK and Rec-pro-UK obeys Michaelis-Menten kinetics.

2) Rec-pro-UK has a similar catalytic efficiency (k_{cat}/K_m) for the activation of plasminogen as natural urokinase, due to the fact that its lower catalytic rate constant is compensated by its much higher affinity for plasminogen. In this respect, pro-UK is unique among the serine proteases.

3) Rec-pro-UK is fully activated to the two-chain enzyme by limited proteolysis by plasmin.

4) In mixtures of plasminogen and Rec-pro-UK, Rec-pro-UK is quickly converted to the two-chain enzyme, by traces of plasmin generated by activation of plasminogen by Rec-pro-UK. Activation of Rec-pro-UK does not occur in the presence of the plasmin inhibitors aprotinin or α_2-antiplasmin.

5) Rec-pro-UK does not activate plasminogen in plasma in the absence of a fibrin clot, due to the presence of a competitive inhibitor. However, within a rather narrow concentration range, specific clot lysis is obtained in the absence of systemic activation of the fibrinolytic system. Preliminary data suggest that fibrin neutralizes the action of the competitive inhibitor.

6) No specific binding of Rec-pro-UK to fibrin has been demonstrated.

A hypothetical mechanism of action for pro-UK which is compatible with these findings, is represented below :

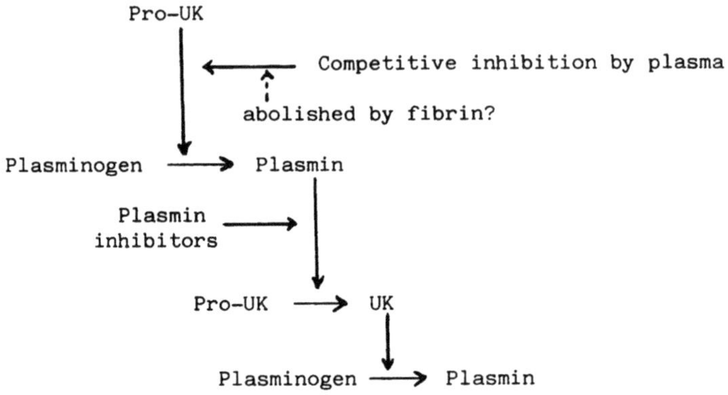

As far as a potential clinical application of pro-UK is concerned, a significant conclusion from the presently available data is that its half-life in vivo is very similar and equally short as that of active urokinase (63), indicating that probably its continuous intravenous infusion will be required. One significant difference between pro-urokinase and urokinase in vivo may be their different reactivity towards the fast-acting inhibitor of tissue-type plasminogen activator and urokinase (35). The concentration of this inhibitor is, however, much lower than the steady state urokinase concentration in plasma required for thrombolysis (59) and therefore we anticipate that the lack of reactivity of pro-UK with this inhibitor does not in itself constitute a significant potential therapeutic advantage.

Our findings in animal models and in human plasma in vitro seem to support the conclusion that t-PA probably has a higher specific thrombolytic activity in man than pro-UK. This anticipated difference in specific activity might, however, not be an impediment to the potential value of pro-UK as a thrombolytic agent, provided that the fibrin-specificity is maintained at therapeutic plasma concentrations.

REFERENCES

1. Collen D. On the regulation and control of fibrinolysis. Thromb. Haemost. 43, 77-89, 1980.

2. Lijnen H.R., Collen D. Interaction of plasminogen activators and inhibitors with plasminogen and fibrin. Seminars in Thrombosis and Haemostasis 8, 2-10, 1982.

3. Collen D., Lijnen H.R. The fibrinolytic system in man. CRC Critical Reviews in Oncology/Hematology. Crc Press, Boca Raton, FL (in press).

4. Sottrup-Jensen L., Petersen T.E., Magnusson S. In : "Atlas of protein sequence and structure", vol. 5, suppl. 3, p. 91, 1978.

5. Wallén P., Wiman B. Characterization of human plasminogen. I. On the relationship between different molecular forms of plasminogen demonstrated in plasma and found in purified preparations. Biochim. Biophys. Acta 221, 20-30, 1970.

6. Wallén P., Wiman B. Characterization of human plasminogen. II. Separation and partial characterization of different molecular forms of human plasminogen. Biochim. Biophys. Acta 257, 122-134, 1972.

7. Robbins K.C., Summaria L., Hsieh B., Shah R.J. The peptide chains of human plasmin. Mechanism of activation of human plasminogen to plasmin. J. Biol. Chem. 242, 2333-2342, 1967.

8. Brockway W.J., Castellino F.J. Measurement of the binding of antifibrinolytic amino acids to various plasminogens. Arch. Biochem. Biophys. 151, 194-199, 1972.

9. Rickli E.E., Otavsky W.I. A new method of isolation and some properties of heavy chain of human plasmin. Eur. J. Biochem. 9, 441-447, 1975.

10. Hoylaerts M., Lijnen H.R., Collen D. Studies on the mechanism of the antifibrinolytic action of tranexamic acid. Biochim. Biophys. Acta 673, 75-85, 1981.

11. Markus G., De Pasquale J.L., Wissler F.C. Quantitative determination of the binding of epsilon-aminocaproic acid to native plasminogen. J. Biol. Chem. 253, 727-732, 1978.

12. Vali Z., Patthy L. Location of the intermediate and high affinity omega-aminocarboxylic acid binding sites in human plasminogen. J. Biol. Chem. 257, 2104-2110, 1982.

13. Wiman B., Wallén P. The specific interaction between plasminogen and fibrin. A physiological role of the lysine binding site in plasminogen. Thromb. Res. 10, 213-222, 1977.

14. Christensen U., Clemmensen I. Kinetic properties of the primary inhibitor of plasmin from human plasma. Biochem. J. 163, 389-391, 1977.

15. Wiman B., Collen D. On the kinetics of the reaction between human antiplasmin and plasmin. Eur. J. Biochem. 84, 573-578, 1978.

16. Wiman B., Boman L., Collen D. On the kinetics of the reaction between human antiplasmin and a low-molecular-weight form of plasmin. Eur. J. Biochem. 87, 143-146, 1978.

17. Wiman B., Lijnen H.R., Collen D. On the specific interaction between the lysine-binding sites in plasmin and complementary sites in α_2-antiplasmin and in fibrinogen. Biochim. Biophys. Acta 579, 142-154, 1979.

18. Lijnen H.R., Hoylaerts M., Collen D. Isolation and characterization of a human plasma protein with affinity for the lysine-binding sites in plasminogen. Role in the regulation of fibrinolysis and identification as histidine-rich glycoprotein. J. Biol. Chem. 255, 10214-10222, 1980.

19. Wiman B., Collen D. Molecular mechanism of physiological fibrinolysis. Nature 272, 549-550, 1978.

20. Rijken D.C., Wijngaards G., Zaal-De Jong M., Welbergen J. Purification and partial characterization of plasminogen activator from human uterine tissue. Biochim. Biophys. Acta 580, 140-153, 1979.

21. Rijken D.C., Collen D. Purification and characterization of the plasminogen activator secreted by human melanoma cells in culture. J. Biol. Chem. 256, 7035-7041, 1981.

22. Collen D., Rijken D.C., Van Damme J., Billiau A. Purification of human tissue-type plasminogen activator in centigram quantities from human melanoma cell culture fluid and its conditioning for use in vivo. Thromb. Haemost. 48, 294-296, 1982.

23. Pennica D., Holmes W.E., Kohr W.J., Harkins R.N., Vehar G.A., Ward C.A., Bennett W.F., Yelverton E., Seeburg P.H., Heyneker H.L., Goeddel D.V., Collen D. Cloning and expression of human tissue-type plasminogen activator cNDA in E. coli. Nature 301, 214-221, 1983.

24. Collen D., Stassen J.M., Marafino B.J., Builder S., De Cock F., Ogez J., Tajiri D., Pennica D., Bennett W.F., Salwa J., Hoyng C.F. Biological properties of human tissue-type plasminogen activator obtained by expression of recombinant DNA in mammalian cells. J. Pharm. Exp. Ther. 231, 146-152, 1984.

25. Zamarron C., Lijnen H.R., Collen D. Kinetics of the activation of plasminogen by natural and recombinant tissue-type plasminogen activator. J. Biol. Chem. 259, 2080-2083, 1984.

26. Wallén P., Bergsdorf N., Rånby M. Purification and identification of two structural variants of porcine tissue plasminogen activator by affinity adsorption on fibrin. Biochim. Biophys. Acta 719, 318-328, 1982.

27. Banyai L., Varadi A., Patthy L. Common evolutionary origin of the fibrin-binding structures of fibronectin and tissue-type plasminogen activator. FEBS Lett. 163, 37-41, 1983.

28. Cash J.D. Control mechanism of activator release. In: "Progress in chemical fibrinolysis and thrombolysis, Vol. 3" (Davidson J.F., Rowan R.M., Samama M.M., Desnoyers P.C., eds.). Raven Press, New York, 1978, p. 65-75.

29. Colucci M., Stassen J.M., Salwa J., Collen D. Identification of plasminogen activator releasing activity in the neurohypophysis. Br. J. Haematol. 58, 337-346, 1984.

30. Comp P.C., Esmon C.T. Generation of fibrinolytic activity by infusion of activated protein C into dogs. J. Clin. Invest. 68, 1221-1228, 1981.

31. Colucci M., Stassen J.M., Collen D. Influence of protein C activation on blood coagulation and fibrinolysis in squirrel monkeys. J. Clin. Invest. 74, 200-204, 1984.

32. Korninger C., Stassen J.M., Collen D. Turnover of human extrinsic (tissue-type) plasminogen activator in rabbits. Thromb. Haemost. 46, 658-661, 1981.

33. Nilsson T., Wallén P., Mellbring G. Turnover of tissue-type plasminogen activator in man. Haemostasis 14, 90, 1984 (abstr).

34. Rijken D.C., Juhan-Vague I., Collen D. Complexes between tissue-type plasminogen activator and proteinase inhibitors in human plasma, identified with an immunoradiometric assay. J. Lab. Clin. Med. 101, 285-294, 1983.

35. Juhan-Vague I., Moerman B., De Cock F., Aillaud M.F., Collen D. Plasma levels of a specific inhibitor of tissue-type plasminogen activator (and urokinase) in normal and pathological conditions. Thromb. Res. 33, 523-530, 1984.

36. Wiman B., Chmielewska J., Rånby M. Inactivation of tissue plasminogen activator in plasma. Demonstration of a complex with a new rapid inhibitor. J. Biol. Chem. 259, 3644-3647, 1984.

37. Kruithof E.K.O., Trom-Thang C., Ransijn A., Bachmann F. Demonstration of a fast-acting inhibitor of plasminogen activators in human plasma. Blood 64, 907-913, 1984.

38. Verheijen J.H., Chang G.I.C., Mullaart E. Inhibition of extrinsic (tissue-type) plasminogen activator by human plasma: Evidence for the occurrence of a fast-acting inhibitor. Thromb. Haemost. 50, 294, 1983 (abstr 930).

39. Kruithof E.K.O., Ransijn A., Bachmann F. Inhibition of tissue plasminogen activator by human plasma. In: "Progress in fibrinolysis, Vol. VI" (Davidson J.F., Bachmann F., Bouvier C.A., Kruithof E.K.O., eds.). Churchill Livingstone, Edinburgh, 1983, p. 365-369.

40. Wijngaards G., Groeneveld E. Temporarily increased inhibition by plasma of plasminogen activator activity in severely ill patients. Haemostasis 12, 571, 1982.

41. Bertina R.M., van Hinsbergh V.W.M., Emeis S.J., van Wijngaarden A. Inhibition of tissue-type plasminogen activator inhibitor activity by activated protein C. Circulation 70, 94, 1984 (abstr 374).

42. Hoylaerts M., Rijken D.C., Lijnen H.R., Collen D. Kinetics of the activation of plasminogen by human tissue plasminogen activator. Role of fibrin. J. Biol. Chem. 257, 2912-2919, 1982.

43. Rånby M. Studies on the kinetics of plasminogen activation by tissue plasminogen activator. Biochim. Biophys. Acta 704, 461-469, 1982.

44. Nieuwenhuizen W., Voskuylen M., Traas D.W., Hoegee-de Nobel, B., Verheijen J.H. Kinetics of the tissue-type plasminogen activator-mediated activation of plasminogen. Influence of CNBr fibrin(ogen), fragment FCB-2 and dif-

ferent forms of plasminogen. In: "Fibrinogen, structure and function" (Henschen A., ed.). Walter de Gruyter, Berlin, 1984 (in press).

45. Rijken D.C., Hoylaerts M., Collen D. Fibrinolytic properties of one-chain and two-chain human extrinsic (tissue-type) plasminogen activator. J. Biol. Chem. 257, 2920-2925, 1982.

46. Tran-Chang C., Kruithof E.K.O., Bachmann F. Tissue-type plasminogen activator increases the binding of Glu-plasminogen to clots. J. Clin. Invest. 74, 2009-2016, 1984.

47. Collen D., Lijnen H.R. New approaches to thrombolytic therapy. Arteriosclerosis 4, 579-585, 1984.

48. Bernik M.B. Increased plasminogen activator (urokinase) in tissue culture after fibrin deposition. J. Clin. Invest. 52, 823-834, 1973.

49. Nolan C., Hall L., Barlow G., Tribby I.I.E. Plasminogen activator from human embryonic kidney cell cultures. Evidence for a proacivator. Biochim. Biophys. Acta 496, 384-400, 1977.

50. Nielsen L.S., Hansen J.G., Skriver L., Wilson E.L., Kaltoft K., Zeuthen J., Danø K. Purification of zymogen to plasminogen activator from human glioblastoma cells by affinity chromatography with monoclonal antibody. Biochemistry 21, 6410-6415, 1982.

51. Sumi H., Kosugi T., Matsuo O., Mihara H. Physicochemical properties of highly purified kidney cultured plasminogen activator (single polypeptide chain-urokinase). Acta Haematol. Japon. 45, 119-128, 1982.

52. Husain S., Gurewich V., Lipinski B. Purification and partial characterization of a single-chain high-molecular-weight form of urokinase from human urine. Arch. Biochem. Biophys. 220, 31-38, 1983.

53. Wun T.C., Ossowski L., Reich E. A proenzyme form of human urokinase. J. Biol. Chem. 257, 7262-7268, 1982.

54. Kohno T., Hopper P., Lillquist J.S., Suddith R.L., Greenlee R., Moir D.T. Kidney plasminogen activator: a precursor form of human urokinase with high fibrin affinity. Biotechnology 2, 628-634, 1984.

55. Sumi H., Toki N., Sasaki K., Mihara H. Comparative properties of single and double polypeptide chains of high molecular weight urokinase. In: "Progress in fibrinolysis, Vol. VI" (Davidson J.F., Bachmann F., Bouvier C.A., Kruithof E.K.O., eds.). Churchill Livingstone, Edinburgh, 1983, p. 165-167.

56. Gurewich V., Pannell R., Louie S., Kelley P., Suddith R.L., Greenlee R. Effective and fibrin-specific clot lysis by a zymogen precursor form of urokinase (pro-urokinase). A study in vitro and in two animal species. J. Clin. Invest. 73, 1731-1739, 1984.

57. Heyneker H.L., Holmes W.E., Vehar G.A. Preparation of functional human urokianse proteins. European Patent Application nr. 83103629.8, Publication nr. 0092182A2, European Patent Office, Munich, West-Germany.

58. Zamarron C., Lijnen H.R., Van Hoef B., Collen D. Biological and thrombolytic properties of proenzyme and active forms of human urokinase. I. Fibrinolytic and fibrinogenolytic properties in human plasma in vitro of urokinase obtained from human urine or by recombinant DNA technology. Thromb. Haemost. 52, 19-23, 1984.

59. Collen D., Stassen J.M., Blaber M., Winkler M., Verstraete M. Biological and thrombolytic properties of proenzyme and active forms of human urokinase. III. Thrombolytic properties of natural and recombinant urokinase in rabbits with experimental jugular vein thrombosis. Thromb. Haemost. 52, 27-30, 1984.

60. Lijnen H.R., Zamarron C., Collen D. Pro-urokinase: Kinetics and mechanism of action. Thromb. Haemost. (in press).

61. Lijnen H.R., Zamarron C., Blaber M., Winkler M., Collen D. Activation of plasminogen by pro-urokinase. I. Mechanism. (submitted for publication).

62. Collen D., Zamarron C., Lijnen H.R., Hoylaerts M. Activation of plasminogen by pro-urokinase. II. Kinetics. (submitted for publication).

ISOLATION AND CHARACTERISATION OF PLASMIC DEGRADATION PRODUCTS OF FIBRINOGEN BY HIGH - PERFORMANCE LIQUID CHROMATOGRAPHY

E. Müller, A. Henschen

Max-Planck-Institute for Biochemistry , 8033 Martinsried / München, FRG

Introduction

The biochemical and clinical importance of the plasmic degradation products of fibrinogen is well recognised. Some of the products play an important pathophysiological role because of their anticlotting properties and have frequently been analysed in patients suffering from fibrinolytic or thrombotic disorders (1,2). The biochemistry of the plasmic degradation of fibrinogen has been studied in great detail, the most commonly used analytical method being gel-electrophoresis. The main degradation products have been purified and characterized by proteinchemical methods (3,4). It is, however, obvious that important information about the exact mechanism of the degradation, the relative order of the cleavages and the properties of the pure components is still partly missing. The main reason for this has been the extreme difficulty to isolate the components of the complex fibrinolytic cleavage mixture in a pure state and to distinguish between closely related molecular species using classical fractionation and analysis methods. This report describes a procedure for the isolation and identification

Fibrinogen - Fibrin Formation and Fibrinolysis, Vol. 4
© 1986 Walter de Gruyter & Co., Berlin · New York - Printed in Germany.

of the plasmic degradation products using more modern separation methods with high resolving power, based on high performance liquid chromatography on improved column materials. Adapting these methods to the separation of all fibrinolytic degradation products present at each stage of the proteolysis it is now possible to obtain a large number of components in a pure state and to identify them. By monitoring the appearance and disappearence of the individual components detailed conclusions may be drawn about the relative order of peptide bond cleavage and the pure components become available for reinvestigations of their functional properties.

Results and Discussion

Human fibrinogen was incubated with human plasmin using various enzyme concentrations and incubation times. Fractionation of the degradation mixture on a size exclusion column resulted in the separation of the fragments X, Y, D, E and many smaller peptides. The formation of the components could be monitored as a function both of time and of enzyme concentration (Fig. 1). At the higher enzyme concentrations, fibrinogen was broken down into the fragments D and E already after an incubation time of less than 10 minutes. D and E fragments were protected during further degradation by the presence of calcium ions in the incubation mixture (5).

The products having higher molecular weights, i.e. X,Y,D and E, were S-carboxymethylated (6) and the constituent peptide chain components separated on a high - performance liquid chromatography reversed phase column. Fig. 2 shows the chromatographies of the D fragment and E fragment components.

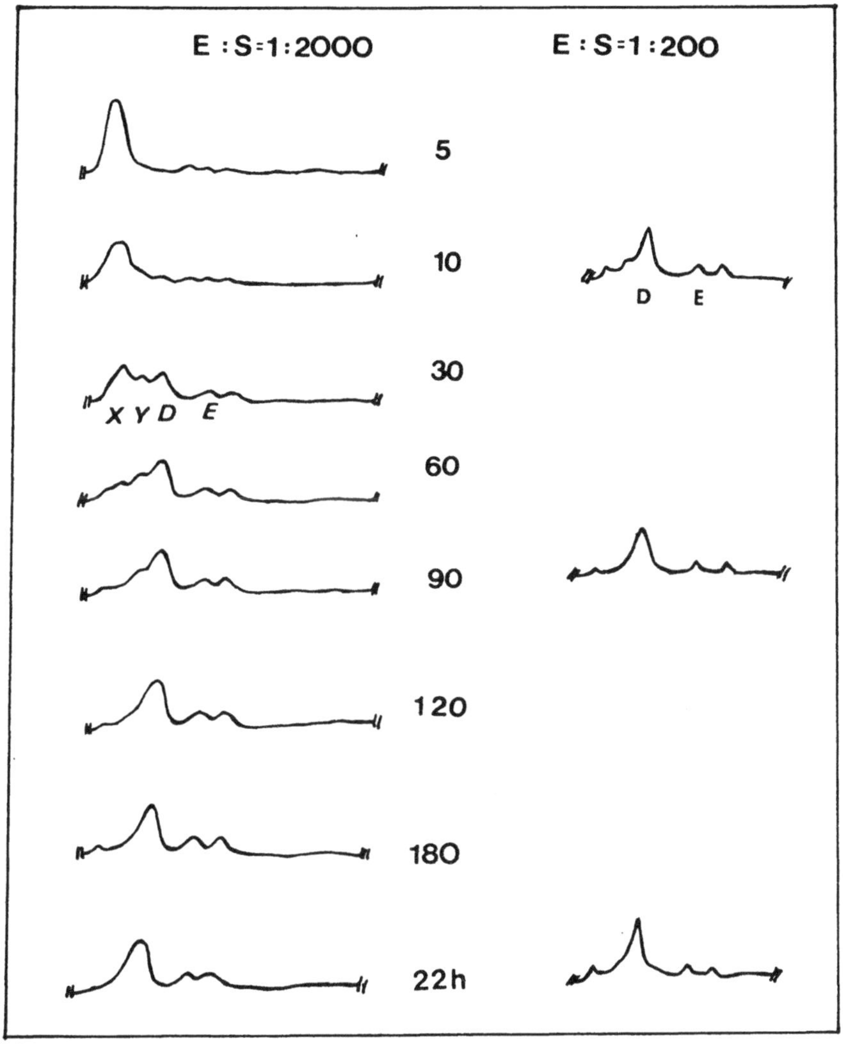

Fig.1: Gel chromatography on a size exclusion column (Sephacryl S-300 sf) of cleavage mixtures obtained with two different enzyme concentrations (E:S = 1:2000 and 1:200 w/w) after various incubation times (numbers indicate the time in minutes).

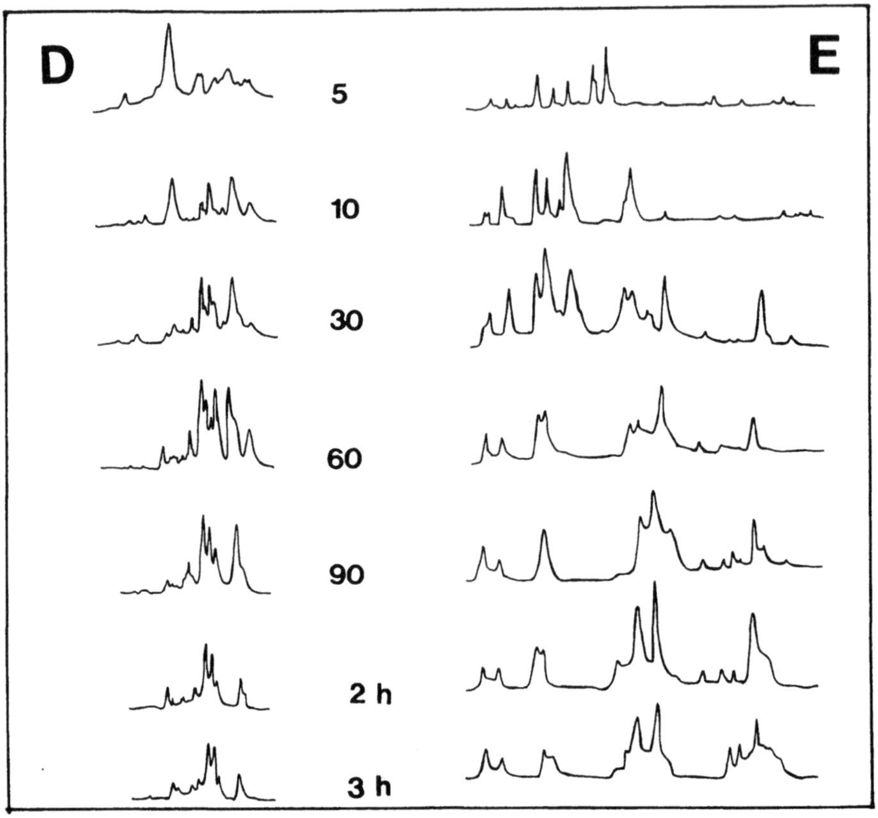

Fig.2: High-performance liquid chromatography on a reversed phase column (Vydac TP 18) of the S-carboxymethylated D and E fragments from cleavage mixtures obtained with the lower enzyme concentrations after various incubation times (numbers indicate the time in minutes).

The products having lower molecular weights were fractionated without previous modification. All components were identified by amino acid analysis and N-terminal amino-acid sequence determination (7,8). The precursor - product relationship of the individual peptides could often be determined. Fig. 3 shows the chromatographies of peptides smaller than the E fragment. All peaks could be related to predictable fragments of the fibrinogen molecule (see Fig. 4).

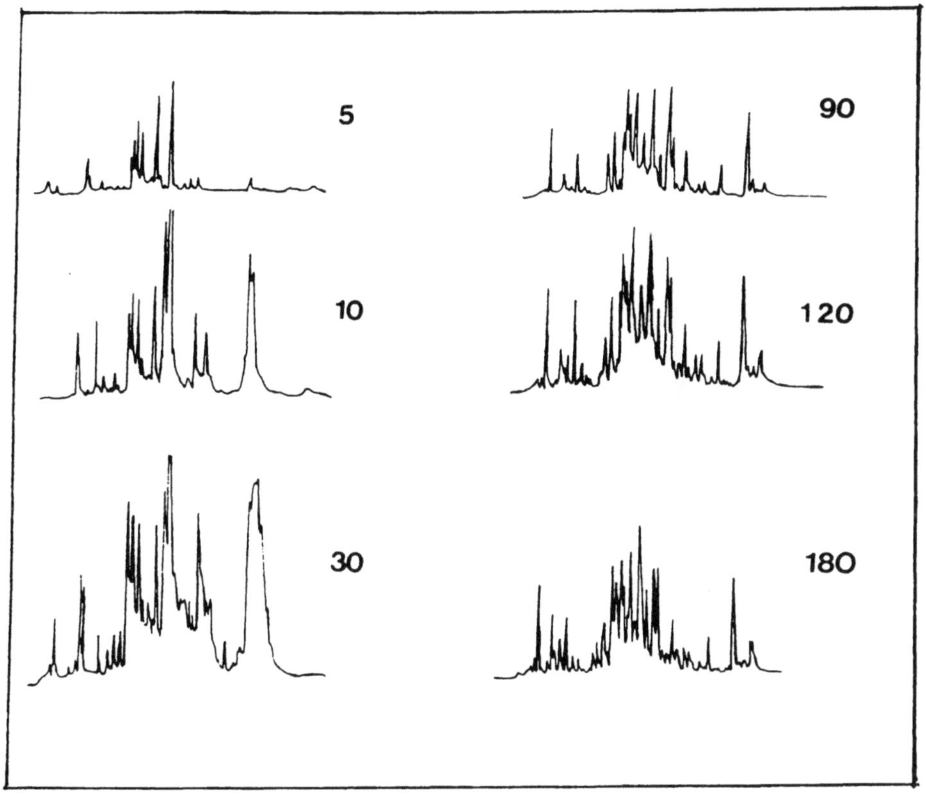

Fig.3: High-performance liquid chromatography on a reversed phase column (Vydac TP 18) of the smaller peptides from cleavage mixtures obtained with the lower enzyme concentrations after various incubation times (numbers indicate the time in minutes).

In an alternative experiment the relationship between the composition of the plasmic cleavage mixture and the increase in thrombin clotting time was studied. An aliquot sample of the plasmic cleavage mixture was used for thrombin clotting time determination ; in another sample the higher molecular weight components were removed by heat precipitation and centrifugation , whereas the soluble lower molecular weight components were analyzed by reversed phase high-performance liquid chromatography (Fig. 5). It was observed that a large number of peptides could be released from fibrinogen without an obvious change in thrombin clotting time.

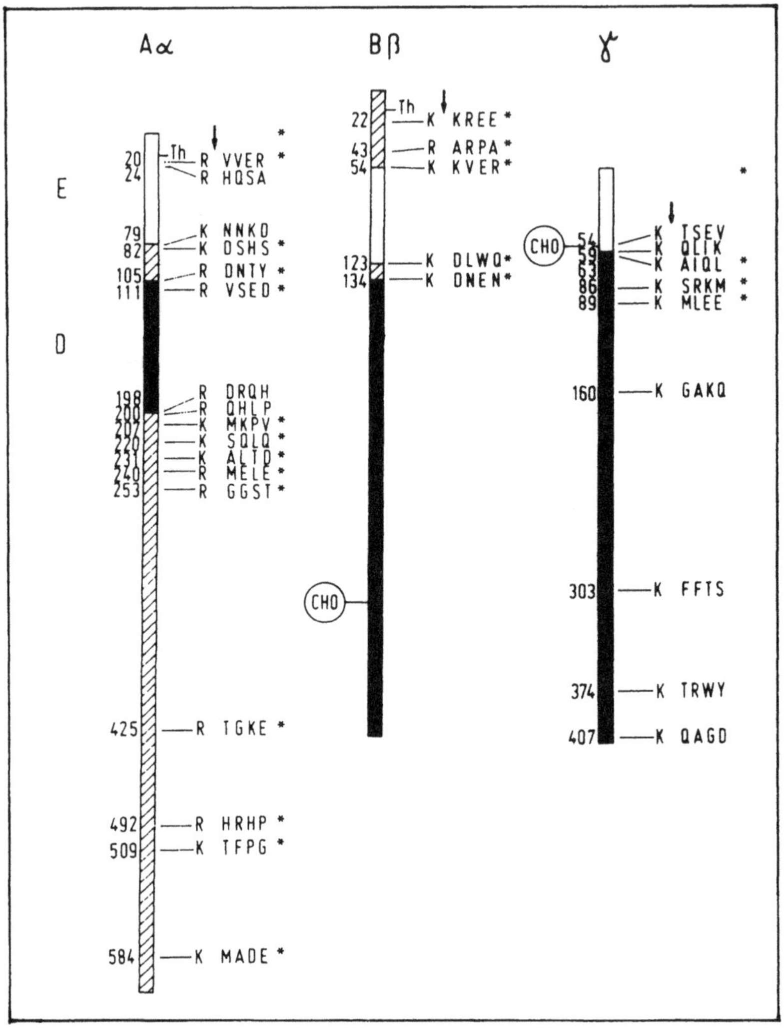

Fig.4: Plasmic cleavage sites in human fibrin(ogen) identified during previous or present investigations. The arrows show the cleavages in the indicated sequences. The numbers give the position of the new N-terminal residues. Fragment E is white and D black. Th denotes a thrombin cleavage site and CHO a carbohydrate linkage site. Sequences so far identified during this study are marked by *.

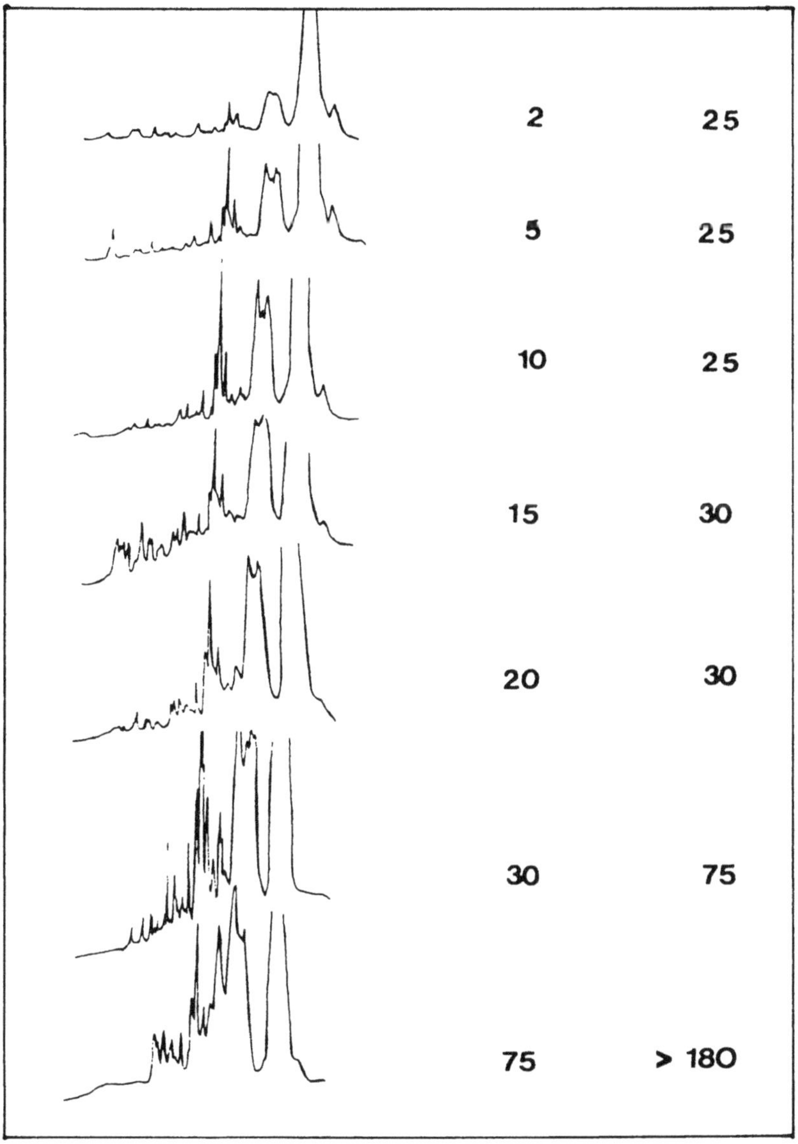

Fig.5: High-performance liquid chromatography on a reversed phase column (Vydac TP 18) of the soluble lower molecular weight peptides in the supernatant of cleavage mixtures obtained after various incubation times (numbers on the left side indicate the incubation time in minutes, numbers on the right side indicate the clotting time after addition of thrombin in seconds).

Only after 30 minutes of incubation an appreciable increase in clotting time was noticed. The peptides released were identified by amino acid analysis and N-terminal sequence determination. They could all be shown to have their origin in the C-terminal part of the Aα-chain and the N-terminal part of the Bβ-chain. The preliminary conclusion is therefore that these peptides could be of minor importance for the clotting function of fibrinogen. However, it will be necessary to confirm the conclusions by analysing the corresponding still clottable parts of the fibrinogen molecule.

References

1. Marder, V.J. and N.R. Shulman. 1968. High molecular weight derivates of human fibrinogen produced by plasmin. II. Mechanism of their anticoagulant activity. J. Biol. Chem. 244, 2120-2124.

2. Larrieu, M.-J., L. Dray, and N. Ardaillou. 1975. Biological effects of fibrinogen - fibrin degradation products. Thromb. Diathes. Haemorrh. 34, 686-692.

3. Furlan, M. and E. A. Beck. 1972. Plasmic degradation of human fibrinogen. Biochim. Biophys. Acta 263, 631-644.

4. Henschen, A. and F. Lottspeich. 1980. Fibrinogen structure and fibrinolysis. Haematologica 65, 535-541.

5. Haverkate, F. and G. Timan. 1977. Protective effect of calcium in the plasmin degradation of fibrinogen and fibrin fragments D. Thromb. Res. 10, 803-812.

6. Henschen, A. and P. Edman. 1972. Large scale preparation of S-carboxymethylated chains of human fibrinogen and fibrin and the occurrence of γ-chain variants. Biochim. Biophys. Acta 263, 351-367.

7. Edman, P. and A. Henschen. 1975. Sequence determination. In: Protein sequence determination. Springer, Berlin. pp. 232-279.

8. Lottspeich, F. 1985. Microscale isocratic separation of phenylthiohydantoin amino acid derivatives. J. Chrom. 326, 321-327.

THE ACCELERATION OF TISSUE-TYPE PLASMINOGEN ACTIVATOR (t-PA)-MEDIATED ACTIVATION OF PLASMINOGEN BY FIBRINOGEN CYANOGEN BROMIDE FRAGMENTS IS SPECIES SPECIFIC

W. Nieuwenhuizen and J. Keyser

TNO Gaubius Institute for Cardiovascular Research,
Herenstraat 5d, 2313 AD Leiden, The Netherlands.

Introduction

The accelerating action of fibrin on t-PA mediated plasminogen activation is well known (1). It has been concluded from kinetic data (2-5) that a ternary complex formed between plasminogen, t-PA and fibrin, plays an essential role in this acceleration (2-5).

Kringles I-IV domain of plasminogen is important in this complex formation (6), and possibly also the heavy chain of two-chain t-PA (7). As for fibrin(ogen) we have shown that a relatively short stretch of the Aα chain i.e. Aα 148-197 is essential in the acceleration of plasminogen activation (8-10).

One approach to gain insight into the mechanism of this system at the molecular level is to look for correlations between differences in primary structures and changes e.g. in the kinetics of the same systems from different species. The primary structures of human plasminogen (11), t-PA (12) and fibrin(ogen) (13,14) are known and those of other species will probably become available within a few years. Rat fibrinogen, for instance, is under study (15).

As a first step in this approach we looked for possible species specificities in the acceleration of t-PA mediated activation by fibrin monomers and fibrin(ogen) CNBr fragments. Correlation of our findings with primary structures will have to await sequence data for the other protein species used in this study i.e. rat, cat, monkey and pig.

Fibrinogen - Fibrin Formation and Fibrinolysis, Vol. 4
© 1986 Walter de Gruyter & Co., Berlin · New York - Printed in Germany.

Materials and Methods

Blood was collected on aprotinin and treated with diisopropylphosphofluoridate (DFP) and plasma prepared as described before (16).

Plasminogens were prepared from fresh plasmas by affinity chromatography (17) on lysine-Sepharose (Pharmacia Fine Chemicals, Uppsala, Sweden), precipitated with ammonium sulphate and dialyzed extensively against 0.1 M Tris.HCl, pH 7.5, containing 0.1% (v/v) Tween 80 (Baker Chemicals).

This procedure yields native (glu-)plasminogen when human plasma is used, and native plasminogens are most likely also obtained from the other plasma species.

All plasminogens showed one band on SDS-PAGE, after staining with Coomassie Brilliant Blue. Their concentration was calculated using an $A_{1cm}^{1\%}$ of 16.1 at 280 nm (18).

Fibrin monomers were prepared as described by Haverkate (19).

CNBr digests of fibrinogens were prepared as described by Blombäck et al. (20). Prior to use they were dialyzed exhaustively against distilled water and freeze-dried. Their concentrations were based on dry weight.

Tissue-type plasminogen activators

- Human t-PA was purified from melanoma cell culture medium as described before (21,22).
- Porcine t-PA was purified from pig heart as described by Wallén et al. (23).
- Rat t-PA: a serum-free 24 hours culture medium of a continuous parietal yolk sac carcinoma cell line was used. This cell line (L-2) was kindly donated by Dr. U. Wewer (University Institute of Pathological Anatomy, Copenhagen, Denmark) and was described in (24). Table 1 summarizes the proteins which were used in all combinations in this study.

Assay system

The assay system, used to assess the acceleration of plasminogen activation, was a continuous spectrophotometric assay using S-2251 (Kabivitrum, Stockholm, Sweden) as a plasmin substrate (25). A constant concentration of 0.11 μM of each of the plasminogens was used. Activities of the t-PA's were expressed in uroki-

Table 1. Proteins used in this study.

t-PA species	plasminogen species	fibrin monomers or CNBr fragments of fibrinogen
Human (22)	human	human
Porcine (23)	porcine	porcine
Rat*	rat	rat
	feline	cat
	monkey (Macaca mulatta)	monkey (Macaca mulatta)

*Culture medium of a continuous parietal yolk sac carcinoma cell line (L-2) kindly donated by Dr. U. Wewer, Copenhagen.

nase equivalent units by comparison of fibrinolytic activities on plasminogen enriched fibrin plates (26). In the present study these were 1.5, 2 and 0.5 units/ml for human, pig and rat t-PA, respectively. The amounts of each fibrin monomer species and of each fibrinogen CNBr digest were varied from 0 to 40 µg/ml, and 0 to 320 µg/ml, respectively. Activation rate is proportional to OD_{405} per t^2 (4,25). Increases in activation rates are expressed as the ratios of the rates of activation in the presence and in the absence of stimulator after correction for the appropriate blanks (4,25).

Results and Discussion

No species specificities are detectable when plasminogen activation is stimulated with intact fibrin monomers, i.e., the activation rates of all five plasminogen species by the three t-PA species increased more than 20-fold in the presence of each of the five monomer species (man, pig, rat, cat, monkey). This indicates that effective interspecies interactions can occur.
Tables 2 and 3 summarize the maximum increases in activation rate of human, monkey, cat, pig and rat plasminogen in the presence of CNBr digests of fibrinogens from all of these same species by t-PA from man, pig and rat.
In these tables +/- indicates a less than 5-fold increase in activation rate; + between 5 and 10-fold; ++ between 10 and

15-fold; +++ between 15- and 20-fold and ++++ 20-fold or more, as compared with the situation without any CNBr digest present.

Table 2. Acceleration of the activation of plasminogens by different t-PA's, in the presence of different fibrinogen CNBr digests.

t-PA species	CNBr digest of fibrinogen from man	pig	rat	monkey	cat
			human plasminogen		
human	++	++	++	++++	++++
pig	++++	+++	+++	++++	++++
rat	++	+++	+++	++	+++
			monkey plasminogen		
human	+++	++	+++	+++	++
pig	+/-	+	+/-	++	+
rat	+++	++	++++	+	+
			cat plasminogen		
human	++++	+++	+++	+++	+
pig	+++	++	++	+++	+
rat	+++	+++	++++	+	+

Our results with fibrin monomers and fibrinogen CNBr fragments allow the following conclusions:

- All structural information for effective interactions is available in t-PA, plasminogen and fibrin monomers of each of the tested species.
- Cleavage of fibrinogen with CNBr leads to the loss of part of structural information. The residual information in the CNBr digests is apparently sufficient to accelerate the activation of human, cat and monkey plasminogen and not for pig and rat plasminogen. A CNBr digest of a fibrinogen can be effective

in the activation of one plasminogen and without effect in the activation of another. This does not change when another t-PA species is chosen.
Therefore, the plasminogen species and not the source of fibrinogen or t-PA seems to dictate if the rate of activation can be increased by the addition of a fibrinogen CNBr digest.

Table 3. Acceleration of the activation of plasminogens by different t-PA's, in the presence of different fibrinogen CNBr digests.

t-PA species	CNBr digest of fibrinogen from man	pig	rat	monkey	cat
			porcine plasminogen		
human	-	-	+/-	+/-	-
pig	-	+/-	+/-	+/-	-
rat	+/-	-	+/-	+/-	-
			rat plasminogen		
human	-	-	+/-	+/-	+/-
pig	+/-	+/-	+/-	+/-	+/-
rat	+	-	+	+/-	+/-

The differences between human, monkey and cat plasminogen on the one hand and porcine and rat plasminogen on the other hand, are much alike the described differences in activation of these plasminogens by streptokinase (27). Also, as far as streptokinase activation is concerned, plasminogens can be divided in different categories: human, monkey and cat plasminogens can be activated with low concentrations of streptokinase, whereas pig and rat plasminogen can not be activated with any concentration of streptokinase (27).
The molecular basis for this parallel between acceleration of t-PA catalyzed activation and activation of different plasminogens by streptokinase is not clear at present. More experimental

data, especially on the interaction between plasminogens and domains of fibrinogen will be needed to understand this similarity in behaviour. Plasminogen conformational changes induced by streptokinase might also be elicited by accelerating fragments of fibrinogen. However, in the case of streptokinase, this leads to plasmin activity, whereas interaction with cyanogen bromide fragments seems to make some plasminogens only more easily t-PA activatable.

Acknowledgements

Thanks are due to Dr. J.J. Emeis for the L-2 cell culture medium; to Mr. D. Jense for his help during the blood sampling; to Mrs. B. Hoegee-de Nobel for her help in part of the experiments and to M.R. and C. Horsting for typing the manuscript.

References

1. Wallén, P. 1977. Activation of plasminogen and tissue activator. In: Thrombosis and Urokinase. (R. Paoletti and S. Sherry, eds.) Academic Press, New York. pp. 91-102.

2. Hoylaerts, M., D.C. Rijken, H.R. Lijnen and D. Collen. 1982. Kinetics of the activation of plasminogen by human tissue plasminogen activator. Role of fibrin. J. Biol. Chem. 257, 2912-2919.

3. Rånby, M. 1982. Studies on the kinetics of plasminogen activation by tissue plasminogen activator. Biochim. Biophys. Acta 704, 461-469.

4. Nieuwenhuizen, W., M. Voskuilen, D.W. Traas, B. Hoegee-de Nobel and J.H. Verheijen. 1984. Kinetics of the tissue-type plasminogen activator-mediated activation of plasminogen. Influence of CNBr fibrin(ogen) fragment FCB-2 and different forms of plasminogen. In: Fibrinogen Vol. 3. (A. Henschen and T. Saldeen, eds.) Walter de Gruyter, Berlin (in press).

5. Nieuwenhuizen, W., M. Voskuilen, D.W. Traas and B. Hoegee-de Nobel. 1984. Kinetics of the tissue-type plasminogen activator (t-PA) mediated activation of different forms of plasminogen (plg). Influence of fibrinogen fragments. VIII International Congress on Thrombosis, Istanbul, June 4-7, Abstract 86.

6. Verheijen, J.H., W. Nieuwenhuizen, D.W. Traas, G.T.G. Chang and E. Hoegee. 1983. Differences in effects of fibrin(ogen) fragments on the activation of 1-glu-plasminogen and 442-val-

plasminogen by tissue-type plasminogen activator. Thromb. Res. 32, 87-92.

7. Rijken, D.C. 1984. Isolation and properties of the light chain of tissue-type plasminogen activator. Haemostasis 14, abstract 18.

8. Verheijen, J.H., W. Nieuwenhuizen, and G. Wijngaards. 1982. Activation of plasminogen by tissue activator is increased specifically in the presence of certain soluble fibrin(ogen) fragments. Thromb. Res. 27, 377-385.

9. Nieuwenhuizen, W., J.H. Verheijen, A. Vermond and G.T.G. Chang. 1983. Plasminogen activation by tissue activator is accelerated in the presence of fibrin(ogen) cyanogen bromide fragment FCB-2. Biochim. Biophys. Acta 755, 531-533.

10. Nieuwenhuizen, W., A. Vermond, M. Voskuilen, D.W. Traas and J.H. Verheijen. 1983. Identification of a site in fibrin-(ogen) which is involved in the acceleration of plasminogen activation by tissue-type plasminogen activator. Biochim. Biophys. Acta 748, 86-92.

11. Castellino, F.J. 1984. Biochemistry of human plasminogen. Seminars in Thrombosis and Haemostasis 10, 18-23.

12. Pennica, D., W.E. Holmes, W.J. Kohr, R.N. Harkins, G.A. Vehar, C.A. Ward, W.F. Bennett, E. Yelverton, P.H. Seeburg, H.L. Heyneker, D.V. Goeddel and D. Collen. 1983. Cloning and expression of human tissue-type plasminogen activator cDNA in E.coli. Nature 301, 214-221.

13. Henschen, A. 1981. Fibrinogen-Blutgerinnungsfaktor I. Biochemische Aspekten. Haemostaseologie 1, 49-61.

14. Doolittle, R.F. 1981. Fibrinogen and fibrin. Sci. Amer. 245, 92-101.

15. Crabtree, G.R. and J.A. Kant. 1982. Organization of the rat γ-fibrinogen gene: alternative mRNA splice patterns produce the γA and γB (γ') chains of fibrinogen. Cell 31, 159-166.

16. Van Ruijven-Vermeer, J.A.M. and W. Nieuwenhuizen. 1978. Purification of rat fibrinogen and its constituent chains. Biochem. J. 169, 653-658.

17. Deutsch, D.G. and E.T. Mertz. 1970. Plasminogen: purification from human plasma by affinity chromatography. Science 170, 1095-1096.

18. Wallén, P. and B. Wiman. 1970. Characterization of human plasminogen. I. On the relationship between different molecular forms of plasminogen demonstrated in plasma and found in purified preparations. Biochim. Biophys. Acta 221, 20-30.

19. Haverkate, F., and G. Timan. 1976. Preparation of highly purified bovine fibrin plates. In: Progress in Chemical fibrinolysis and Thrombolysis, Vol. 2. (J.F. Davidson, M.M.

Samama and P.C. Desnoyers, eds.) Raven Press, New York. pp. 67-71.

20. Blombäck, B., M. Blombäck, B. Hessel and S. Iwanaga. 1967. Structure of N-terminal fragments of fibrinogen and specificity of thrombin. Nature (London) 215, 1445-1448.

21. Rijken, D.C., G. Wijngaards, M. Zaal-De Jong and J. Welbergen. 1979. Purification and partial characterization of plasminogen activator from human uterine tissue. Biochim. Biophys. Acta 580, 140-153.

22. Rijken, D.C. and D. Collen. 1981. Purification and characterization of the plasminogen activator secreted by human melanoma cells in culture. J. Biol. Chem. 256, 7035-7041.

23. Wallén, P., M. Bergsdorf and M. Rånby. 1982. Purification and identification of two structural variants of porcine tissue plasminogen activator by affinity adsorption on fibrin. Biochim. Biophys. Acta 719, 318-328.

24. Wewer, U. 1982. Characterization of a rat yolk sac carcinoma cell line. Developm. Biol. 93, 416-421.

25. Verheijen, J.H., E. Mullaart, G.T.G. Chang, C. Kluft and G. Wijngaards. 1982. A simple sensitive spectrophotometric assay for extrinsic (tissue-type) plasminogen activator applicable to measurements in plasma. Thromb. Haemostas. 48, 266-269.

26. Haverkate, F. and D.W. Traas. 1974. Dose-response curves in the fibrin plate assay. Fibrinolytic activity of proteases. Thromb. Diath. Haemorrh. 32, 356-365.

27. Marcum, J.A. and D.L. Kline. 1983. Mini-review: Species specificity of streptokinase. Comp. Biochem. Physiol. 75B, 389-394.

ROLE OF FIBRIN POLYMERIZATION IN FIBRINOLYSIS: COMPARISON BETWEEN POLYMERISABLE AND UNPOLYMERISABLE FIBRINS IN THE POTENTIATING EFFECT OF PLASMINOGEN ACTIVATION BY TISSUE-TYPE PLASMINOGEN ACTIVATOR (tpA).

J. Soria, C. Soria, O. Bertrand, M. Mirshahi, F.W. Dunn, E. Svenson,
P. Desvignes, P. Bonnet, M. Samama, J.P. Caen.
Hôtel Dieu (Service des Prof. Bernadou, Fabiani, Samama), Paris.
Hôpital Lariboisière (Services des Prof. Caen, Rousselet), Paris.

Activation of plasminogen to the active enzyme plasmin by tissue plasminogen activator(tpA) is potentiated by fibrin or derivatives such as fibrin monomer (4), fragment D (9) and cyanogen bromide treated-fibrinogen (10). Because of the defective potentiating effect of fibrin from dysfibrinogenia with abnormal fibrin polymerisation (as described the first time for fibrinogen Dusard (6)), we wanted to determine the role of fibrin polymerisation in potentiating tpA-induced plasminogen activation. The present investigation was therefore undertaken in order to examine whether the potentiating effect of fibrin monomer on plasminogen activation by tpA is dependent of fibrinopeptides release only or fibrin polymerisation subsequent to fibrinopeptides release. In order to study the role of fibrin polymerisation, we compared the potentiating effect on tpA-induced plasminogen activation of normal des-A fibrin with that of des-A fibrin from fibrinogen ALES. Fibrinogen ALES is an homozygous dysfibrinogenemia characterized by an absence of polymerisation after reptilase addition, despite a normal release of fibrinopeptide A. On the contrary, fibrin clot is formed when thrombin is added to fibrinogen ALES. The anomaly is located on the γ chain and therefore it is suggested that fibrinogen abnormality in fibrinogen ALES is located on the polymerising site a (reptilase expressed the polymerisation site A in the amino-terminal part of the α chain, which interacts with preexisting complementary site located in the carboxyl terminal part of the γ chain of another fibrin monomers (site a).

Material and Methods

Reagents :

Plasminogen = Lys plasminogen (substrene) was purchased from Choay Lab (Paris). The small quantity of plasmin present in the reagent was eliminated by

© 1986 Walter de Gruyter & Co., Berlin · New York - Printed in Germany.

aprotinin agarose adsorption. The chromogenic substrate S2251 was obtained from Kabi (Stockholm). The tpA was isolated from human melanoma cells in culture (5). It was kindly given by D. Lijnen (Univ. of Leuven). The activity was expressed in urokinase equivalent units by comparison of the fibrinolytic activity on fibrin plates. The specific activity was about 90,000 IU/mg.
Buffer : 0.1 M phosphate buffer pH 7.3 containing 10 mM EDTA, 0.1% NaN_3. and 0.1% triton X100 in order to avoid unspecific adsorption. 0.1% tween 80 was added for the preparation of tpA solution.

Fibrinogen - Normal and ALES fibrinogens were isolated from citrated plasmas according to the technique of BLOMBACK (1).
Fibrinopeptide A (fpa) determination was performed by an immunoenzymological procedure (7) using asserachrom fpa (Diagnostica Stago-Asnières, France).

Obtention of Des-A fibrin : Normal or patient fibrinogen was incubated with reptilase (Diagnostica Stago) for 2 hours at 37°C.
Clot formation occurred in less than 1 minute with normal fibrinogen.To dissolve the clot, urea was added until a final concentration of 7M. None occurred when using fibrinogen ALES for incubation time of more than 3 hours.
Comparison of the potentiating effect of tpA-induced plasminogen activator of: normal fibrinogen, des-A normal fibrin, des-A fibrin ALES (unpolymerisable), in the presence or absence of urea.
To 0.1ml of lys plasminogen at 85 µg/ml in phosphate buffer were added 0.1 ml of tpA at various concentrations, 0.1ml S2251 at 3mM in water, followed by the addition of either 10 µl of reptilase (control) or 10 µl of each potentiator to be tested at several concentrations (fibrinogen, fibrinogen in 7 M urea, des-A normal fibrin dissolved in 7 M urea, des-A ALES fibrin in the presence or absence of urea). Incubation was done at 37°C in a microtiter plate and the absorbance at 405 nm was measured every hour using an Elisa autoreader (Dynatech).
When des-A normal fibrin was tested in the absence of urea, normal fibrinogen was incubated at 37°C with tpA, plasminogen, S2251 and reptilase. After incubation, tubes were centrifuged and the absorbance at 405 nm of the supernatant measured. (Concentration of tpA-plasminogen and fibrin derivative are similar to those used in the presence of urea).

Comparison between normal and ALES fibrin clot lysis induced by tpA.
Normal or patient fibrinogen enriched in plasminogen was clotted by thrombin in the presence of calcium and of 3 concentrations of tpA. (25 -12 and 6 ng/ml final concentration).Incubation of the clots was done at 37°C and clot lysis time was determined.

Results

1. Release of fibrinopeptide A from reptilase-treated fibrinogen.
Despite the absence of fibrin clot, after treatment of fibrinogen ALES with reptilase the amount of fpa released per mg of fibrinogen is similar to that obtained with normal fibrinogen incubated in the presence of reptilase (results not shown).

2. Potentiating effect on tpA-induced plasminogen activation of normal fibrinogen, des-A normal fibrin, des-A unpolymerisable fibrin ALES (in the presence or absence of urea). Plasminogen activation by tpA is determined by amidolytic activity on S2251. As shown on fig 1, this is very low in controls (reptilase) or in the presence of untreated fibrinogen.
On the contrary, generation of great amount of plasmin occurs when normal Des-A fibrin is added either in the presence or absence of urea. To be noted , however,in presence of normal fibrinogen dissolved in 7 M urea a small amount of plasmin in formed.
Results shown in fig 2 compare the potentiating effect of normal des-A fibrin monomer dissolved in urea, to those of des-A fibrin ALES in the presence or absence of urea. In the absence of urea, des-A fibrin ALES, incapable of polymerisation, does not stimulate plasminogen activation by tpA. When urea is added to des-A fibrin ALES, however, a generation of plasmin occurs. This still remains smaller than the plasmin generation obtained with normal des-A fibrin.

3. Comparison between normal and ALES fibrin clot lysis induced by tpA.
Contrary to what preceeds with reptilase a clot forms when thrombin is added to the abnormal fibrin ALES. In the presence of tpA, clot lysis occurs at the same rate for normal and abnormal fibrin clot. This shows that plasmin is generated normally when fibrin ALES is allowed to polymerise. (results not shown).

Discussion

The activation of plasminogen by tpA is greatly increased in the presence of fibrin. It has been suggested that fibrin facilitates the interactions between tpA and plasminogen(4). The potentiating effect of fibrin is decreased in some cases of dysfibrinogenemia presenting severe thrombotic disorder as described in Dusard Syndrome (6). These dysfibrinogenemia are characterized by an abnormal qualitative fibrin polymerisation: all fibrinogen is clottable, but

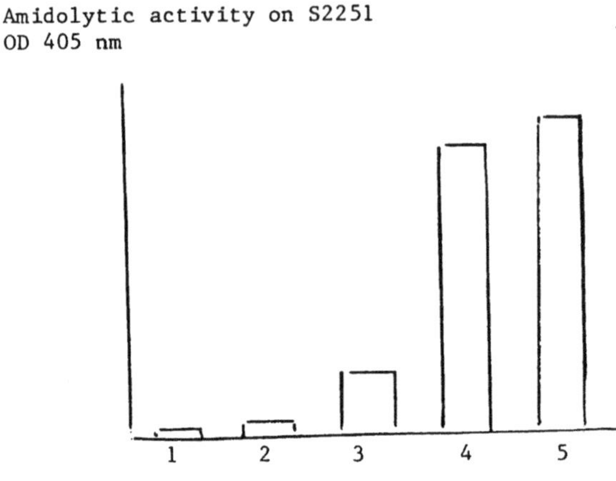

Figure 1

Plasminogen activation by tpA - Comparison between the potentiating effect induced by -

1. reptilase (control)
2. normal fibrinogen
3. normal fibrinogen in 7 M urea
4. des-A normal fibrin in 7 M urea
5. des-A normal fibrin clot

Conditions used
- -0.1 ml tpA (0.4 ng/ml)
- -0.1 ml plasminogen
- -10 µl potentiator (2.5 mg/ml)
- -100 µl S2251

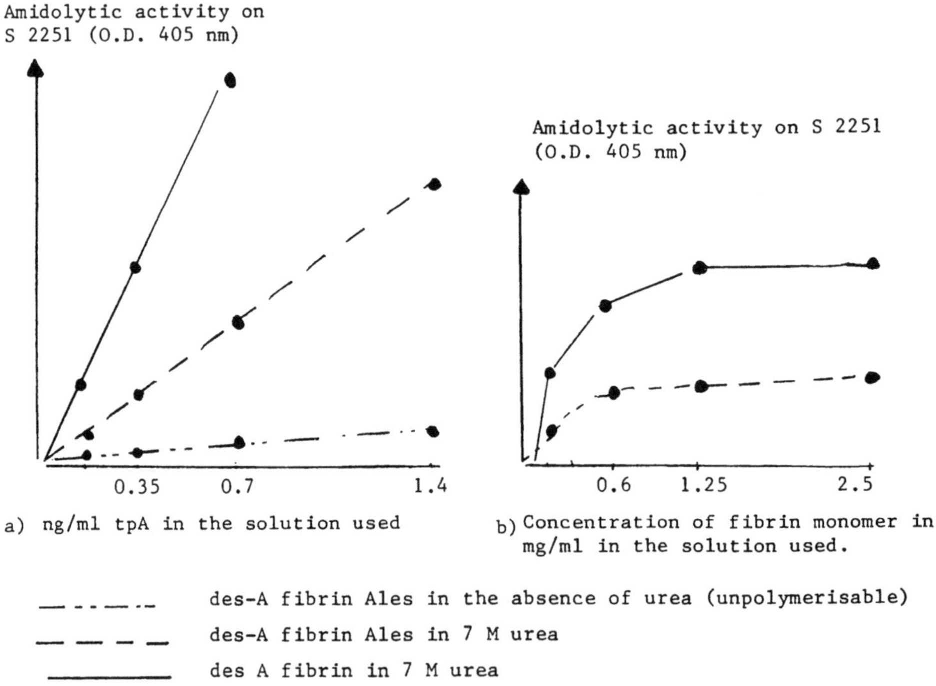

Figure 2 : Stimulating effect of des-A Normal fibrin and des-A fibrin Ales on tpA-induced plasminogen activation.

the structure of the clot is abnormal. Therefore, this study was carried out to analyze the importance of fibrin polymerisation in the potentiating effect of fibrin in tpA -induced plasminogen activation.

In order to study the role of fibrin polymerisation, we compared the potentiating effect on the activation of plasminogen by tpA of normal des A fibrin monomer (which polymerized during the incubation) with that of unpolymerisable fibrin monomer. We have had the opportunity to use des-A fibrin monomer prepared from fibrinogen ALES (homozygous case of dysfibrinogenemia uncapable of polymerization after reptilase addition despite a normal release of fibrinopeptide A as shown by immunoenzymological procedure).

The results show that des-A fibrin monomer from ALES does not have a potentiating effect on the activation of plasminogen by tpA. A potentiating effect appears however, when des-A fibrin monomers from ALES are treated by urea but remains smaller than that observed with normal des-A fibrin. This seems not specific since normal fibrinogen dissolved in urea induces also a stimulating effect on plasminogen activation.

Potentiating effect of fibrin ALES appears normal however when fibrin ALES is allowed to polymerise. Polymerisation occurs when thrombin is added to fibrinogen ALES. This polymerisation is due to the interaction between the site B unmasked by thrombin, and preexisting site b located in the carboxyl terminal part of another fibrin monomer. TpA-induced clot lysis occurs at the same rate for normal and patient fibrin. This indicates that plasmin generations occurs similarly in the presence of normal or ALES fibrin and therefore fibrin ALES is efficient in stimulating plasminogen activation.

These results clearly indicate that in physiological conditions, fibrin polymerisation is essential to its potentiating effect on plasminogen activation by tpA. These results are in good correlation with those already reported by E. Svenson and L.C. Petersen (8).

We suggest that in dysfibrinogenemia, responsible for spontaneous thrombotic episodes, and in which an abnormal polymerisation was discovered, the abnormal fibrin does not reveal the site involved in the potentiating effect on tpA-induced plasminogen activation. It is also possible that an abnormal clot organization intervenes secondarily: the site responsible of the stimulating effect on tpA-induced plasminogen activation being hidden in the abnormal fibrin.

References

1. Blomback, B., M. Blomback 1956. Purification of human and bovine fibrinogen. Archiv. for Kemi. 10, 415-443.

2. Hoylaerts M., D.C. Rijken, H.R. Lijnen, D. Collen. 1982. Kinetics of the activation of plasminogen by human tissue-plasminogen activator. J. Biol. Chem. 257, 2912-2919.

3. Olexa S.A., A.Z. Budzynski. 1981. Localization of a fibrin polymerizing site. Journal of Biol. Chem. 256, 3544-3549.

4. Ranby M., B. Norman, P. Wallen. 1982. A sensitive assay for tissue plasminogen activator. Thrombosis Research. 27, 743-749.

5. Rijken D.C., D. Collen. 1981. Purification and characterization of the plasminogen activator secreted by human melanoma cells in culture. J.Biol. Chem. 256, 7035-7041.

6. Soria J., C.Soria, J.P.Caen. 1983. A new type of congenital dysfibrinogenemia with defective fibrin lysis. Dusard Syndrome = Possible relation to thrombosis. Brit. Journ. Haemat. 53, 575-586.

7. Soria J, C. Soria, J.J.Ryckewaert. 1980. A solid phase immuno-enzymological assay for the measurement of human fibrinopeptide A.Thrombos. Res. 20, 425-435.

8. Svenson E., and L.C. Peterson. 1985. Polymerisation of fibrin as a prerequisite to the stimulating effects in fibrinolysis. In Fibrinogen Workshop. London.

9. Verheijen J.H, W. Nieuwewhuizen W, Wijngaards G. 1982, Activation of plasminogen by tissue activator is increased specifically in the presence of certain soluble fibrin(ogen) fragments. Thrombosis Research. 27, 377-388.

10. Verheijen J.H., E. Nullaart, GTG Chang, C. Kluft, G. Vingaard. 1982. A simple sensitive spectrophotometric assay for extrinsic (tissue type) plasminogen activator applicable to measurement in plasma. Thromb. Research. 48, 266-269.

ROLE OF FIBRIN AND ITS DEGRADATION PRODUCTS IN THE ACTIVATION OF PLASMINOGEN BY STREPTOKINASE AND UROKINASE

A. Takada, Y. Takada

Department of Physiology, Hamamatsu University, School of Medicine, Hamamatsu-shi, Shizuoka 431-31, Japan

Introduction

Much attention has been paid to the roles of fibrin and its degradation products in the activation process of human plasminogen(plg). It is well established that the activity of tissue plg activator (t-PA) is significantly enhanced in the presence of fibrin(1, 2). It is also suggested that the precursor form of urokinase(pro-UK) has also enhanced activity in the presence of fibrin (3). The effects of fibrin on the activation of plasminogen by urokinase(UK) and streptokinase (SK) have been controversial for years. In 1970, we have reported (4, 5) that there is a factor in the human plasma which potentiates the activation rate of plasminogen by SK. This factor was first called SK-activatable proactivator of plasminogen, and later renamed as SK-potentiator (6. 7). As to the effects of fibrin, we have also reported that the activation rate of a native form of plasminogen (Glu-plg) by UK was enhanced in the presence of fibrin and fibrinogen, but that of a modified form (Lys-plg) was not influenced in their presence (8, 9).

In the present paper we further describe the physicochemical characteristics of SK-potentiator and the fibrin induced enhancement of UK activation of Glu-plg.

Materials and Methods

Purification of Human Plasminogen and SK-potentiator(7)

Out-dated human plasma was dialyzed against 20 volumes of water overnight, and insoluble materials were removed by centrifugation.

Fibrinogen - Fibrin Formation and Fibrinolysis, Vol. 4
© 1986 Walter de Gruyter & Co., Berlin · New York - Printed in Germany.

The supernatant was applied to lysine-Sepharose column in the presence of aprotinin. PH of the pass through fractions was adjusted to 5.2, and the precipitate was passed through Sepharose 4B, DE23 and Sephadex G-200 columns to get SK-potentiator. Plasminogen was eluted from lysine-Sepharose column with 0.2 M epsilon aminocaproic acid (EACA). One unit of SK-potentiator was tentatively determined when 1 μmol of TAMe (Tosyl arginine methyl ester) was hydrolyzed in 30 min by the mixture of plasminogen(0.4 casein unit(cu)/ml), SK (10 u/ml) and SK-potentiator in excess of the hydrolysis of TAMe in the absence of SK-potentiator (6).

Hydrolysis of TAMe (6, 10)

Plasminogen was mixed with SK-potentiator, SK(Kabikinase, AB KABI, Stockholm, Sweden) and TAMe. After incubation for 30 min at 37°C, Hesterin reagents were added, and absorbance was measured at 530 nm.

Hydrolysis of S-2251(H-D-Val-Leu-Lys-pNA:AB KABI, Stockholm, Sweden)

Glu-plg was activated by UK(Kowa Co. Ltd., Tokyo, Japan) in the plasma or clotted plasma, or in the presence of fibrinogen(grade L: AB KABI, Stockholm, Sweden) or fibrin (fibrinogen plus thrombin: Green Cross Co. Ltd., Osaka, Japan) in the purified system. The hydrolysis of S-2251 was quenched by the addition of 50 % acetic acid. In the case of continuous monitoring by Beckman DU8B spectrophotometer, acetic acid was not added.

Results

The Enhancement of the Activation of Plasminogen by SK in the Presence of SK-potentiator

Fig. 1 shows the results of experiments in which 0.1 ml of SK(10 u) and 0.2 ml of various amounts of plasminogen were mixed with 0.5 ml of TAMe (10 μmol) in the presence or absence of 0.2 ml of SK-potentiator (42 u) and incubated for 30 min at 37°C, then hydrolysis of TAMe was measured. Plasminogen was hardly activated by SK in the absence of SK-potentiator, whereas significant amounts of TAMe was hydrolyzed in its presence, indicating the larger extent of the activation of plasminogen.

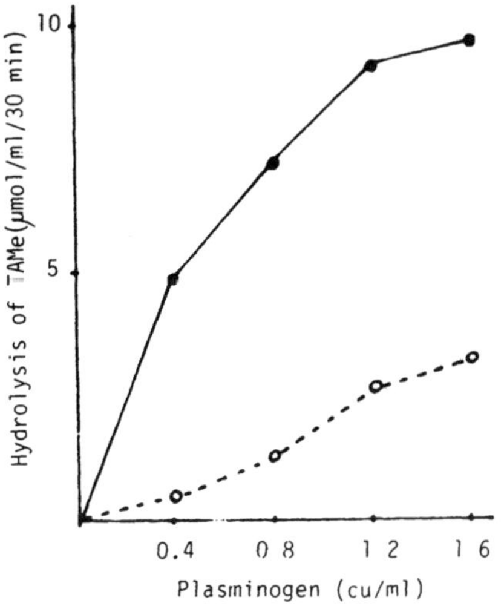

FIG. 1

Hydrolysis of TAMe by SK and various amounts of plasminogen in the presence (●——●) or absence (o------o) of SK-potentiator.

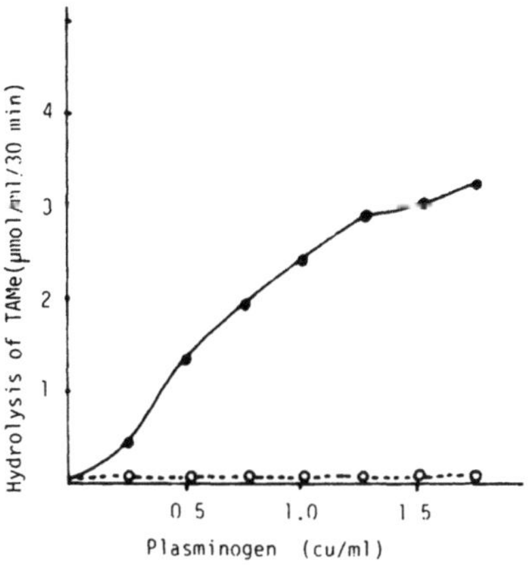

FIG. 2

Hydrolysis of TAMe by plasminogen after preincubation of the equimolar mixture of SK and plasminogen in the presence (●——●) or absence (o----o) of SK-potentiator.

In order to show the enhancement of the activation of plasminogen by the equimolar complex of SK, plasminogen and SK-potentiator, or the complex of SK and plasminogen, 2 ml of SK (200 u) and 2 ml of plasminogen (0.086 cu) were mixed with 2 ml of either SK-potentiator (420 u) or tris buffer. After 5 min incubation at 37°C, 0.3 ml of the mixture was added to 0.2 ml of plasminogen (2 cu/ml) and 0.5 ml of TAMe (10 µmol). Fig. 2 shows that the mixture of SK and plasminogen in the present concentration did not activate plasminogen, but the mixture of SK, plasminogen and SK-potentiator activated plasminogen significantly.

Characterization of SK-potentiator

Fig. 3 shows the results of SDS-polyacrylamide gel electrophoresis (SDS-PAGE) of human fibrinogen and SK-potentiator. There are three bands, α, β, γ chains, on SDS-PAGE of fibrinogen, while SK-potentiator shows two bands corresponding to β and γ chains of fibrinogen. The molecular weight was determined to be about 240,000 (7).

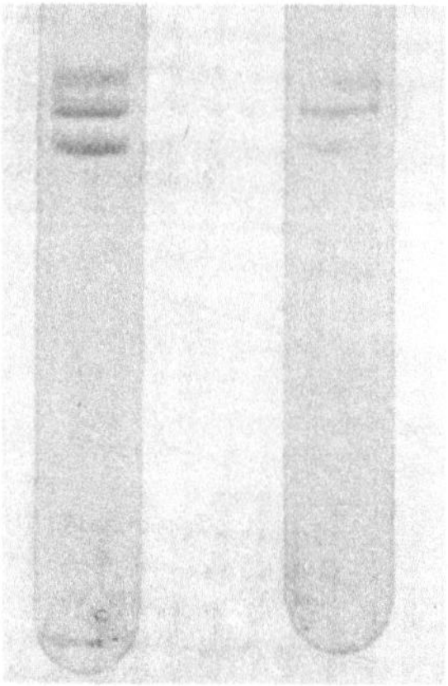

FIG. 3

SDS-PAGE of fibrinogen(left) and SK-potentiator(right).

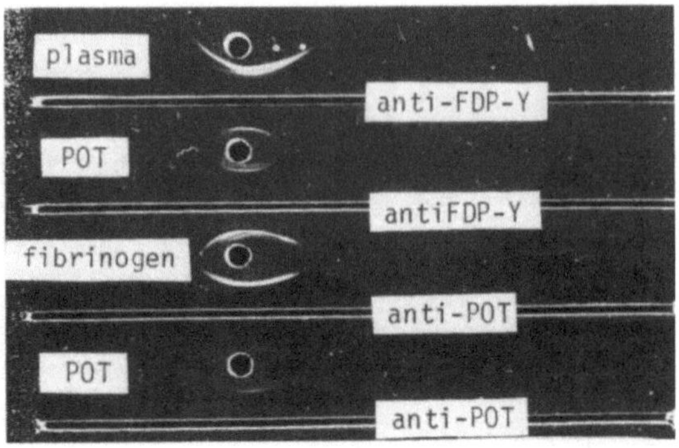

FIG. 4

Immunoelectrophoresis of SK-potentiator in comparison to fibrinogen and plasma.

Each well contains SK-potentiator (POT), fibrinogen or plasma. Each trough contains anti-FDP-Y, or anti SK-potentiator(anti-POT).

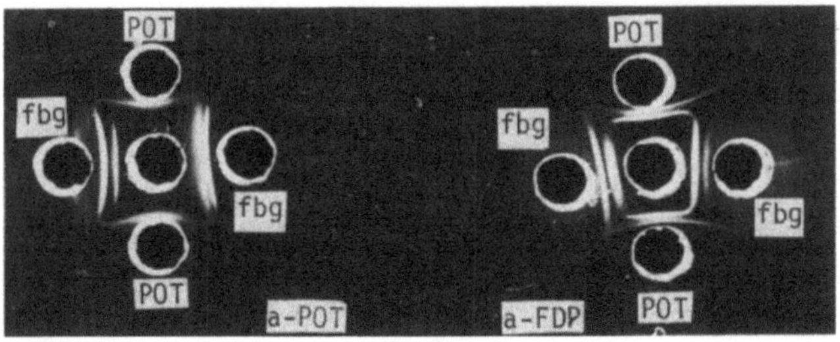

FIG. 5

Immunodiffusion of SK-potentiator (POT) and fibrinogen (fbg). Left center well contains anti-SK-potentiator (a-POT) and right center well contains anti-FDP-Y (a-FDP).

In immunoelectrophoresis (Fig. 4), SK-potentiator crossreacts with anti-FDP-Y at γregion. Fig. 5 shows that anti-SK-potentiator had one precipitin line against SK-potentiator but two lines against fibrinogen, and that anti-FDP-Y has two precipitin lines against both fibrinogen and SK-potentiator. These data show that fibrinogen and SK-potentiator have at least one antigenic determinant not in common, but share one determinant with each other.

Effects of Fibrin(ogen) and SK-potentiator on the Activation of Glu-plg by Various Units of SK

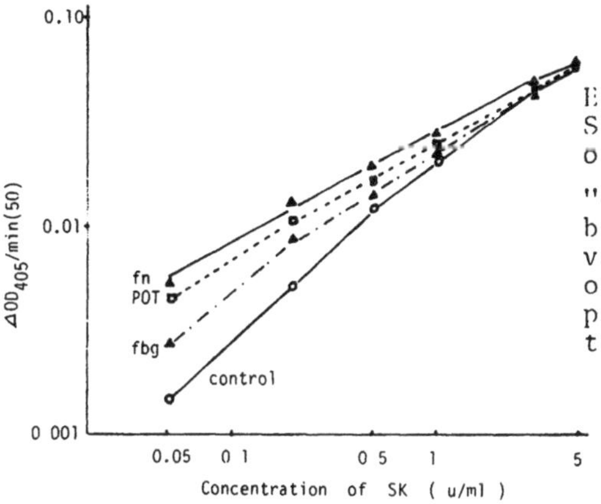

FIG. 6

Effects of fibrin, fibrinogen and SK-potentiator on the activation of Glu-plg by various units of SK.

"control" indicates ΔOD_{405}/min(50) by the mixture of Glu-plg and various units of SK. "fn", "POT" or "fbg" indicates that in the presence of fibrin, SK-potentiator or fibrinogen, respectively.

0.1 µM of Glu-plg was activated by various units of SK in the presence of fibrin, fibrinogen or SK-potentiator, and the hydrolysis of S-2251 was measured. In order to compare activator activities, ΔOD_{405}/min at 50 % hydrolysis (ΔOD_{405}/min(50)), which was constant for some incubation periods was taken. Fig. 6 shows that potentiating effects of these substances were larger at smaller SK units. The presence of SK at larger units than 2.5 u/ml(equimolar to 0.1 µM of Glu-plg) resulted in little enhancement of the activator activity formed by SK, Glu-plg and potentiating substances.

Effects of Fibrin, Fibrino and Their Degradation Products on SK-activation of Glu-plg

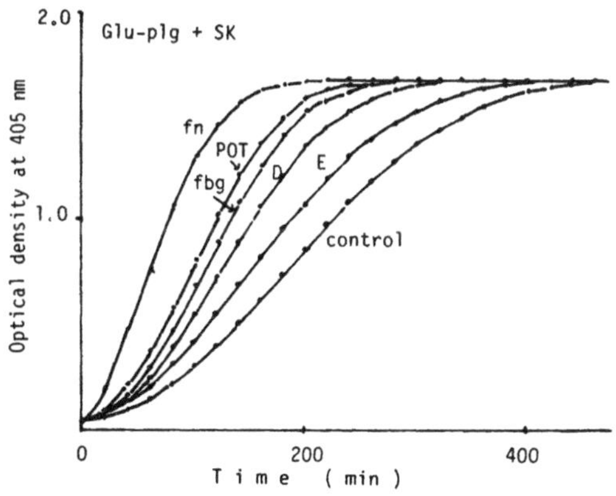

FIG. 7

Effects of fibrin, fibrinogen and their degradation products on the activation of Glu-plg by SK.

"control" indicates the hydrolysis of S-2251 by the mixture of Glu-plg and SK. Other lines indicate that in the presence of fibrin(fn), SK-potentiator(POT), fibrinogen(fbg), fragment D(D), and fragment E(E), respectively.

Fig. 7 shows the results of experiments in which 0.1 μM of Glu-plg was activated by 0.5 u/ml of SK in the presence of 0.1 μM of fibrin, fibrinogen and their degradation products. Enhancing effects of of these agents were in the order of fibrin > SK-potentiator > fibrinogen > D > E.

Effects of the Activation of Plasminogen by UK in the Human Plasma or Clotted Plasma

0.3 ml of human plasma was mixed with 0.1 ml of various units of UK, 0.1 ml of thrombin (50 u/ml) and 0.5 ml of S-2251 (0.36 mM), and incubated for 10 min at 37°C. As controls 0.1 ml of buffer was added instead of thrombin. OD_{405} was measured to know the hydrolysis of S-2251. Fig. 8A shows that more S-2251 was hydrolyzed in the clotted plasma than in the plasma after the activation of plasminogen by UK. Fig. 8B shows the results of experiments in which 0.1 ml of $CaCl_2$ (0.3 M) was used instead of thrombin. Coagulation caused by the addition of $CaCl_2$ resulted in a better activation of plasminogen by UK than in the plasma.

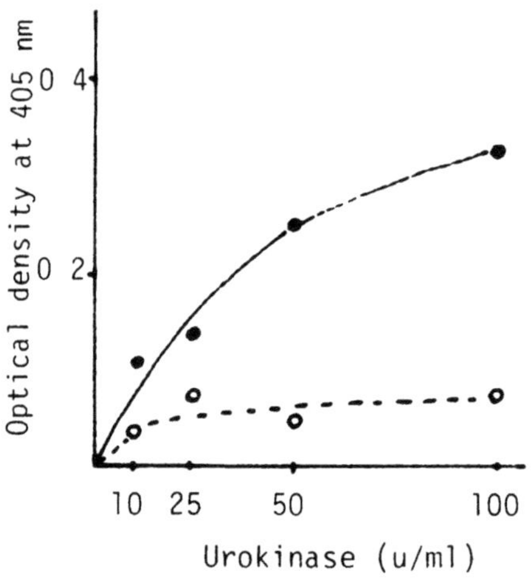

FIG. 8A

Activation of plasminogen by UK in the plasma (o---o) and the clot formed by the addition of thrombin (●—●).

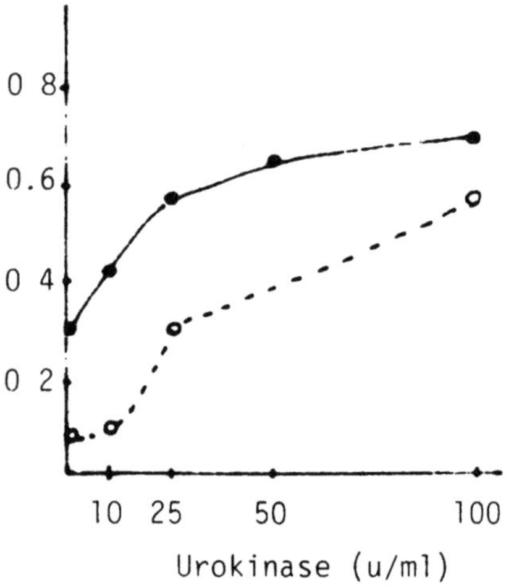

FIG. 8B

Activation of plasminogen by UK in the plasma (o---o) and the clot formed by the addition of $CaCl_2$ (●—●).

Effects of Fibrinogen and Fibrin on the Activation of Glu-plg by UK

0.1 ml of Glu-plg (1 μM) was mixed with 0.1 ml of UK(1,000 u/ml), 0.1 ml of fibrinogen (3 μM) and 0.1 ml of human thrombin(10 u/ml) in the presence of 100 μg of S-2251 (total volume: 1 ml) and the mixture was incubated for various time intervals, then 1.5 ml of 50 % acetic acid solution was added to stop the reaction before OD_{405} was measured. Fig. 9 shows that Glu-plg was far better activated by UK in the presence of fibrin than fibrinogen, although the latter still enhanced its activation to less extent.

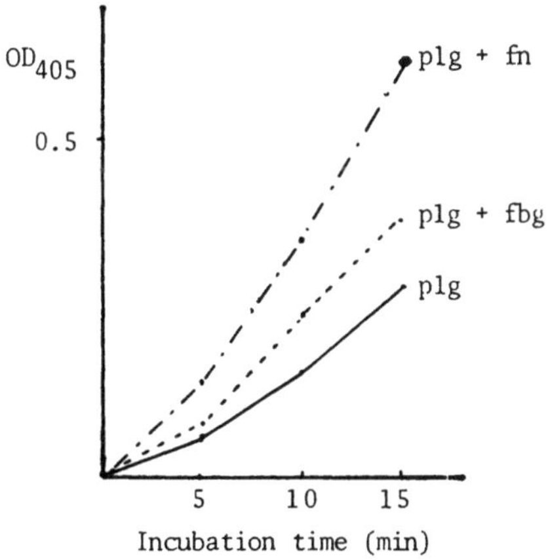

FIG. 9
Effects of fibrin and fibrinogen on the activation of Glu-plg by UK.
"plg" indicates the hydrolysis of S-2251 by the mixture of Glu-plg and UK, and "plg + fn" or "plg + fbg" indicates that in the presence of fibrin or fibrinogen, respectively.

Effects of Various Concentration of Fibrinogen or Fibrin on the Activation of Glu-plg by UK

0.1 μM of Glu-plg was activated by 1 u/ml of UK in the presence of various concentration of fibrinogen. Figs. 10 A and 10B show that increase in the concentration to 0.4 μM (4 times more than Glu-plg) resulted in increase in the extent and the rate (ΔOD_{405} per min) of the hydrolysis of S-2251. Further increase in the concentration of fibrinogen resulted in no or less increase in the hydrolysis of S-2251.

Figs. 11A and 11B show that increase in the extent and rate of the hydrolysis of S-2251 after Glu-plg(0.1 μM) was activated by 1 u/ml of UK in the presence of various concentration of fibrin. Increase

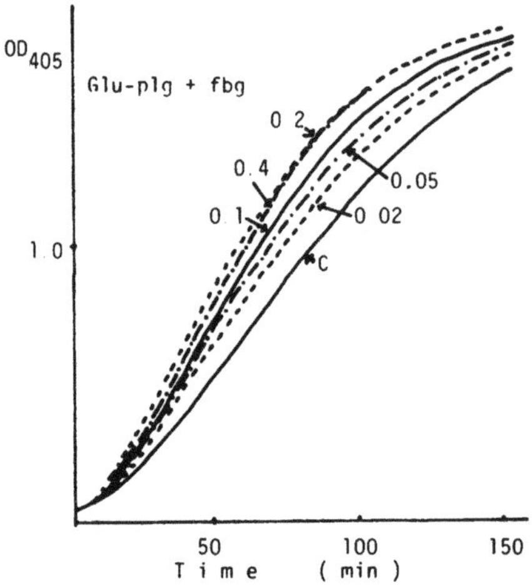

FIG. 10A

Effects of various concentration of fibrinogen on the activation of Glu-plg by UK.

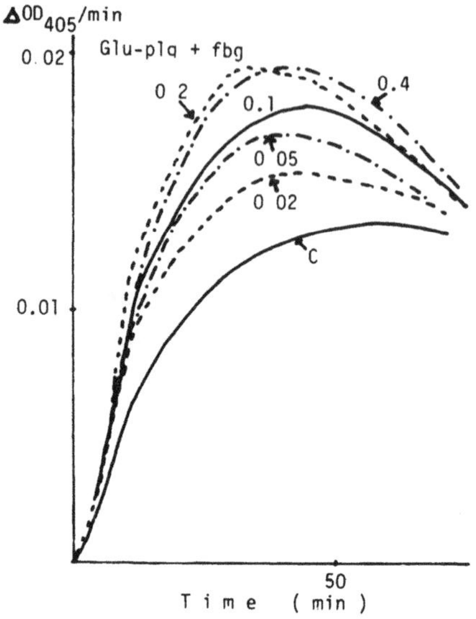

FIG. 10B

Increase in the hydrolysis of S-2251 per min($\triangle OD_{405}$/min) at various incubation times.

Numbers in these figures indicate the concentration of fibrinogen (μM).

in the concentration of fibrin resulted in increase in the rate of S-2251 hydrolysis.

Fig. 12 compares the effects of fibrinogen and fibrin on the enhancement of the activation of Glu-plg by UK. We compared the peak values of $\triangle OD_{405}$/min. $\triangle OD_{405}$/min in the presence of fibrinogen or fibrin was divided by $\triangle OD_{405}$/min in their absence to know the ratio of the increase.

Fig. 13 shows the results of experiments in which 0.1 μM of Lys-plg was activated by 1 u/ml of UK in the presence of fibrinogen and fibrin, or in their absence. In contrast to the results of Glu-plg the activation of Lys-plg by UK was hardly influenced by the presence or absence of fibrinogen or fibrin.

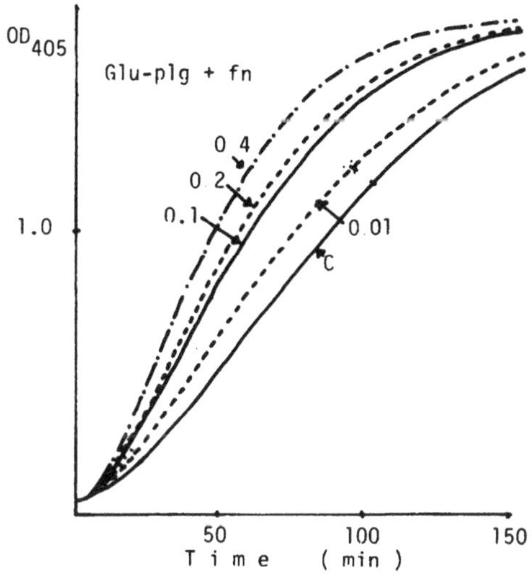

FIG. 11A

Effects of various concentration of fibrin on the activation of Glu-plg by UK.

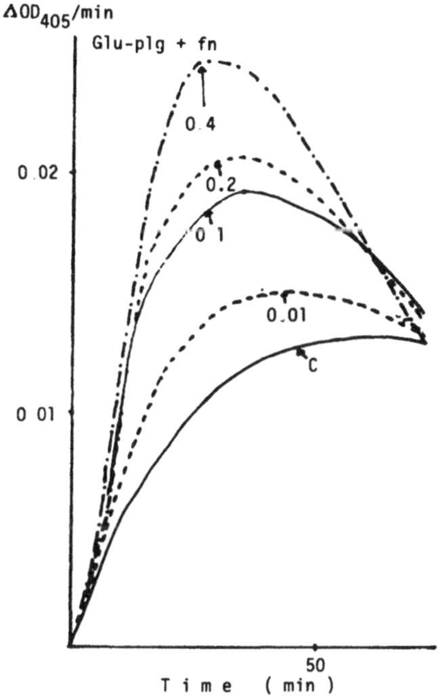

FIG. 11B

Increase in the hydrolysis of S-2251 per min(ΔOD_{405}/min) at various incubation times.

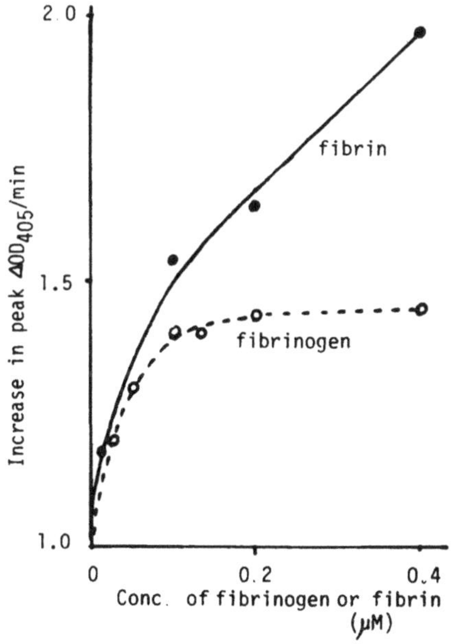

FIG. 12

Effects of various concentration of fibrin or fibrinogen on the enhancement of the activation of the activation of Glu-plg by UK.

Ordinate indicates increase in peak ΔOD_{405}/min, which is the peak value of ΔOD_{405}/min in the presence of fibrin or fibrinogen divided by that in their absence.

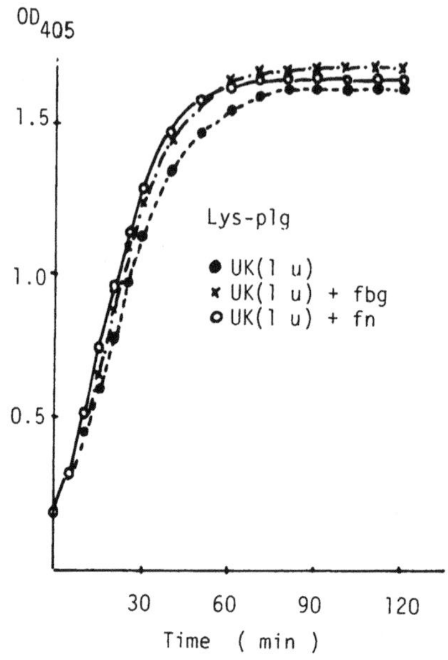

FIG. 13
Time course of the hydrolysis of S-2251 by the mixture of Lys-plg and UK in the presence of fibrinogen(fbg) or fibrin(fn).

Discussion

As stated in Introduction, roles of fibrin in the activation of the fibrinolysis system have lately been studied extensively. In the past, the participation of fibrin or its degradation products has been very controversial. As to the activation of plasminogen by SK, Müllertz and Lassen (11) proposed a scheme in which proactivator in human plasma was activated by SK and converted to activator which activates plasminogen of all animal species. After searching for the proactivator it was concluded that proactivator was plasmin itself (12). It is now well established that SK forms an equimolar complex with human plasminogen or plasmin, which activates plasminogen of all animal species (13). In 1970, we have reported that there is a factor in human plasma which potentiates the activation of plasminogen by SK (4, 5) and is called SK-activatable proactivator. The factor turned out to be early degradation products of fibrinogen (7), renamed as SK-potentiator. Fig. 2 shows that SK-plasminogen complex in the presence of SK-potentiator activated plasminogen significantly whereas SK-plasminogen complex did not activate plasminogen in its absence. Since SK-potentiator did not enhance the activator activity of SK-plasminogen complex once SK-plasminogen (or -plasmin) complex was formed, the mechanisms of the potentiation by SK-potentiator appears to be the formation of a trimolecular complex between SK, plasminogen and SK-potentiator. It was suggested that a binding site of SK-potentiator on SK-plasminogen complex was not the lysine binding sites(LBS) but the other site not interfered by tranexamic acid (14). We, therefore, concluded that a trimolecular complex between SK, plasminogen and SK-potentiator is a better activator than a dimolecular complex. Comparison of various fibrinogen degradation products indicates that effectiveness of the enhancement was in the order of fibrin $>$ SK-potentiator $>$ fibrinogen $>$ D $>$ E (Fig. 7). Since fibrinogen preparation used is contaminated with a partially degraded fragment of fibrinogen (especially with its α chain degraded), enhancing effects of this fibrinogen may be larger than native fibrinogen without any degradation.

Effects of fibrin or its degradation products on the activation of plasminogen by UK have also been controversial. There have been many reports (1, 2) indicating that the activation of plasminogen by t-PA is significantly enhanced in the presence of fibrin but that its activation by UK is not influenced in the presence of fibrin. As indicated in Fig. 8A, the addition of UK and thrombin to the plasma in the presence of S-2251 resulted in the larger extent of the hydrolysis of S-2251 than the addtion of UK to the plasma did, indicating that Glu-plg was activated better in the presence of fibrin than fibrinogen. Using enzyme immunoassay of FDP, we indicated that fibrin was degraded faster by UK in the clotted plasma than in the plasma (15). These observations may be explained by the fact that Glu-plg was activated better by UK in the presence of fibrin and that $\alpha_2$antiplasmin (α_2AP) did not inhibit plasmin effectively in the presence of fibrin (16, 17). Figs. 9, 10 and 11 show that purified Glu-plg was activated better by UK in the presence of fibrin than fibrinogen, the latter being able to enhance the activation to less extent. On the other hand, the activation rate of Lys-plg was not influenced much in the presence of fibrinogen or fibrin (Fig. 13).

It is well established that Glu-plg changed its conformation upon the interaction of its LBS with lysine analogues, but that Lys-plg did not change the conformation (18, 19). It was also shown that conformationally altered Glu-plg was more easily activated by activators than a native Glu-plg (18, 19). Since fibrin was shown to bind with LBS (20), it is possible that the enhanced activation of Glu-plg in the plasma or purified system may be due to the interaction of Glu-plg with fibrin and its conformational changes.

Recently Müllertz et al (21) and Thorsen et al (22) indicated that the form of plasminogen in the plasma was Glu-form, and that it was activated by activators to Glu-plasmin in the plasma. In the clotted plasma, more easily activatable Lys-form was formed by plasmin. Lys-forms were shown to be largely bound on fibrin. Suenson et al (23) indicated that initial plasmin-degradation of fibrin resulted in the exposure of a high affinity binding site for Glu-plg. Finally, Lijnen et al (24) showed that cyanogen-bromide digested fibrinogen enhanced the activation of Glu-plg by UK. These observations seem to indicate followings. Small amounts of Glu-plg bound with fibrin resulted in the conformational changes and the better activation by UK, and the resulting Glu-plasmin degraded fibrin to some extent, exposing the high affinity site for Glu-plg on fibrin. Glu-plg now bound with fibrin effectively, and changed conformations and activatability. Plasmin thus formed not only lyzed fibrin but also released N-terminal peptides from Glu-plg bound with fibrin. Such conversion of Glu-plg to Lys-plg further accelerated fibrinolysis. These hypotheses solved a long lasting puzzle why Glu-plg with a very low affinity for fibrin could be activated better in the presence of fibrin.

In conclusion, Glu-plg in the plasma or purified system was far better activated by UK or SK in the presence of fibrin. Mechanisms of the enhancement may be different between those of SK- and UK-activations of Glu-plg.

References

1. Wallen, P. 1978. In: Progress in Chemical Fibrinolysis and Thrombolysis, Vol. 3(J.F. Davidson, R.M. Rowan, M. Samama and P.C. Desnoyers, eds.) Raven Press, New York. pp. 167-181.

2. Hoylaerts, M., Rijken, D.C., Lijnen, H.R. and Collen, D. 1982. J. Biol. Chem. 257, 2912-2919.

3. Gurewich, V., Pannel, R., Louie, S., Kelly, P., Suddith, R.L. and Greenlee, R. 1984. J. Clin. Invest. 73, 1731-1739.

4. Takada, A., Takada, Y. and Ambrus, J.L. 1970. J. Biol. Chem. 245, 6389-6396.

5. Takada, A., Takada, Y. and Ambrus, J.L. 1972. Biochim. Biophys. Acta 263, 610-618.

6. Takada, A. and Takada, Y. 1978. Thrombos. Res. 13, 325-335.

7. Takada, A., Mochizuki, K. and Takada, Y. 1980. Thrombos. Res. 19, 485-492.

8. Takada, A., Urano, T. and Takada, Y. 1979. Thrombos. Haemostas. 42, 901-908.

9. Takada, A. and Takada, Y. 1980. Thrombos. Res. 18, 167-176.

10. Roberts, P.S. 1958. J. Biol. Chem. 232, 285-291.

11. Müllertz, S. and Lassen, M. 1953. Proc. Soc. Exp. Biol. Med. 82, 264-268.

12. Kline, D.L. and Fishman, J.B. 1961. 236, 2807-2812.

13. Castellino, F.J. 1981. Chemical Reviews 81, 431-446.

14. Smith, J.H., Morris, J.P., Chibber, B.A. and Castellino, F.J. 1984. Thrombos. Res. 34, 499-506.

15. Urano, T., Takada, Y. and Takada, A. 1984. Thrombos. Res. 36, 429-435.

16. Wiman, B. and Collen, D. 1978. Nature 272, 549-550.

17. Takada, A., Ito, T. and Takada, Y. 1980. Thrombos. Haemostas. 43, 20-23.

18. Violand, B.N., Byrne, R. and Castellino, F.J. 1978. J. Biol. Chem. 253, 5395-5401.

19. Markus, G., Priore, R.L. and Wissler, F.C. 1979. J. Biol. Chem. 254, 1211-1216.

20. Váli, Z. and Patthy, L. 1984. J. Biol. Chem. 259, 13690-13694.

21. Müllertz, S., Thorsen, S. and Sottrup-Jensen, L. 1984. Biochem. J. 223, 169-177.

22. Thorsen, S., Müllertz, S., Suenson, E. and Kok, P. 1984. Biochem. J.223, 179-187.

23. Suenson, E., Lutzen, O. and Thorsen S. 1984. Eur. J. Biochem. 140, 513-522.

24. Lijnen, H.R., Van Hoef, B. and Collen, D. 1984. Eur.J.Biochem. 144, 541-544.

V. Interactions with Cells

THE ROLE OF FIBRINOGEN IN PLATELET AGGREGATION

G. Marguerie
INSERM U 217, Centre d'Etude Nucléaire, Grenoble, France

M.H. Ginsberg, E.F. Plow
Research Institute of Scripps Clinic, La Jolla, CA 92037, U.S.A.

Introduction

Formation of efficient plugs at sites of injury of a vessel wall is contingent upon modification of the adhesive properties of the membrane of platelets. These alterations are generally accomplished via a multi step mechanism encompassing: 1) adhesion and spreading of the cells to the subendothelium matrix; 2) activation of the platelet by specific agonists; and 3) interaction of the activated platelet with cofactors which modify the adhesive properties of the cell to form aggregates. A number of biochemical events have been associated with this phenomenon. This includes calcium distribution, prostaglandin synthesis, actin polymerization, microtubules disassembly, and changes in adenylate cyclase activity. While these reactions have been identified their sequence and interrelationship in the transition reaction between a circulating and an aggregating platelet have yet to be delineated. It is well established, however, that a specific stimulus and an exogenous cofactor with adhesive properties are necessary for aggregation to occur. Early studies on patients with congenital afibrinogenemia have provided evidence that fibrinogen fulfills the role of essential cofactor in this reaction. Platelets from these patients fail to aggregate or aggregate weakly in response to ADP or epinephrine and normal aggregation is restored upon addition of fibrinogen in the plasma of these patients. These observations have been confirmed for many years but the molecular basis for the participation of fibrinogen in platelet aggregation was uncertain. Over the past years the bulk of information which has been obtained now clearly establishes that the cofactor function of fibrinogen involves

Fibrinogen - Fibrin Formation and Fibrinolysis, Vol. 4
© 1986 Walter de Gruyter & Co., Berlin · New York - Printed in Germany.

specific and inducible receptors for this molecule on the membrane of the platelet.

Interaction of Fibrinogen with Platelet

The essential features for fibrinogen binding to platelet have been characterized. The molecule does not interact with the non stimulated platelet, whereas binding is observed when the cell is challenged with ADP and the binding sites exhibit the characteristics of a receptor system (1-3). The interaction is saturable with respect to both ADP and fibrinogen concentration, divalent ion dependent, specific for the native molecule and occurs in buffer system as well as in a plasma milieu (Table 1) (4). We have established in the past that the binding of fibrinogen to this receptor system is part of a multistep reaction which entails: 1) the initial stimulation of the cell, 2) the induction of the receptor, 3) the binding of fibrinogen and 4) the stabilization of the fibrinogen receptor complex (3).

A large variety of physiologic and pharmacologic stimuli other than ADP support fibrinogen binding. These include collagen, thrombin, epinephrine, platelet aggregating factor (PAF), calcium ionophore, arachidonic acid and prostaglandin derivatives. With all stimuli a single class of receptor is induced on platelet, with an average density of 45,000 ± 10,000 sites per platelet and an affinity constant of 10^6 to 10^7 M^{-1}. Moreover, binding of fibrinogen can be

Table 1. Summary of Parameters for the Interaction of Fibrinogen with Platelet in Buffer and in Plasma

	Buffer	Plasma
Number of sites per platelet	45,000 ± 10,000	32,000 ± 10,000
Affinity constant, Ka (M^{-1})	2×10^6	1.8×10^6
Rate constant of association $k_{on}^{37°C}$ (M^{-1}-min^{-1})	$0,26 \times 10^6$	$0,40 \times 10^6$
Divalent requirement	yes	yes
Stabilization	yes	partial

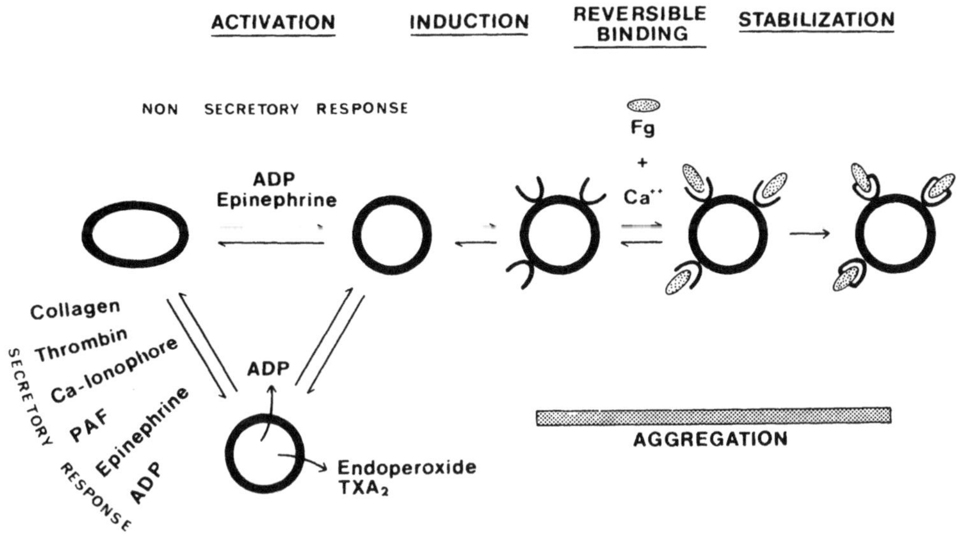

Figure 1. Secretory and Non Secretory Dependent Mechanisms for the Introduction of the Platelet Fibrinogen Receptor

correlated with the platelet aggregatory response to these stimuli. On this basis we have suggested that binding of fibrinogen to the cell is a pathway common to all stimuli for platelet aggregation and can occur via secretory and non secretory dependent reactions (Figure 1). The existence of such a mechanism provides a molecular basis for the role of fibrinogen in platelet function and the regulation of aggregation by this cofactor (5).

Molecular Nature of the Fibrinogen Receptor

Two major surface membrane glycoproteins have been implicated in fibrinogen receptor function. GPIIb has a molecular weight of approximately 136,000 when non reduced and is made up with two disulfide linked subunits (molecular weights 116,000 and 23,000). GP III consists of a single polypeptide chain of Mr = 95,000. These two glycoproteins have now been purified (6) and it was shown that they are associated into a calcium dependent heterodimer in a 1:1 stoichiometry (7). Although direct evidence that these two glycoproteins represent the binding site for fibrinogen has yet to be published, a large body of information suggests that they may participate in the receptor function: 1) Thrombasthenic platelets generally lack both glycoproteins and fail to bind fibrinogen (2, 8); 2) monoclonal and polyclonal antibodies to these glycoproteins inhibit fibrinogen binding (9,10); 3) using monoclonal antibodies 40,000 copies of these glycoproteins can be identified on the membrane of the platelet, a number which accommodates with the number of fibrinogen receptor (11); 4) fibrinogen interacts specifically with the arc of the GPIIb/GPIII complex in a crossimmunoelectrophoresis system (12); and 5) GPIIb/III complex interacts with fibrinogen adsorbed on plastic wells (13).

These observations point to a key role of the GPIIb/III complex in fibrinogen binding. Independently, each of these lines of evidence may be subject to alternative explanation. For instance it has been shown that thrombasthenic platelets also fail to interact with fibronectin and von Willebrand factor (14,15). Thus the defect underlying thrombasthenia may be more complex than a sole absence of the fibrinogen receptor. Monoclonal and polyclonal antibodies may block receptor induction rather than receptor function per se. Nevertheless most of the studies suggest that the complex GPIIb/III rather than the individual glycoproteins functions as the fibrinogen receptor.

Recently photosensitive heterobifunctional reagents were used to crosslink the fibrinogen molecule to the membrane of the stimulated platelet (16,17). One of the advantages of the photoaffinity labelling is that binding can be performed under conditions which preserve the functional integrity of the cell. In our own studies we have used the N-succinimidyl-6-(4'-azido-2'-nitrophenylamino) hexanoate reagent (SANAH) (15). Identification of the membrane component to which fibrinogen was crosslinked was determined by immunoprecipitation of the complex with antibodies specific to membrane glycoproteins. The cocmplex was specifically precipitated by an anti GPIIb/III but not by an anti GPIb. Those studies provided a direct evidence for a proximal relationship between fibrinogen and the GPIIb/III complex. It should be mentioned, however, that such an approach does not identify the receptor per se since the crosslinking reaction may occur between adjacent molecules. Thus it is still premature to exclude a model in which a different membrane component would reside in close proximity with the GPIIb/III complex.

Recognition Sites Within the Fibrinogen Molecule

Two series of observations have first established that the native structure of the fibrinogen molecule is a prerequisite for optimal binding. From aggregation studies it was shown that fragment X from plasmic digests were less potent than fibrinogen in supporting aggregation, whereas fragments Y and D were totally ineffective. Fragment X had a decreased affinity for platelet relative to fibrinogen. Secondly, analysis of the molecule which interacted with platelet indicated that fibrinopeptides A were present, establishing that activation by thrombin was not necessary for fibrinogen-platelet interaction (1).

Further insights to the structural requirement for fibrinogen binding were recently provided by Hawiger and his group and by our laboratories and progress has been made in identifying sites of interaction within the fibrinogen molecule in the past two years.

We have isolated a D fragment of high molecular weight (Mr = 100,000) from a prolonged plasmic digest of fibrinogen in the presence of calcium. This fragment inhibited fibrinogen binding to the platelet, whereas further digestion of this fragment in the absence of calcium, to generate a fragment D of 80,000 molecular weight abolished this inhibition (19). Since the transition between the two fragments results primarily from the proteolysis of the C-terminal part of the chain, this portion of the molecule was thought to be important for interaction with the platelet. Recently in an elegant series of studies, Kloczewiack et al have shown that synthetic peptides from this region were active in inhibiting fibrinogen binding (20). In our studies (21) a dodecapeptide corresponding to the C-terminal sequence of the γ-chain was synthesized and we have confirmed the observations of Koczewiack et al. Thus it is now apparent that the C-terminal part of the γ-chain represents a site which is recognized by the activated platelet.

A second domain within the structure of the molecule may also be implicated in fibrinogen platelet interaction. Hawiger et al have initially indicated that aggregated A α-chain support platelet agglutination (22). In our studies using heterobifunctional reagents we found that the A α-chain was crosslinked to the GPIIb/III complex and that the structural integrity of the C-terminal part of this chain was a requesite for crosslinking (17). Thus the A α-chain may also possess a contact site which is recognized by the activated platelets. This proposal is consistent with the observation that fragment X is a weak cofactor of aggregation and support the concept that fibrinogen is a multivalent molecule which exhibits multiple recognition sites.

Molecular Mechanisms for Platelet Aggregation

Several mechanisms can be hypothesized to understand the role of fibrinogen in the aggregation phenomenon (Figure 2). Since fibrinogen is a dimeric molecule a direct bridging between two adjacent platelets by the molecule can be hypothesized. Alternatively, fibrinogen molecules may self-associate on the surface membrane and generate a fibrin-like bridge between two aggregating platelets. Interaction of fibrinogen may be directly mediated by the GPIIb/III complex which may represent fibrinogen receptor. Models, however, in which binding of fibrinogen is mediated by other membrane associated components cannot be excluded. Interaction of the molecule with receptor in close proximity to the GPIIb/III complex may in fact stimulate the aggregation activity of this complex. At the present time these mechanisms are only speculative and will be discriminated by the isolation of the receptor entity and the study of the direct interactions between fibrinogen and this receptor in a fluid phase system.

Relationship Between the Fibrinogen Receptor and Other Adhesive Proteins

Beside fibrinogen, two other glycoproteins are important for platelet adhesion and spreading: fibronectin and von Willebrand factor.

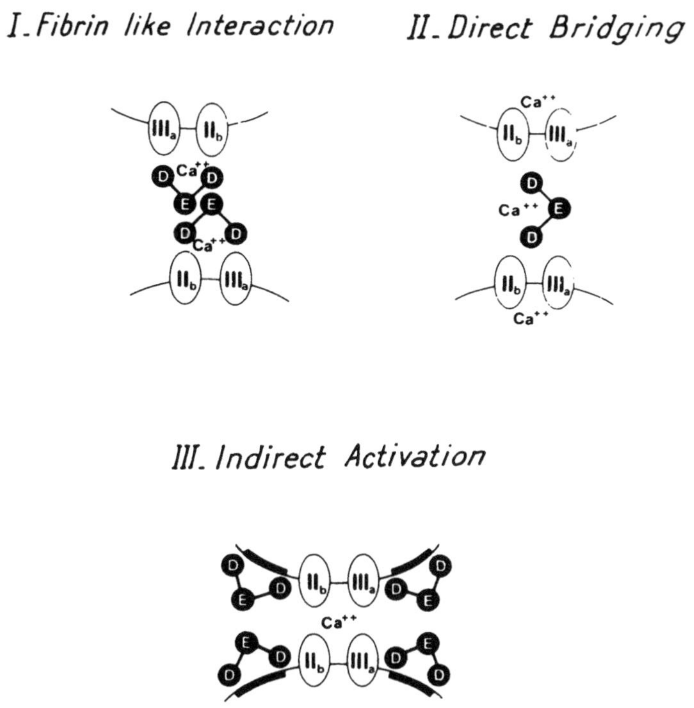

Figure 2. Alternative mechanisms for the participation of fibrinogen in aggregation

I: Direct bridging between two adjacent platelets
II: Self association in a fibrin-like bridge between adjacent platelets
III: Interaction of fibrinogen with receptors in close proximity to GPIIb/III complex and activation of this complex.

Like fibrinogen these two glycoproteins exhibit a multimeric structure, bind calcium and interact with specific receptor sites on the surface of the membrane of activated platelets (23). For the three proteins, binding is calcium dependent and is inhibited by ADP scavengers. The recent observation that thrombasthenic platelets do not interact with fibrinogen (2), fibronectin (24) and von Willebrand factor (25) have raised the possibility that these glycoproteins may interact with the same set of receptor or with inter-related receptors. In our most recent studies we have observed that plasmic degradation fragment D of high molecular weight which inhibit the binding of fibrinogen, also inhibit interaction of von Willebrand factor to thrombin and ADP stimulated platelet (26). In addition synthetic dodecapeptides similar to the C-terminal portion of the γ-chain, which inhibited the binding of fibrinogen, were also potent inhibitors of fibronectin and von Willebrand factor binding (21). Finally, monoclonal antiplatelet antibodies, reacting against GPIIb and GPIII inhibit the binding of all three proteins (27).

Taken together these observations provide evidence that the three adhesive proteins interact with the same recognition site on activated platelets, implying that these glycoproteins share structural features necessary for the recognition of the molecules by the cell. Alternatively this common site may not be the unique receptor for these glycoproteins but rather be a part of a more complex multivalent structure expressing common as well as specific sites. Further studies are required to understand the exact relationship between those glycoproteins on the surface membrane and their respective role in platelet function.

Acknowledgements

These studies were supported by grants INSERM 805029 and NIH HL16411 and NATO 1852.

References

1. Marguerie, G.A., E.F. Plow, T.S. Edgington. 1979. J.Biol. Chem. 254, 5357.
2. Bennett, J.S., G. Vilaire. 1979. J.Clin.Invest. 64, 1393.
3. Marguerie, G.A., T.S. Edgington, E.F.Plow. 1980. J.Biol.Chem. 255, 154.
4. Marguerie, G.A., N. Thomas-Maison, M.J. Larrieu, E.F. Plow. 1982. Blood 59, 91.
5. Marguerie, G.A., E.F. Plow. 1983. Ann.N.Y.Acad.Sci. 408, 556.
6. Jennings, L.S., D.R. Phillips. 1982. J.Biol.Chem. 257, 10458.
7. Fujimura, K., D.R. Phillips. 1983. J.Biol.Chem. 258, 10247.
8. Nurden, A.T., J.P. Caen. 1974. Br.J.Haematol. 28, 233.
9. Coller, B.S., E.I. Peerschke, L.E. Scudder, C.A. Sullivan . 1983. J.Clin.Invest. 72, 278
10. Lee, H., A.T. Nurden, A. Thomaidis, J.P. Caen. 1981. Br.J. Haematol. 48, 47.

11. McEver, R.P., N.L. Baetziger, P.W. Majerus. 1980. J.Clin. Invest. 66, 1311.

12. Gogstad, G.O., F. Brosstad, M.B. Krutnes, L. Hagen, N.O. Solum. 1982. Blood 60, 663.

13. Nachman, R.L., L.L.K. Leung. 1982. J.Clin.Invest. 69, 263.

14. Ginsberg, M.H., J. Forsyth, A. Lightsey, J. Chediak, E.F. Plow. 1983. J.Clin.Invest. 71, 619.

15. Ruggeri, Z.M., R. Bader, L. de Marco. 1982. Proc.Natl.Acad. Sci.U.S.A. 79, 6038.

16. Bennett, J.S., G. Vilaire, D.B. Cines. 1982. J.Biol.Chem. 297, 8049.

17. Marguerie, G.A., N. Thomas-Maison, M. Ginsberg, E.F. Plow. 1984. Eur.J.Biochem. 139, 5.

18. Niewiarowski, S., A.Z. Budzynski, B. Lipinski. 1977. Blood 49, 635.

19. Marguerie, G.A., N. Ardaillou, G. Cherel, E.F. Plow. 1982. J.Biol.Chem. 257, 11872.

20. Kloczeviak, M., S. Timmons, T.J. Lukas, J. Hawiger. 1984. Biochemistry 23, 1767.

21. Plow, E.F., A.H. Srouji, D. Meyer, G.A. Marguerie, M.H. Ginsberg. 1984. J.Biol.Chem. 259, 5388.

22. Hawiger, J., S. Timmons, M. Kloczeviak, D.D. Strong, R.F. Doolittle. 1982. Proc.Natl.Acad.Sci.U.S.A. 79, 2068.

23. Plow, E.F., G. Marguerie, M.H. Ginsberg. 1984. In: The Biology of Platelets (D.K. Philips and M.A. Shuman, eds.), in press.

24. Ginsberg, M.H., J. Forsyth, A. Lightsey, J. Chediak, E.F. Plow. 1983. J.Clin.Invest. 71, 619.

25. Ruggeri, Z.M., R. Bader, L. de Marco. 1982. Proc.Natl.Acad. Sci.U.S.A. 79, 6038.

26. Pietu, G., G. Cherel, G. Marguerie, D. Meyer. 1984. Nature 308, 648.

27. Plow, E.F., E. McEver, B. Coller, V.L. Woods, G. Marguerie, M.H. Ginsberg, in press.

PLATELET-ASSOCIATED FIBRINOGEN : CONFORMATIONAL CHANGE OF FIBRINOGEN INDUCED BY ITS ADSORPTION TO PLATELET-SURFACE.

C. Soria, J. Soria, M. Mirshahi, C. Boucheix, A. Thomaïdis, A. Bernadou, M. Samama, J.P. Caen.
Hôpital Lariboisière, (Services des Professeurs Caen et Rousselet),
Hôtel-Dieu, (Services des Professeurs Bernadou, Fabiani, Samama), Paris, France.

Introduction

It is well recognized that ADP-induced platelet aggregation requires the binding of fibrinogen to a specific platelet membrane receptor (6, 10). The mechanism of aggregation related fibrinogen birding however is not yet known.

Since unstimulated platelets adhere directly to fibrinogen-coated surfaces and since as shown previously fibrinogen undergoes a conformational change subsequent to polystyrene adsorption (12), we were interested to determine whether the configuration of platelet-bound fibrinogen might be different from that of soluble fibrinogen and similar to fibrinogen bound to a synthetic surface. For this purpose, we compared the binding of three different monoclonal antibodies (MCAb) to either fibrinogen in solution or to fibrinogen bound to ADP-stimulated platelets (2, 8, 11).

The first MCAb (DSB) recognizes an epitope present in fragment D and which is also accessible on fibrinogen either immobilized or in solution. The second MCAb (F_1E_1) interacts very strongly with immobilized fibrinogen and fragment D (immobilized or in solution) but very little with fibrinogen in solution. Therefore, it is speculated that the immobilization of fibrinogen leads to the exposure of an epitope which is present on fragment D (immobilized or in solution) but which is partly hidden in the fibrinogen molecule in solution. Therefore, this antibody is suited for the detection of a conformational change in fibrinogen which occurred subsequently to its adsorption on a solid phase (anticonformation MCAb). The third MCAb (F_2C_5) is a D neo MCAb because it interacts only with fragment D and not with fibrinogen (in solution or immobilized). The characteristics of these three MCAb are summarised in Table I.

Fibrinogen - Fibrin Formation and Fibrinolysis, Vol. 4
© 1986 Walter de Gruyter & Co., Berlin · New York - Printed in Germany.

MCAb used	Reactivity of MCAb with epitopes accessible on			
	Fibrinogen		Fragment D	
	in solution	immobilized on polystyrene	in solution	immobilized on polystyrene
antifibrinogen (DSB)	+++	+++	+++	+++
anticonformation (F_1E_1)	±	+++	+++	+++
anti D neo (F_2C_5)	-	-	+++	+++

TABLE I : Characteristics of the 3 MCAb used

Material and methods.

Platelet preparation.

Blood 5,5 volumes was collected on 1 volume ACD solution (318 mM citric acid, 62 mM trisodium citrate and 133 mM glucose) and centrifuged for 10 minutes at 100 g and 20°C in order to obtain platelet rich plasma (PRP). Washed platelets were prepared according to the technique of Patscheke and Worner (9) but without adding heparin to the buffer solution.

Monoclonal antibodies (MCAb) were obtained by immunization of BALB/C mice with cross-linked fibrin degradation products.Hybridization between mouse immune spleen cells and myeloma cells were performed according to the technique of Kohler and Milstein (5) modified by Fazekas de Saint Groth and Scheiddeger (4). Hybridoma supernatants were tested between day 11 and day 13 by immunoenzymological procedure (2, 8, 11). Cells of the selected wells were cloned by limiting dilution. The selected clones were also injected intraperitoneally into mice in order to produce ascitic fluid. Purified Ig were isolated from ascitic fluid according to Boschetti et al (1).

Fibrinogen binding to platelets.

It was assessed at room temperature according to the technique of Marguerie (6, 7) : 1 x 10^9 platelets/ml were incubated with 100 µg/ml of fibrinogen (Kabi lab.) and 10 µM ADP. After 20 minutes incubation 250 ul of the mixture was removed and layered on 1 ml cold sucrose (20% W/V)in albumine tyrode buffer. The tubes were centrifuged at 12,000 g for 2 minutes to separate the free fibrinogen from platelet- bound fibrinogen. After discarding the supernatant, each pellet was reconstituted with 250 µl PBS containing 0.1 % bovine serum albumin (BSA).

Fibrinogen-MCAb interaction.

The capacity of soluble fibrinogen, fragment D or platelet-bound fibrinogen to inhibit the binding of the three different MCAbs to fragment D-coated plates was determined as already described elsewhere (2, 8, 11). For these assays, purified Ig MCAb were used. Optimal dilution was determined previously by testing serial dilutions of purified Ig solution on fragment D coated plates. The dilution choosen was that which gave 90 % of maximal binding.

A two step procedure was carried out :

- First step : serial dilutions of fibrinogen in PBS containing 0.1% BSA or suspension of ADP-treated platelets previously incubated with fibrinogen were incubated for 2 hours at room temperature with each of the three different MCAb. Then, after centrifugation tween 20 was added to the supernatant in order to obtain 0.05 % tween 20 (preincubation mixture).

- Second step : 100 µl of each preincubation mixture were added to fragment D-coated wells (fibrinogen coated plates were used for some experiment). After 1 hour incubation at 37°C, the plates were washed 4 times. The quantity of mouse Ig bound to the plates was then determined using a peroxidase-labeled Ig anti mouse Ig. After washing the amount of immune peroxidase bound to each well was measured by adding to each well orthophenylene diamine and perhydrol. The colour development was stopped after 3 minutes by adding sulfuric acid and absorbance was recorded at 492 nm using an Elisa autoreader.

Results (figure 1)

Fibrinogen in solution prevented the binding of DSB MCAb (antifibrinogen) to fragment-D coated wells. A linear dose response curve exists between concentration of fibrinogen (log scale) and the decrease in Ig binding to fragment D-coated well (optical density OD). The amount of fibrinogen present in the suspension of ADP-stimulated platelet subsequent to fibrinogen incubation, was 12 µg/ml.

Neither fibrinogen in solution nor platelets bound fibrinogen inhibited the binding of D neo MCAb (F_2C_5) to fragment D coated plates.

Fibrinogen in solution prevented very poorly the binding of anticonformation MCAb (F_1E_1) to either fragment D-coated plates or fibrinogen-coated plates : (up to 25 µg/ml fibrinogen in solution is unable to prevent any binding). Fragment D in solution, however, even at very low concentration was able to inhibit the binding of this MCAb to either fibrinogen or fragment D-coated plates. The anticonformational MCAb reacted similarly with either 12 µg/ml of fibrinogen bound to the stimulated platelets (as calculated using DSBMCAb) or with 350 µg/ml of fibrinogen in solution.

Discussion

This study was undertaken in order to explore the functional role of fibrinogen in ADP-induced platelet aggregation. Due to the facts that platelets adhere to fibrinogen-coated surface and fibrinogen conformation is modified after its absorption to polystyrene, we analyzed in the present work, the conformational change of fibrinogen which bound to platelets. For this purpose we analyzed the capacity of platelet bound-fibrinogen to interact with a MCAb which reacts very poorly with fibrinogen in solution but which reacts very strongly with polystyrene bound-fibrinogen. It is speculated that the binding of fibrinogen to polystyrene yields an epitope which becomes accessible and which is already exposed on fragment D (immobilized or in solution) but which is poorly exposed in undegraded fibrinogen in solution. Therefore, the three MCAb used allows to detect a conformational change in fibrinogen which is induced by its absorption to a solid phase. Using an anti

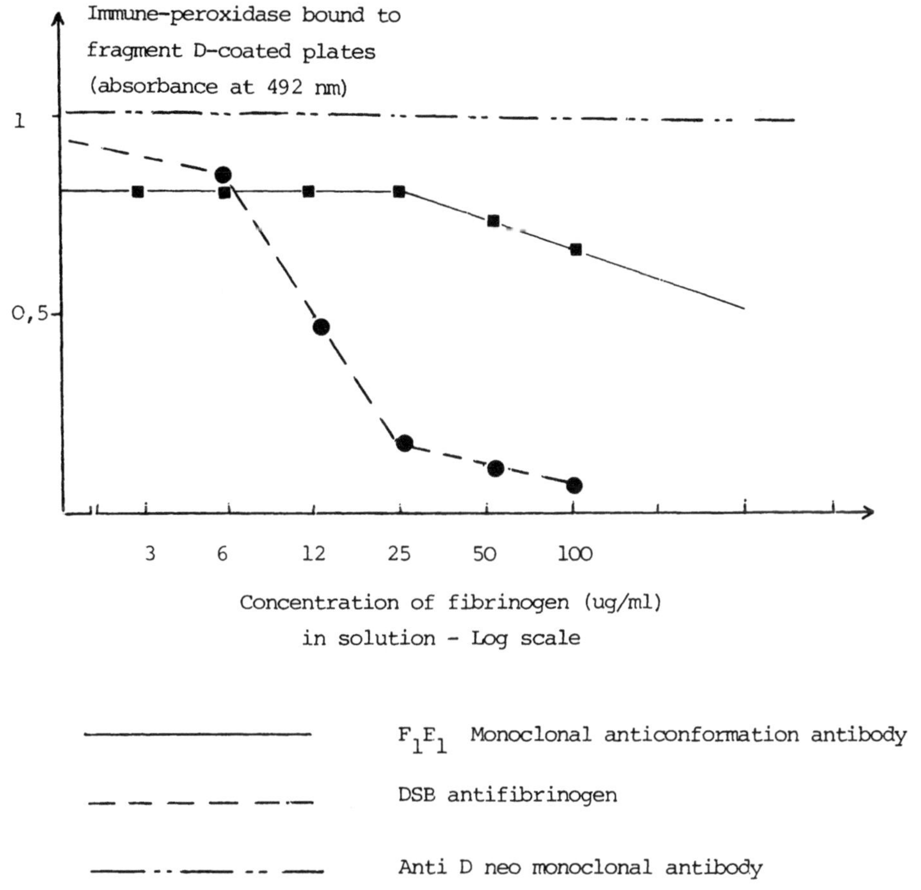

Figure 1 : Competitive inhibition of the binding of 3 different monoclonal antibodies to fragment D-coated plates, by fibrinogen in solution.

D neo MCAb we have checked that platelet bound fibrinogen was not degraded in our experimental conditions. This control was important because the anti-conformation MCAb interacts with fragment D. We have found that after centrifugation, 12 µg fibrinogen remained bound to 1 ml of suspension of platelets previously activated by ADP and incubated in the presence of fibrinogen in excess. This amount of fibrinogen which bound to platelets reacted similarly with anticonformational MCAb as 350 µg/ml of fibrinogen in solution. Therefore, as shown previously with fibrinogen immobilized to polystyrene, it is demonstrated that a conformational change of fibrinogen also occurs when it binds to the platelet surface. Further work however will be necessary to determine if this conformational change is essential for ADP induced-platelet aggregation.

References

1. Boschetti, E., Corthier, G., Monsigny, M. : 1982. An improved chromatography method for the purification of IgG and monoclonal antibodies. Special FEBS meeting on cell function and differentiation. Athenes. Abst. 146.

2. Boucheix, C., Mirshahi, M., Soria, J., Soria, C., Perrot, J.Y., Bernadou, A., Rosenfeld, C. 1982. Monoclonal antibodies for domains which are differentially exposed in fibrinogen, fibrinogen degradation products or fibrin degradation products. Protides of Biological fluid. (H. Peeter Editor). Pergamon Press. 30 : 399-452.

3. Fair, D.S., Edgington, T.S., Plow, E.F. 1981. Immunochemical mapping of the conformation of human fibrinogen. The 95-264 segments is sequestered in native fibrinogen but progressively exposed by plasmic cleavage. J. Biol. Chem., 256 : 8018-8023.

4. Fazekas de Saint Groth, S., Scheidegger, D. : Production of monoclonal antibodies : strategy and tactis. J. Immunol. Meth., 35 : 1-21.

5. Kohler, G., Milstein, C. 1975. Continuous cultures of fused cells secreting antibody of predefined specificity. Nature, 256 : 495-497.

6. Marguerie, G.A., Edgington, T.S., Plow, E.G., 1980. Interaction of fibrinogen with its platelets receptor as part of a multistep reaction in ADP-induced platelet aggregation. J. Biol. Chem., 255 : 154-161.

7. Marguerie, G.A., Plow, E.F., Edgington, T.S. 1979. Human platelets possess an inducible and saturable receptor specific for fibrinogen. J. Biol. Chem., 254 : 5357-5363.

8. Mirshahi, M., Soria, J., Soria, C., Boucheix, C., Perrot, J.Y., Niewenhuizen, W., Haverkate, F., Bernadou, A., Samama, M., Rosenfeld, C. 1983. Characterization of differently expressed epitopes in fibrinogen, fibrinogen degradation products and fibrin degradation products using monoclonal antibodies. Thromb. Haemostasis, 50 : 3 (abstract).

9. Patscheke, H., Worner, P. 1978. Platelet activation detected by turbidimetric shape change analysis. Thromb. Research, 12 : 485-496.

10. Peerschke, E.L., Zucker, M.B., Grant, R.A., Egan, J.J., Johnson, M.M. 1980. Correlation between fibrinogen binding to human platelets and platelet aggregability. Blood, 55 : 841-847.

11. Soria, J., Soria, C., Boucheix, C., Mirshahi, M., Perrot, J.Y., Bernadou A., Samama, M. 1983. Immunochemical differentiation of fibrinogen, fragment D or E and cross linked fibrin degradation produts using monoclonal antibodies. Fibrinogen, functional aspects and metabolism (Editors : Haverkate. Henschen. Niewenhuizen and Straub). Walter de Gruyter. Berlin. New-York. 2 : 227-233.

12 Soria, J., Soria, C., Mirshahi, M., Boucheix, C., Aurengo, A., Perrot, J.Y., Bernadou, A., Samama, M., Rosenfeld, C. : Conformational change in fibrinogen induced by adsorption to a surface. Journal of Colloid and Interface Science. In press.

MIGRATION OF CULTURED ENDOTHELIAL CELLS IN RESPONSE TO FIBRINOGEN

E. Dejana, L.R. Languino, S. Colella, A. Erroi, A. Mantovani

Istituo di Ricerche Farmacologiche Mario Negri, via Eritrea 62, 20157 Milano, Italy

G. Marguerie

Institut de Pathologie Cellulaire, Institut National de la Sante et de la Recherche Medicale, U143, Hopital de Bicetre, 94270 Le Kremlin Bicetre, France.

Luk Maes

Faculty of Medicine, V.U.B. Brussels, Belgium.

Introduction

Endothelial cells (EC) migration and proliferation are fundamental processes for vessel wall repair at sites of injury and tumors neovascularization. It has been suggested that fibrinogen (fg) or its physiological derivatives influence the motility and growth of EC (1-5); however, direct evidence supporting this concept are still lacking. We have recently reported that fg can specifically associate to EC (6). The association to the cells appears to be specific, time dependent and saturable with respect to time and fibrinogen concentration. We have also shown, using a modification of the Boyden chamber technique, that fg interaction with EC enhances the motility of these cells *in vitro* (6). In this study we report data on the specificity and the structural requirement of the fg molecule in inducing EC migration.

Results and Discussion

We studied the effect of fg on EC migration in a Boyden chamber.

Fibrinogen - Fibrin Formation and Fibrinolysis, Vol. 4
© 1986 Walter de Gruyter & Co., Berlin · New York - Printed in Germany.

This technique and its application to cultured EC has been already described in details (6). The experiments reported were made using bovine aortic EC; similar results were obtained using human umbilical vein EC. As shown in fig. 1 EC were seeded in the upper well of the chamber.

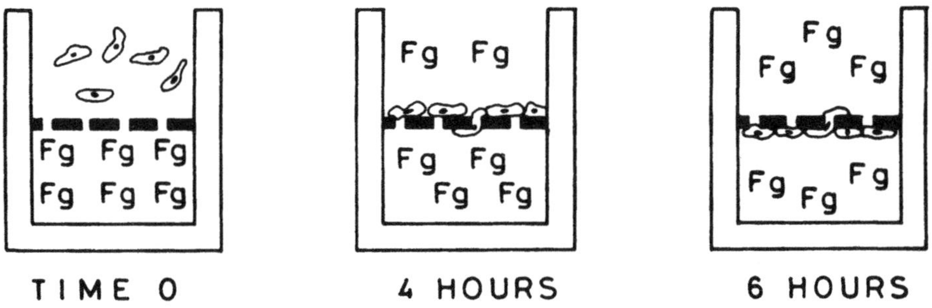

Figure 1
Schematic drawing of a Boyden chamber. At time 0 EC in suspension were seeded in the upper compartment of the assay chamber. Fg was added in the lower compartment. At 4h and 6h the cells adhere to the filter and migrate from the upper to the lower compartment.

Highly purified human fg or other substances being tested for chemotactic activity were placed into the lower compartment of the chamber. The upper and the lower compartments were separated by a polycarbonate filter with 5 µm pores. As represented in fig. 1 and described previously (6), EC adhere to the upper part of the filter and migrate through the pores toward the concentration gradient of the chemotactic agent. Fig. 2 is a scanning electron micrograph of the cells passing through the pores of the filter.

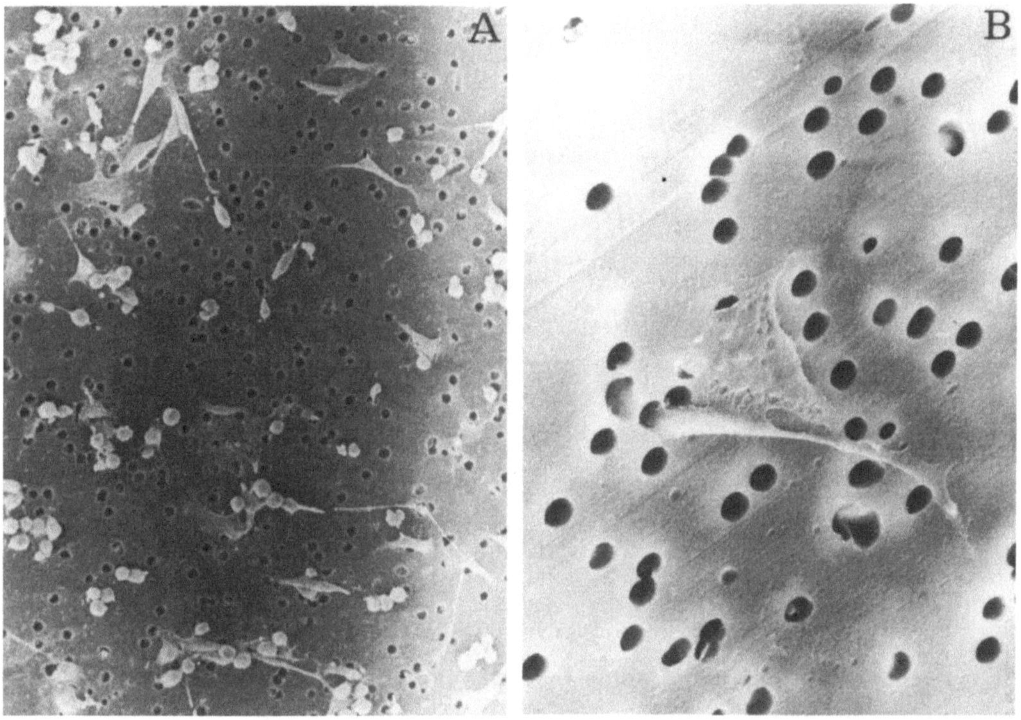

Figure 2

Scanning electron micrographs of EC migrating through the pores in response to fg (1000 µg/ml). A) magnification x 300; B) magnification x 1300.

Fg, added to the lower compartment, induced EC migration in a concentration dependent way as shown in Fig. 3. Migration of EC was very low in absence of fg, it became significantly ($p < 0.01$ Duncan's test) detectable at 40 µg/ml fg and increased raising the fg concentration to 1000 µg/ml fg.

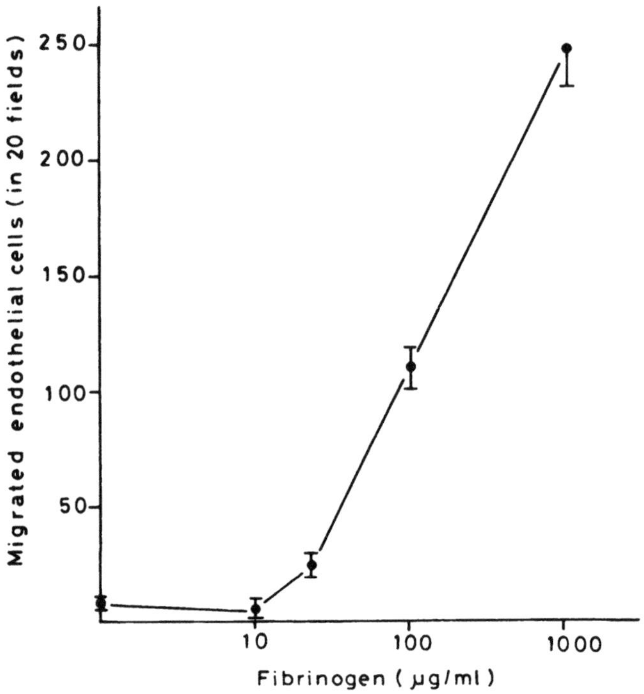

Figure 3

Effect of increasing fg concentration on EC migration. At 6h of incubation the cells adhering to the lower surface of the filter were stained and counted, as described previously in details (6).

As reported previously (6) the concentration gradient of fg between the two chambers was annulled in about 6h, the number of migrated cells increased with time and reached a plateau in the same period. Conditions routinely used for assays included 1000 µg/ml fg with 6h incubation. To investigate whether the induction of migration was in fact attributable to fg and not to possible degradation products of this molecule we used different approaches. As shown in fig. 4, when fg was dialyzed, the same chemotactic effect was observed, thus excluding the contribution of contaminating small active peptides.

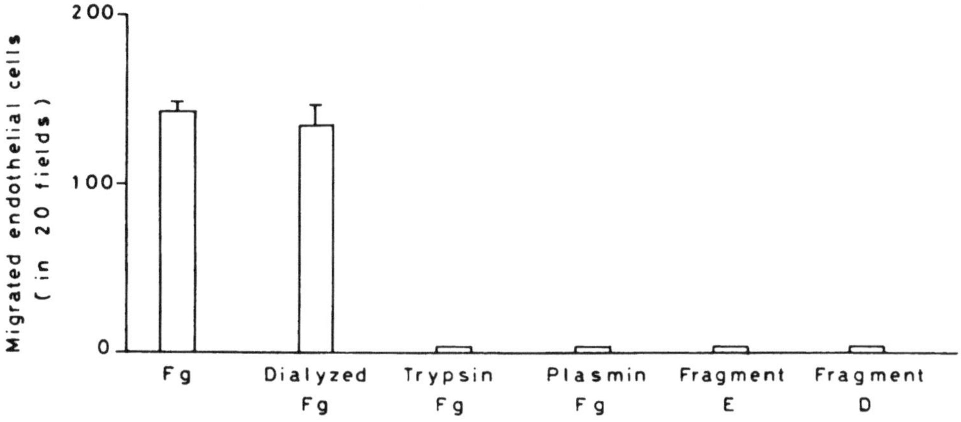

Figure 4
Effect of dialysis, trypsin and plasmin treatment of fg and of purified fragments E and D (both used at final concentration of 2.000 µg/ml) on EC migration. Fg treatments and fragment E and D purification were performed as described (10).

Overnight trypsin or plasmin digestion of fg completely abolished this effect. Purified plasmin derived fragments E (50.000 M.W.) and D (100.000 M.W.), corresponding respectively to the amino and carbossiterminal part of the molecule, did not induce migration. These results indicate that the native molecule of fg is required to induce EC migration. Large and small peptides derived from fg digestion did not appear to play a major role in this activity.

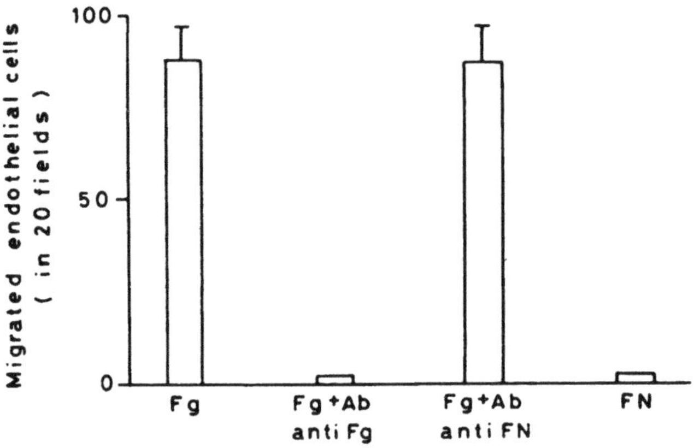

Figure 5

Effect of anti fg and anti FN antibodies on fg induced EC migration. FN alone was tested at 300 μg/ml.

The fg preparation, used in this study, contained less than 0.5 μg/mg of contaminating fibronectin (FN), as tested by double antibody radioimmunoassay (7). This plasma protein, however, is known to be associated to EC matrix and it has been reported to induce EC migration (8). In order to investigate whether contaminating FN might play a role in inducing EC migration, we tested a highly purified FN preparation (9) in our system. As shown in fig. 5 FN was completely ineffective in promoting EC migration.

In the figure 5 we report the data obtained with 300 μg/ml of FN but the same results were obtained in a range of concentration from 5 to 1000 μg/ml (data not shown). In addition, preincubation of fg with a specific antibody against FN, did not modify fg induced cell migration, while an antibody against fg completely abolished it. The preparation and the characterization of the antibodies has been previously described in details (10). The results reported here indicate that fg induces EC migration in a concentration dependent way and that this effect is not due to degradation products of the molecule or to FN contaminating the fg preparation. The relevance of these observations to EC behaviour in vivo remains to be established. It has been shown that fg associates to vascular endothelium in an experimental system *in vivo* (11). The observation that EC migrate from lower to higher concentration of fg is compatible with several reports indicating that when fibrin is present *in vivo* EC mobility is increased (1,12). Other authors have shown that whole fibrin is indeed able to induce retraction and disorganization of cultured EC in monolayer (2,4,5). It is likely that whatever property is involved in fibrin stimulation of EC contraction migration and proliferation, it is contained in the native molecule of fg.

Acknowledgements

This work was supported by NATO (project 0572/82) by the Italian National Research Council (contracts 84.00882.51 and 84.00656.44) and by the Commission of the European Communities (contract STI

029 JC). L.R. Languino is a fellow of Pepsico Foundation, Purchase, N.Y.

References

1. Nicosia, R.F., R. Tchao, J. Leighton. 1982. Histotypic angiogenesis in vitro: Light microscopic, ultrastructural, and radioautographic studies. In Vitro 18, 538-549.

2. Kadish, J.L., C.E. Butterfield, J. Folkman. 1979. The effects of fibrin on cultured vascular endothelial cells. Tissue Cell. 11, 99-108.

3. Dang, C.V., W.R. Bell, D. Kaiser, A. Wong. 1985. Disorganization of cultured vascular endothelial cell monolayers by fibrinogen fragment D. Science 227, 1487-1490.

4. Rowland, F.N., M.J. Donovan, P.T. Picciano, D.L. Kreutzer. 1984. Fibrin-mediated vascular injury: Demonstration of vascular endothelial cell retraction in response to soluble fibrin-associated factors. J. Exp. Pathol. 1, 217-240.

5. Schleef, R.R., C.R. Birdwell. 1984. Biochemical changes in endothelial cell monolayers induced by fibrin deposition in vitro. Arteriosclerosis 3, 14-20.

6. Dejana, E., L.R. Languino, N. Polentarutti, G. Balconi, J.J. Ryckewaert, M.J. Larrieu, M.B. Donati, A. Mantovani, G. Marguerie. 1985. Interaction between fibrinogen and cultured endothelial cells. Induction of migration and specific binding. J. Clin. Invest. 75, 11-18.

7. Plow, E.F., C. Birdwell, M.H. Ginsberg. 1979. Identification and quantitation of platelet-associated fibronectin antigen. J. Clin. Invest. 63, 540-543.

8. Bowersox, J.C., N. Sorgente. 1982. Chemotaxis of aortic endothelial cells in response to fibronectin. Cancer Res. 42, 2547-2551.

9. Engwall, E., E. Rouslahti. 1977. Binding of soluble form of fibroblast surface protein, fibronectin, to collagen. Int. J. Cancer 20, 1-5.

10. Marguerie, G.A., N. Ardaillou, G. Cherel, E.F. Plow. 1982. The binding of fibrinogen to its platelet receptors: Involvement of the D domain. J. Biol. Chem. 257, 11872-11875.

11. Witte, S. 1983. The endothelial lining as studied by a fluorescent labeling technique in situ. Thromb. Res. Suppl. V, 93-104.

12. Dvorak, H.F., A.M. Dvorak, E.J. Manseau, L. Wiberg, W.H. Churchill. 1979. Fibrin gel investment associated with line 1 and line 10 solid tumor growth, angiogenesis, and fibroplasia in guinea pigs. Role of cellular immunity, myofibroblasts, microvascular damage, and infarction in line 1 tumor regression. JNCI 62, 1459-1472.

CHARACTERISTICS OF THE INTERACTIONS OF FIBRINOGEN AND SOLUBLE FIBRIN WITH CULTURED ENDOTHELIAL CELLS

U. Delvos, K.T. Preissner, G. Müller-Berghaus

Clinical Research Unit for Blood Coagulation and Thrombosis of the Max-Planck-Gesellschaft at the Justus-Liebig-Universität, Giessen, W.-Germany

Introduction

Two findings prompted us to study the interactions between fibrin and fibrinogen and endothelial cells in culture. Firstly, the observation that polymerized fibrin can induce morphological alterations of cultured endothelial cells (1) suggesting an intimate interaction with the enthelial cell surface and secondly, that the clearance of soluble fibrin generated in the course of disseminated intravascular coagulation is preferentially achieved by highly vascularized organs such as liver and spleen (2,3). Although evidence has been accumulated that macrophages are involved in this process (4,5), endothelial cells may play an additional role in clearing soluble fibrin as has earlier been proposed (6). When thrombin is formed in blood, fibrinogen is rapidly converted to fibrin by removal of the fibrinopeptides A and after a lag phase the fibrinopeptides B are cleaved off. The generated fibrin ("fibrin-monomer") either polymerizes to a clot or can be kept soluble and transported in the circulating blood by an interaction with fibrinogen and/or its degradation products. In the present investigation, an excess of fibrinogen was used to keep fibrin in its soluble state. For this reason the interaction of fibrinogen with intact monolayers of cultured bovine endothelial cells was characterized first, before the behaviour of soluble fibrin towards the endothelial cells was attempted.

Fibrinogen - Fibrin Formation and Fibrinolysis, Vol. 4
© 1986 Walter de Gruyter & Co., Berlin · New York - Printed in Germany.

Materials and Methods

Bovine aortic endothelial cells were isolated, subcultured and characterized as previously described (7). Eight different cell strains from passage four to twelve were used in this study. Experiments were performed with cells plated into 35 mm diameter multiwell plates that had reached confluency. Prior to use cells were washed with serum free medium (SFM) containing 10 mg/ml bovine serum albumin (BSA).

Bovine fibrinogen was purified according to Blombäck and Blombäck (8) and rendered plasminogen-free by chromatography on lysine-Sepharose (9).

Protein labelling: The iodine monochloride method according to McFarlane (10) was adopted to label fibrinogen with ^{131}I and ^{125}I, respectively.

Preparation of soluble fibrin: Two different forms of soluble fibrin were prepared. DesAA-fibrin was formed from iodinated fibrinogen by incubation with batroxobin, whereas desAABB-fibrin was formed when thrombin was used. A monomeric solution of desAA- or desAABB-fibrin was obtained when a clot that had been formed in the presence of EDTA was dissolved in 3 M buffered urea (pH 7.4) (11). Thrombin and batroxobin were inhibited by a five-fold excess of hirudin and an anti-batroxobin antibody, respectively. Afterwards, urea and EDTA were rapidly removed by gel-filtration on a Sephadex G-25 column that had been equilibrated with 10 mg/ml BSA, 5 ATU/ml hirudin and 100 KIU/ml aprotinin in SFM. Immediately before the fibrinmonomer solution was applied to the column an at least 20-fold excess of fibrinogen was added to maintain the fibrin in solution.

Binding studies: All experiments were performed at 37°C with a final calcium concentration of 2.5 mM in SFM or in the presence of 10 mg/ml BSA. Final incubation volume was 1 ml, pH was maintained at 7.4. Incubation was terminated by fast removal of the supernatant followed by three washes with warm saline containing 2.5 mM calcium ions. Subsequently, cell-layers were solubilized in 0.25 N NaOH containing 1% SDS and repeatedly washed. Radioactivities of the combined solutions representing the bound and unbound material were determined.

Results

Endothelial cells could bind fibrinogen in a calcium-dependent fashion therefore the calcium concentration was maintained at 2.5 mM. When the binding of fibrinogen to endothelial cells was followed with time, a constant increase in binding was observed. Binding was not saturable. This was also the case when BSA (10 mg/ml) was added to the incubation mixtures to prevent binding that might be non-specific. The binding capacity of bovine endothelial cells could not be exceeded. Addition of increasing amounts of labelled fibrinogen to the cells did not lead to a saturation of binding.

Competition experiments together with displacement experiments were performed to evaluate the specificity of the fibrinogen endothelial cell interaction. These investigations could not

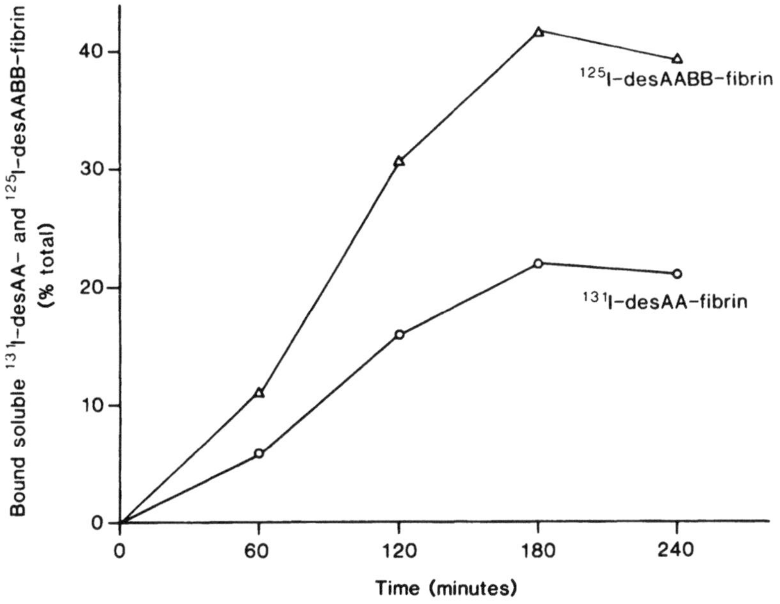

Figure 1: Competition of soluble ^{131}I-desAA- and ^{125}I-desAABB-fibrin for binding to bovine aortic endothelial cells followed for four hours (n = 3). From: Delvos et al (12).

establish that a specific binding site for the fibrinogen molecule is responsible for its binding to cultured endothelial cells. Taken together, a weak and unspecific interaction of fibrinogen with intact layers of bovine aortic endothelial cells was found (13). Thus, fibrinogen appeared to be a suitable protein to keep fibrin in solution and to study the interaction of soluble fibrin with cultured endothelial cells. Soluble fibrin generated from labelled fibrinogen, obtained in monomeric form in urea, and kept in solution by excess fibrinogen bound to cultured bovine endothelial cells. Binding was dependent on the presence of calcium ions. In contrast to the results obtained with fibrinogen, binding was saturable after 4 to 5 hours. The different forms of fibrin, desAA- and desAABB-fibrin, showed different affinities to the cells. This finding held also true,

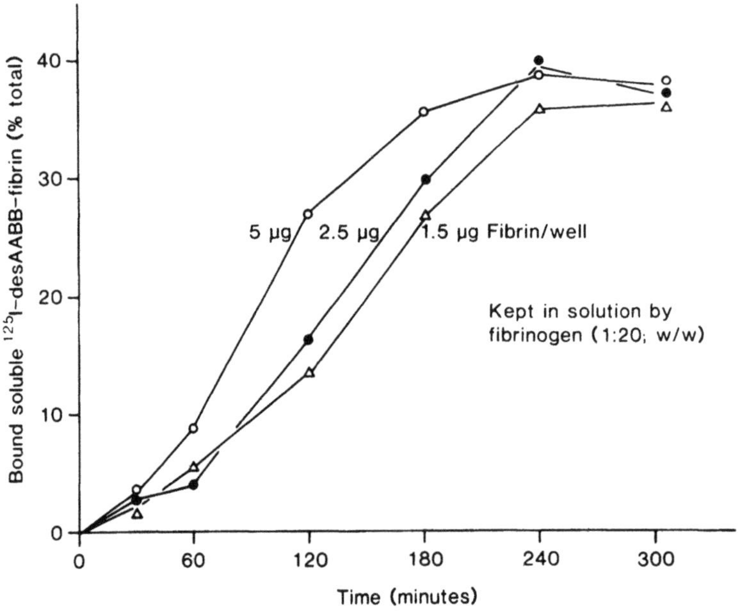

Figure 2: Time course of the binding of soluble ^{125}I-desAABB-fibrin to bovine aortic endothelial cells. Different amounts of fibrin were added without changing the ratio of 1:20 to the solubilizing protein fibrinogen (n = 4). From: Delvos et al (12).

when differently labelled desAA- and desAABB-fibrin were added in identical concentrations and competed for the binding to the cells (Fig. 1). The course of binding was dependent on the total amount of fibrin present in the culture dish. At a constant ratio to fibrinogen (1:20, w/w) binding of desAABB-fibrin to the cells was accelerated the more fibrin was present (Fig. 2). When, however, the amount of solubilizing protein, i.e. fibrinogen, was increased in the incubation mixture, binding could be substantially slowed down (Fig. 3). Furthermore, when after incubation with labelled soluble fibrin unbound material was washed off and again labelled soluble fibrin was added, the newly added fibrin could be bound to the cells. Under these conditions saturation of binding to the cells was achieved at a higher level compared to the controls.

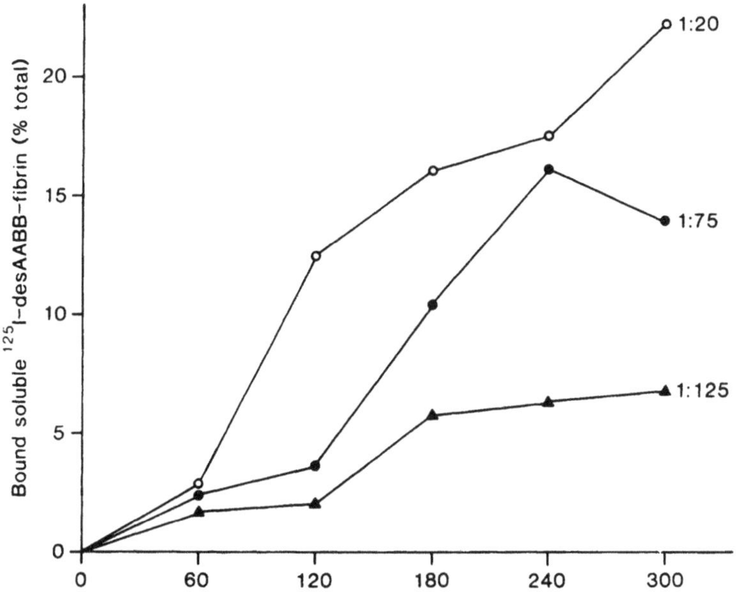

Figure 3: Time course of binding of soluble ^{125}I-desAABB-fibrin to bovine aortic endothelial cells. Dependence of binding on the ratio of soluble fibrin to fibrinogen is depicted (n = 3). From: Delvos et al (12).

Discussion

Our data indicate that soluble fibrin formed in urea and kept in solution by excess fibrinogen interacts avidly with cultured bovine endothelial cells. The findings are highly suggestive that polymerization of the soluble fibrin molecules is taking place at the cell-surface. The different affinities of the different forms of fibrin to the endothelial cell-layer are compatible with this assumption. As documented by ultracentrifugation studies (14), desAA-fibrin is forming polymers of considerably smaller size compared to desAABB-fibrin. The availability of additional polymerisation sites (15) after removal of the fibrinopeptides B may lead to the generation of these larger polymers composed of desAABB-fibrin that formed at the endothelial cell surface.

These in vitro observations are also in accordance with in vivo studies in rabbits that revealed an increase in size of the circulating fibrin monomers with time until a dissociation from the solublizing proteins occurred (11,16).

At the present it remains unclear whether a specific receptor site for the fibrin molecule is involved in the initial binding to the cells.

Acknowlegdement

The excellent technical assistance of Barbara Schneider and Iris Stehl is gratefully acknowleged. This study was supported by the Stiftung Volkswagenwerk, Hannover.

References

1. Kadish, J.L., C.E. Butterfield, J. Folkman. 1979. Tissue & Cell. 11, 99.

2. Sherman, L.A., J. Lee, A. Jacobson. 1977. Br.J.Haematol. 37, 231.

3. Nieuwenhuizen, W., J.J. Emeis, A. Vermond. 1982. Biochem. Biophys.Res.Commun. 105, 1122.

4. Sherman, L.A., J. Lee. 1977. J.Exp.Med. 145, 77.

5. Gonda, S.R., J.R. Shainoff. 1982. Proc.Natl.Acad.Sci.USA 79, 4565.

6. Kisker, C.T., J.C. Hoak, B.J. Taylor, G.L. Fry. 1977. Blood 50, 273 (Abstr)

7. Delvos, U., C. Gajdusek, H. Sage, L.A. Harker, S.M. Schwartz. 1982. Lab.Invest. 46, 61.

8. Blombäck, B., M. Blombäck. 1956. Ark.Kemi. 10, 415.

9. Deutsch, D.G., E.T. Mertz. 1970. Science. 170, 1095.

10. McFarlane, A.S. 1958. Nature 182, 53.

11. Müller-Berghaus, G., I. Mahn, G. Köveker, F.D. Maul. 1976. Br.J.Haematol. 33, 61.

12. Delvos, U., K.T. Preissner, G. Müller-Berghaus. 1985. (submitted for publication)

13. Delvos, U., K.T. Preissner, G. Müller-Berghaus. 1985. Thromb. Haemostas. 53, 26.

14. Preissner, K.T., R. Rötker, E. Selmayr, H. Fasold, G. Müller-Berghaus. 1985. Biochim.Biophys.Acta (in press)

15. Olexa, S.A., A.Z. Budszynski. 1980. Proc.Natl.Acad.Sci.USA 77, 1374.

16. Kröhnke, I., I. Mahn, W. Krell, G. Müller-Berghaus. 1980. Br.J.Haematol. 45, 131.

MECHANISM OF FIBRIN-INDUCED DISORGANISATION OF CULTURED HUMAN ENDOTHELIAL CELLS

B. Weimar, U. Delvos, C. Schubring*, G. Müller-Berghaus

Clinical Research Unit for Blood Coagulation and Thrombosis of the Max-Planck-Gesellschaft at the Justus-Liebig Universität, and * Department of Obstetrics and Gynecology, Evangelisches Krankenhaus, Giessen, W.-Germany

Introduction

Deposition of fibrin on the vascular endothelium may occur *in vivo* after thrombotic events and in disease states accompanied by disseminated intravascular coagulation. Fibrin deposits on endothelial cells have also been implied to play a role in the initiation of atherosclerosis (1). Contact of a fibrin clot with a confluent monolayer of cultured vascular endothelial cells leads to morphological alterations of the cell monolayer as was first described for endothelial cells derived from bovine aorta (2). After exposure to fibrin the cells separated in part from adjacent cells and uncovered intercellular spaces that enlarged with time. 24 hours later the cells were aggregated to tightly packed endothelial cell strands and clusters separated by large cell free areas. This disorganisation of the cell monolayer was reversible, i.e. a normal monolayer of cells was reestablished when the clot was removed or lysed with plasmin. These findings indicated that the changes do not simply reflect cell damage by the overlying fibrin gel. Similar morphological alterations were described using collagen gels. Electron microscopical analysis showed pronounced interdigitations at the remaining cell-cell contacts, while the contacts between untreated endothelial cells in culture were minimal (3). The failure of gels of methylcellulose or agarose to cause any alterations when placed on top of endothelial cell monolayers indicated that mechanical pressure and impaired diffusion of metabolites can not explain the phenomenon. Thus, the present study was undertaken to elucidate the

Fibrinogen - Fibrin Formation and Fibrinolysis, Vol. 4
© 1986 Walter de Gruyter & Co., Berlin · New York - Printed in Germany.

mechanism of fibrin induced disorganisation of cultured human endothelial cell monolayers focussing on the structural requirements within the fibrin clot.

Materials and Methods

Human endothelial cells were isolated from umbilical veins according to Jaffe et al. (4) and were grown to confluency in multiwells of 16 mm diameter. The culture medium (Waymouth MB 752/1) was supplemented with 30% fetal calf serum (FCS), 10µg/ml insulin 20 U/ml heparin, 200 U/ml penicillin, 200 µg/ml streptomycin, and 2 mM glutamine. Cells were identified by morphological and immunological criteria. Experiments were exclusivly performed with primary cultures. FCS was replaced in all experiments by serum free medium (SFM) containing 0.1% human serum albumin.

Fibrinogen was purified from human plasma by the glycine precipitation procedure according to Blombäck and Blombäck (5). Two additional purification steps were performed using lysine-Sepharose and gelatin-Sepharose to remove plasminogen and fibronectin, respectively (6,7). The effectiveness of these procedures was evaluated by functional and immunological assays.

Fragment D-cate was purified from a plasmin digest of human fibrinogen in a calcium containing buffer (8). The fragments were separated by chromatography on QAE-Sephadex (9).

Soluble fibrin was prepared by three different methods using either fibrinogen, D-cate or the synthetic tetrapeptide Gly-Pro-Arg-Pro to keep fibrin in solution (10,11,12).

Antibodies against human fibrinogen were raised in goats. The resulting antiserum was subjected to sodium sulphate precipitation, followed by ion exchange chromatography of the dissolved precipitate on DEAE-Sephacel, to isolate the IgG-fraction. Preformed fibrin clots were incubated with this IgG-fraction to prepare antibody-loaded clots.

Several modifications of the fibrin clots were performed: Denaturation was achieved by incubation of preformed clots with glutaraldehyde or formaldehyde or boiling for 15 min. Clots were

dehydrated by incubation with absolute ethanol. Sialic acids in the glycosyl-side chains of the fibrinogen molecule were removed using neuraminidase, before a clot of asialo-fibrin was formed (13). Non-crosslinked fibrin was prepared by clotting fibrinogen in the presence of 200 mM iodoacetamide.
Collagen gels were prepared from acid dissolved bovine type I collagen. A cold solution was rapidly titrated to pH 7.4, supplemented with the appropriate amount of Waymouth MB 752/1 medium and diluted with SFM to a final concentration of 1 mg collagen/ml. This solution was pipetted into multiwells with endothelial cells and allowed to gel by raising the temperature to 37°C.

Results

Exposure of a fibrin clot to a confluent monolayer of cultured human endothelial cells led to morphological alterations of the cell monolayer that occurred in a similar time course as it was described with bovine endothelial cells (Fig. 1 A/B). Fibrin clots prepared from highly purified fibrinogen, free of plasminogen and fibronectin, induced the same morphological alterations as clots from fibrinogen preparations of lower purity. There was no difference when either a solution of fibrinogen was clotted over an endothelial cell monolayer, or when a preformed clot was put on top of the cells. Clots of desAA- as well as desAABB-fibrin led to disorganisation of endothelial cell monolayers. Thrombin or reptilase alone had no effect on endothelial cell morphology. In addition, incubation of cells with fibrinopeptides A and B left their morphology unaltered.
Disorganisation was reversible when the clot was removed or lysed with plasmin. However, with prolonged incubation time the cells became increasingly attached to the overlying fibrin clot and after about 24 hours virtually all the cells remained attached to the clot when it was removed. Furthermore, when such a clot was turned around together with the attached cells the cells reorganised to a monolayer of normal cobblestone appearance on top of this clot.

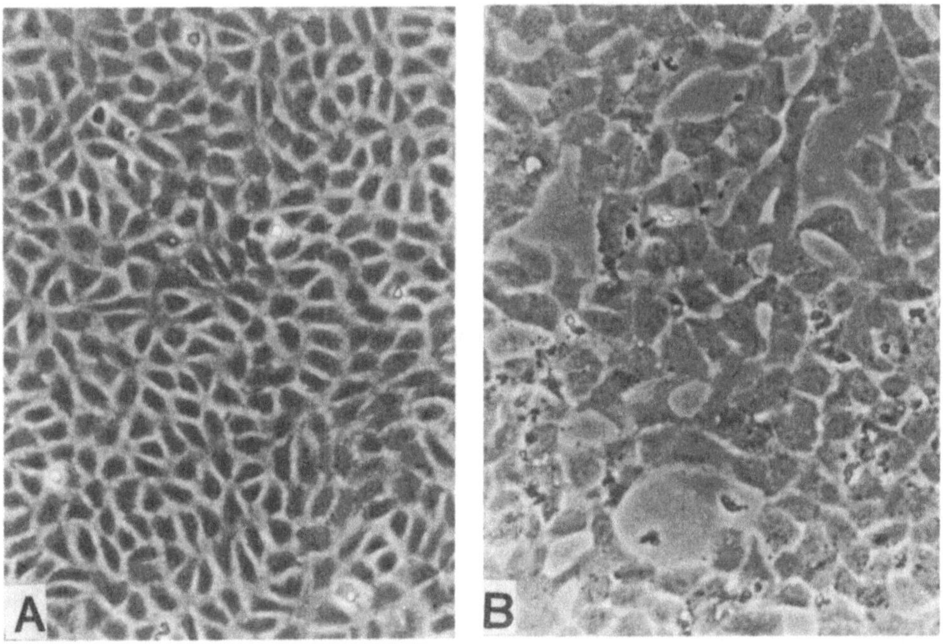

Figure 1: A) Phase contrast micrograph of human umbilical vein endothelial cells after seven days in primary culture. The cells form a typical monolayer of closley aposed, polygonally shaped endothelial cells. B) After exposure to a fibrin clot for 24 h the same cells form a network of tightly packed strands and clusters, separated by cell free areas (Magnification x 75). From: Weimar et al (14).

Damage of the tertiary structure of a fibrin clot by boiling or treatment with denaturing agents could not affect the ability of fibrin to induce disorganisation of endothelial cells. In addition, loading of a clot with large amounts of antibodies against fibrinogen, that should mask a large number of epitopes of the fibrin molecule, had no blocking effect. Preparations of asialofibrin and non-crosslinked fibrin behaved similar as native fibrin when placed on top of endothelial cells.
In contrast, soluble fibrin, kept in solution by either fibrinogen, D-cate or the synthetic peptide Gly-Pro-Arg-Pro, did not cause any visible alterations of an endothelial cell monolayer. Table 1 gives an overview of the results obtained.

Table 1

Effects of Modified Fibrin Clots and Soluble Fibrin on Disorganisation of Endothelial Cell Monolayers

Source of fibrin	Disorganisation
Preformed clot	
- denatured with glutaraldehyde	+
- denatured with formaldehyde	+
- denatured by 15 min boiling	+
- dehydrated with ethanol	+
- loaded with antibodies against fibrinogen	+
Non crosslinked fibrin	+
Asialo-fibrin	+
Soluble fibrin kept in solution by:	
- fibrinogen	∅
- fragment D-cate	∅
- Gly-Pro-Arg-Pro	∅

Under the assumption that disorganisation of endothial cell monolayers by fibrin was obviously not dependent on the fibrin structure, we have tested other materials for their ability to induce disorganisation of endothelial cells. Similar to bovine endothelial cells, collagen induced disorganisation of human endothelial cells. When collagen was heat-denatured to gelatin the ability to polymerize as well as the ability to induce disorganisation was lost. Gels of agarose and mixtures of agarose and fibrinogen did not cause any alterations of endothelial cell monolayers. However, when a solution of bovine thrombin was poured over an agarose/fibrinogen gel on top of endothelial cells, disorganisation did occur.

Alterations of the monolayer similar to fibrin induced changes could be induced by glass. In these experiments small pieces of glass coverslips (0.18 mm thick) were incubated with endothelial cells. Similar to fibrin the cells attached to the overlying glass coverslip, and when this glass coverslip was turned around together with the attached cells, a normal monolayer was restored on top of the glass. The results are summarized in Table 2.

Table 2

Effects of Agarose, Collagen and Glass on Disorganisation of Endothelial Cell Monolayers*

Material	Disorganisation
Agarose	Ø
Agarose + fibrinogen	Ø
Agarose + fibrinogen + thrombin	+
Collagen type I, gel	+
Collagen type I, denatured	Ø
Glass	+

* Data represent the uniform response of the cells in three series of experiments, each of them carried out four times (N=12).

Discussion

Human endothelial cells in culture undergo similar morphological changes in response to fibrin, as it was earlier described for bovine endothelial cells. Components that are involved in fibrin formation, such as the released fibrinopeptides, the clotting agents (thrombin or reptilase) and the polymerization process itself, were found to be not responsible for the induction of disorganisation by fibrin.
Every modification of fibrin tested, including denatured fibrin clots and clots that were loaded with large amounts of antibodies against fibrinogen, induced disorganisation of the cell monolayers, whereas soluble fibrin did not affect the monolayer morphology independent of the solubilizing agent employed in the experiment (Fibrinogen, D-cate and Gly-Pro-Arg-Pro). Recently, a deleterious effect of the fibrinogen fragment D on cultured bovine endothelial cells has been described (15). This observation could not be confirmed by our experiments. The exposure of the fibrinogen degradation product D-cate to the human endothelial cells had no effect on the architecture of the cell monolayer although even larger amounts of purified fragment D-cate

(up to 2 mg/ml) were used in our study. This suggests that the induction of disorganisation is not triggered by a defined component of the fibrin molecule. This conclusion is further supported by the ability of glass to induce disorganisation of endothelial cell monolayers.
As a common feature, that was invariably found when disorganisation was induced, the cells attached to the overlying material. Thus, cell attachment to the overlying material seems to be a prerequisite for the subsequent alterations of the cell monolayer in the process of disorganisation.
Fibronectin that mediates cell attachment in vitro (16) and binds to fibrinogen and collagen (17) may be involved in the attachment of the cells to the overlying material. It was demonstrated in vitro as well as in vivo that fibronectin is associated with the intercellular junctions and the basement membrane of vascular endothelial cells, but is absent on the luminal side of the cells (18, 19). Absence of fibronectin on the luminal side of endothelial cells could well account for the inability of endothelial cells to grow on top of each other and may explain the strict contact inhibition of this cell type.
We should like to speculate that fibronectin becomes exposed on the former luminal part of the endothelial cell membrane. This could enable the cells to grow in part on top of each other resulting in the formation of tightly packed cell strands and clusters.

Acknowledgements

We express our gratitude to the nursery staff of the delivery room for their cooperation and help in obtaining umbilical cords. This study was supported by the Stiftung Volkswagenwerk, Hannover.

References

1. Kadish, J.L. 1979. Atherosclerosis 33, 409.
2. Kadish, J.L., C.E. Butterfield, J. Folkman. 1979. Tissue & Cell 11, 99.
3. Delvos, U., C. Gajdusek, H. Sage, L.A. Harker, S.M. Schwartz. 1982. Lab.Invest. 46, 61.
4. Jaffe, E.A., R.L. Nachman, C.G. Becker, C.R. Minick. 1973. J.Clin.Invest. 52, 2745.
5. Blombäck, B., M. Blombäck. 1956. Ark.Kemi 10, 415.
6. Deutsch, D.G., E.T. Mertz. 1970. Science 170, 1095.
7. Miekka, S.I., K.C. Ingham, D. Menache. 1982. Thromb.Res. 27, 1.
8. Haverkate, F., G. Timan. 1977. Thromb.Res. 10, 803.
9. Chen, J.P., H.M. Shurley, M.F. Vickroy. 1974. Biochem.Biophys.Res.Commun. 61, 66.
10. Haverkate, F., G. Timan, W. Nieuwenhuizen. 1979. Eur.J.Clin. Invest. 9, 253.
11. Kröhnke, I., I. Mahn, W. Krell, G. Müller-Berghaus. 1980. Br.J.Haematol. 45, 131.
12. Laudano, A.P., R.F. Doolittle. 1980. Biochemistry 19, 1013.
13. Kuyas, C., A. Haeberli, P.W. Straub. 1982. Thromb.Haemostas. 48, 19.
14. Weimar, B., U. Delvos, G. Müller-Berghaus. 1985. (submitted for publication)
15. Dang, C.V., W.R. Bell, D. Kaiser, A. Wong. 1985. Science 227, 1487.
16. Mosesson, M.W., D.L. Amrani. 1980. Blood 56, 145.
17. Engvall, E., E. Rouslathi, E.J. Miller. 1978. J.Exp.Med. 147, 1584.
18. Birdwell, C.R., D. Gospodarowicz, G.L. Nicolson. 1978. Proc.Natl.Acad.Sci. USA 75, 3273.
19. Linder, E., A. Vaheri, E. Rouslathi, J. Wartiovaara. 1975. J.Exp.Med. 142, 41.

THE FIBRINOGEN: RED CELL INTERACTION AND ITS INFLUENCE ON BLOOD RHEOLOGY.

M.W. Rampling
Department of Physiology and Biophysics, St Mary's Hospital Medical School, London W2

Introduction

One of the factors which limits the rate of flow of a fluid is its viscosity, hence the viscosity of blood must be a factor determining flow rates in the vascular circulation. However, this would be of relatively little interest were it not for the fact that the viscosity of whole blood can vary dramatically in disease (1). So much is this so that it is now thought to affect the course of a number of diseases, and haemorheological manipulation is being used clinically in an attempt to alleviate their symptoms (1).

Studies of the viscometric properties of whole blood show them to be complex (2), but a particularly interesting property is that of shear-thinning, that is to say if the viscosity of whole blood is measured at various shear rates its value is found to decrease as the shear rate rises (see Fig 1). The cause of this phenomenon is thought to be related to two properties of erythrocytes : their tendency, in whole blood, to adhere together to produce characteristic aggregates known as rouleaux, and their inherent deformability. Thus it is assumed that at low shear rates the large rouleaux present produce high viscometric drag, however as the shear rate increases the shearing forces progressively break up the rouleaux and viscosity falls. Eventually these forces become sufficient to deform the cells into stream-lined shapes and the viscosity falls even further (3). Evidence in favour of these ideas is shown in Fig 1 where it can be seen that the suspension in protein-free buffer (which does not induce cellular aggregation) shows no low shear rate viscosity change. However, at higher shear rates, where cellular stream-lining occurs, the viscosity does still fall. Fig 1 also shows that the low shear rate phenomenon can be ellicited by serum (as can rouleaux-formation) though to a substantially lesser extent than whole plasma. It is now known that these rouleaux-related effects are due to large plasma proteins, but that fibrinogen is by far the most effective (4).

Fibrinogen - Fibrin Formation and Fibrinolysis, Vol. 4
© 1986 Walter de Gruyter & Co., Berlin · New York - Printed in Germany.

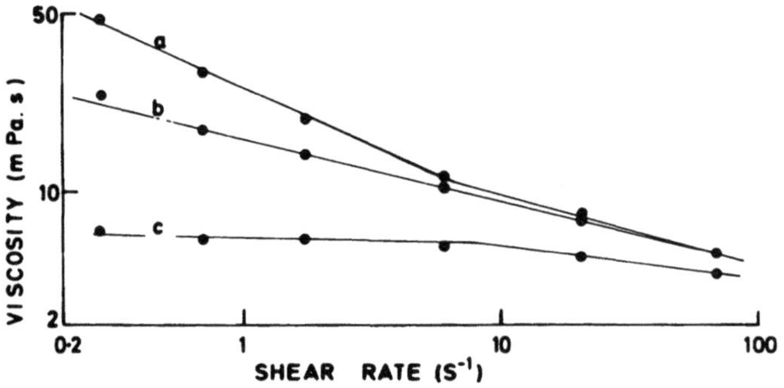

Fig 1. Viscosity : shear rate relationships for cells from the same sample of normal blood suspended in (a) autologous plasma (b) autologous serum (c) isotonic phosphate-buffered saline. Haematocrit 45%, fibrinogen concentration 254 mg/dl.

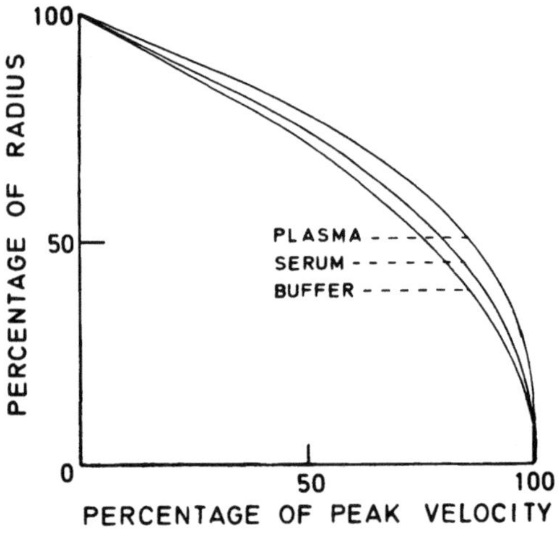

Fig 2. Calculated velocity profiles for the suspensions of Fig 1 flowing in a tube of radius 1 mm length 4 cm under a driving pressure of 4Pa. The abscissa is normalised to the peak velocity in each case, which is 1.2, 1.9 and 3.9 mm/s for the plasma, serum and buffer suspension respectively.

In view of these considerations and the great variability in the concentration of fibrinogen that can occur in diseased conditions, it seems reasonable to suppose that the shear-rate dependence of blood viscosity will have an effect on blood flow. Some idea of its magnitude can be obtained using a computational technique developed by Rampling and Challoner (5). This allows velocity profiles and flow rate : driving pressure relationships of erythrocyte suspensions flowing in cylindrical tubes to be determined from the observed viscosity : shear rate relationships of the suspensions. Using this technique, typical velocity profiles for the suspensions of Fig 1 have been calculated and are illustrated in Fig 2. It can be seen that the profile becomes blunted in the presence of serum and the more so in the presence of plasma, and that the peak velocity falls substantially as the blunting increases. These effects are due to the high effective viscosities of the protein-containing suspensions in the low shear rate central regions of the tube. Fig 3 shows the results of corresponding calculations of the volume flow rate : driving pressure relationships for the same suspensions in a small vessel.

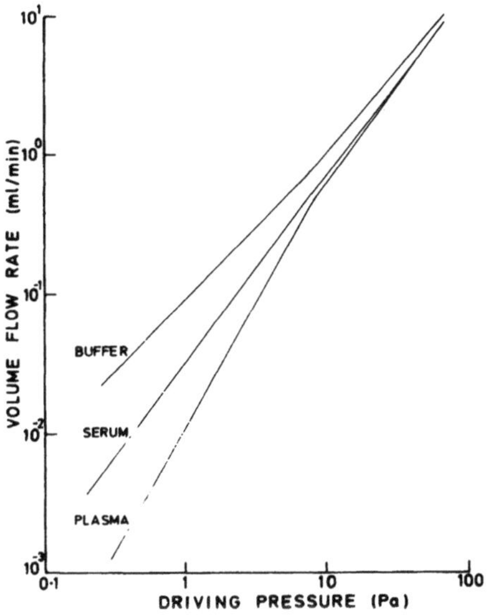

Fig 3. Calculated volume flow rate : driving pressure relationships for the suspensions of Fig 1 flowing in a tube of radius 1 mm and length 4 cm.

It can be seen that at low driving pressures the effects of the plasma proteins, and especially of fibrinogen, are very significant, and in pathological bloods where the fibrinogen concentration is elevated these effects will be more pronounced still (5). Thus it is clear that they are likely to be of physiological and patho-physiological significance. An investigation has, therefore, been made of the physico-chemistry of the fibrinogen : red cell interaction, and some of the results are reported below.

Adsorption of Fibrinogen to Erythrocyte Membranes.

The most extensive studies of rouleaux-formation have been made using dextran or polylysine as aggregating agents (6). They give compelling evidence that these agents act by a bridging mechanism whereby they cross-link between adjacent cell membranes. The necessary characteristics of the cross-linking agents are that they should have adsorption sites at opposite ends of the molecule, and their molecular length should be enough to allow cross-linking to occur at such a distance that the repulsive forces that exist between the cells are less that those of the adhesive molecules. It is generally assumed, by analogy, that fibrinogen acts in a similar way, and its long dimeric structure would fit in with such a role (7). Clearly this hypothesis necessitates that fibrinogen exhibit adhesive properties towards the red cell membrane, and this has been shown to be the case (8, 9). Indeed, using ^{125}I-fibrinogen, Rampling (9) was able to quantitate the adsorption of fibrinogen and found that, up to a suspending phase concentration of 1000 mg/dl, the amount adherent to the red cells was directly proportional to the concentration in the suspending phase. This would imply that in whole blood in vivo some 2% of circulating fibrinogen travels in association with the red cells. The adsorption was also found to be independent of temperature in the range 10-37°C.

Fibrinogen and Rouleaux Size.

The method used to study the relationship between the size of rouleaux and the prevailing fibrinogen concentration was based on that of Chien et al (10). Washed normal erythrocytes were suspended in phosphate-buffered saline as a control non-aggregating sample, or in the same buffer but with added fibrinogen (purified Human Fibrinogen, Kabi Pharmaceuticals, Stockholm). The suspensions were all made up to a haematocrit of 1%. Drops of each suspension were placed on a Neubauer slide under a microscope and allowed to aggregate for 5 minutes. After this time the number of cellular units in a given area of the slide was counted; a cellular unit was either a single cell or a single rouleau. The average number of cells per rouleau was then calculated as:

$$\frac{\text{number of cellular units per unit area in control sample}}{\text{number of cellular units per unit area in test sample}}$$

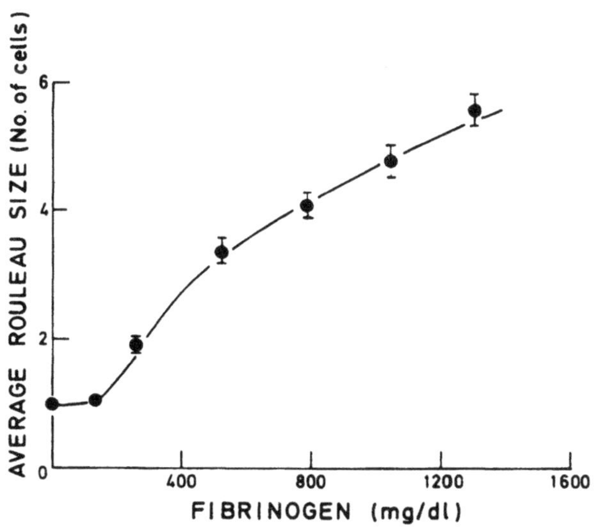

Fig 4. Rouleaux size (average number of cells) as a function of fibrinogen concentration. Haematocrit 1% in phosphate-buffered saline.

Typical results, for one subject, are shown in Fig 4. It can be seen that no significant aggregation occurs until the fibrinogen concentration reaches about 100 mg/dl. Presumably only at this level does enough fibrinogen adsorb to the cells to overcome inherant repulsive forces. However beyond it there is a continuous increase in aggregate size up to a concentration of at least 1200 mg/dl, with no sign of saturation.

Another method of investigating rouleaux formation is the use of the erythrocyte sedimentation rate (ESR), which is generally considered to be raised in the presence of elevated aggregation (11). A number of workers have shown that the ESR increases continuously as fibrinogen concentration rises up to 1000 mg/dl and beyond (12, 13, 14). These workers have also studied the effects of plasmin-derived degradation products of fibrinogen (FDP) on the ESR. They found that the early FDP enhance ESR, while the late fragments are without effect, corresponding to microscopic observations which show that while early FDP produce rouleaux, late fragments do not. Rampling (9) performed adsorption studies on FDP's, similar to those described above, and found that they would all adhere to the erythrocyte membrane. He concluded that only the early fragments are aggregating since only they are dimeric and large enough to cross-link the cells over such a distance that cellular repulsion could be overcome. A curious finding (12, 14) here, however, was that adding any of the FDP's to fibrinogen-containing suspensions enhanced the effect of fibrinogen. Why the non-aggregating terminal FDP's should do this is unclear.

Fibrinogen and Low Shear Rate Viscosity

Rampling et al (14) have studied the effects of addition of purified fibrinogen on the viscometric characteristics of erythrocytes suspended in isotonic phosphate buffer. The measurements were made on a Contraves LS30 Viscometer using a bob-in-cup head. Typical data, for one subject, is shown in Fig 5. It can be seen that at high shear rate, where the shearing forces lead to complete disaggregation of cells, fibrinogen is without effect. However, at low shear rates the viscosity increases almost linearly up to at least 1000 mg/dl, and the effects are more pronounced the lower the shear rate. Clearly there is remarkable correlation between these results and those of fibrinogen adsorption to red cells. The effect of changing temperature from about 10 to 37°C on low shear rate viscosity was also studied. This showed that while the viscosity of the whole suspension decreased with rising temperature, the relative viscosity did not change (15). Since the relative viscosity represents the viscous effect of only the cellular compartment, this implies that the degree of aggregation in this dynamic system does not change with temperature; again correlating with adsorption results. Finally, just as the FDP enhanced the ESR effect of fibrinogen, so they were also found to exaggerate its influence on low shear rate viscosity.

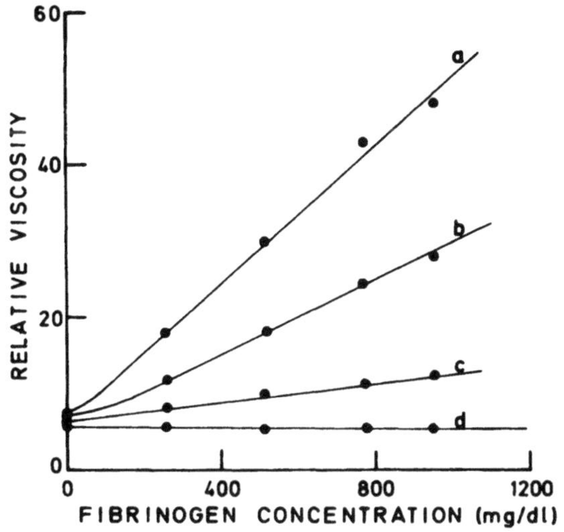

Fig 5. Relative viscosity : fibrinogen concentration relationships for erythrocytes suspended in phosphate-buffered saline. Haematocrit 45%. Shear rates (a) 0.277 (b) 0.945 (c) 5.96 (d) 69.5 S^{-1}

Conclusion

The presence of fibrinogen clearly has a profound effect on the low shear rate viscosity of red cell suspensions, its magnitude increasing progressively with prevailing fibrinogen over the whole range of concentration found in vivo in health and in disease. Furthermore, data such as shown in Fig 3 and elsewhere (5) indicate that this phenomenon is likely to affect the rate of blood flow in vivo particularly at low driving pressures.

The cause of this low shear rate phenomenon is usually considered to be related to the adhesion forces that hold erythrocytes together in rouleaux, and these in turn are considered to result from bridging between cells by adherent fibrinogen molecules. The correspondence between the data on adhesion, rouleaux size and low shear rate viscosity reported above is compatible with this hypothesis.

Acknowledgement

The authors' work described above was supported by the Wellcome Trust.

References

1. Lowe, G.D.O., J.C. Barbenel, C.D. Forbes. 1980. Clinical Aspects of Blood Viscosity and Cell Deformability. Springer-Verlag, Berlin-Heidelberg-New York.

2. Dintenfass, L. 1971. Blood Microrheology - Viscosity Factors in Blood Flow, Ischaemia and Thrombosis. Butterworth, London.

3. Meiselman, H.J. 1980. In: Erythrocyte Mechanics and Blood Flow (G.R. Cokelet, H.J. Meiselman and D.E. Brooks, eds.). Alan R. Liss, New York, pp 75-117.

4. Chien, S., S. Usami, R.J. Dellenback, M.I. Gregersen. 1970. Am. J. Physiol. 219, 143.

5. Rampling, M.W., T. Challoner. 1983. Biorheology, 20, 141.

6. Chien, S. 1980. In: Advances in Chemistry Series, No 188, Biochemistry: Ions, Surfaces, Membranes (H. Blank ed.). American Chemical Society. p. 1-38.

7. Doolittle. 1981. In: Haemostasis and Thrombosis (A.L. Bloom, D.P. Thomas eds.). Churchill Livingstone, London-Melbourne-New York, pp 163-191.

8. Brooks, D.E., R.G. Greig, J. Janzen. 1980. In: Erythrocyte Mechanics and Blood Flow (G.R. Cokelet, H.J. Meiselman, D.E. Brooks eds.). Alan R Liss, New York, pp 119-140.

9. Rampling, M.W. 1981. Acta. Biol. Med. Germ. 40, 373.

10. Chien, S., S. Usami, R.J. Dellenback, M.I. Gregersen, L.B. Nanningen, M.M. Guest. 1967. Science 157, 829.

11. Fahraeus, R. 1929. Physiological Rev. 9, 241.

12. Hermann, H., G. Ruhenstroth-Bauer. 1975. Blut. 30, 51.

13. Marsh, N.A. 1979. Thrombosis Haemostasis 42, 157.

14. Rampling, M.W., P. Whittingstall, O. Linderkamp. 1984. Clinical Haemorheology 4, 533.

15. Rampling, M.W., P. Whittingstall. 1985. Proceeding British Soc. Haematol., Warwick, March 1985, Paper 13.

HAEMORHEOLOGIC EFFECTS OF PLASMIN AND THROMBIN-INDUCED FIBRINOGEN DERIVATIVES: AN IN VITRO STUDY.

G. Palareti, M. Poggi, S. Coccheri

Departement of Angiology and Blood Coagulation, University Hospital
S. Orsola, 40138 Bologna, Italy.

Introduction

The fibrinogen (Fgn) molecule, besides its central role in blood coagulation, has an important effect in determining the rheologic behaviour of blood. Not only Fgn is the main single determinant of plasma viscosity (1) but it also induces the formation of red blood cell (RBC) aggregates that greatly increase whole blood viscosity at low shear conditions (2), thus contributing to the non-newtonian rheology of blood. These effects, though not yet fully elucidated, have been attributed to the high molecular weight and asymmetrical shape of Fgn (3), and have widely been studied in conditions of health and disease. In fact an increase in Fgn concentration frequently occurs in a number of acute and chronic diseases, sometimes reaching very high levels, and is responsible for thrombophylic states (4-7) as well as for changes in blood flow.

The Fgn molecule undergoes specific changes both during coagulation, with formation of fibrin monomers (FM) polymerizing to soluble fibrin monomer complexes (SFMC), and during fibrino(geno)lysis, with formation of fibrin(ogen) degradation products (FDP). Ob-

Fibrinogen - Fibrin Formation and Fibrinolysis, Vol. 4
© 1986 Walter de Gruyter & Co., Berlin · New York - Printed in Germany.

viously SFMC, as well as their complexes with Fgn and early FDP are much larger in size than the parent molecule and its plasmin degradation products. There has been little investigation, so far, on the rheological properties of these circulating Fgn derivatives, in comparison to those of the native Fgn molecule. The aim of this in vitro study was to investigate some effects of plasmin and thrombin Fgn derivatives on the viscosity of plasma and Fgn solutions, both without and with resuspended erythrocytes.

Materials and Methods

Fgn solutions (FgnS) were prepared using human Fgn (Grade L, Kabi, Sweden) dissolved in phosphate saline buffer (PBS), 292 mOsm, pH 7.4, containing bovine albumin 200 mg%, at a final concentration of 280+/-40 mg%. Before use FgnS, as well as plasma samples, were filtered through 0.22 um filters (Millex-GS, Millipore, France).
Blood was obtained from six healthy male donors and anticoagulated with Citrate phosphate dextrose (CPD, 8) at the v/v proportion 1:8. In one case blood sample anticoagulated with EDTA-K2 (final concentration 1.5 mg/ml) was also obtained. Samples were centrifuged at 2000 g at 4 C for 15 min. Plasma was then separated, recentrifuged for 10 min and filtered through 0.22 um filters. After buffy coat remotion by aspiration RBC were washed three times in albuminated PBS and added to FgnS or plasma, as was the case, at a haematocrit level of 45%. To obtain heat-defibrinated plasma some plasma fractions were incubated for 10 min at 56 C, then centrifuged at 2000 g for 20 min and the precipitate discarded. No residual Fgn was found, with either the clotting or the immunologic method; Staphylococcal Clumping test for FDP (Boehringer- Biochemia- Robin, BBR, Milan, Italy) was positive at about the level of 10 mg%.

Fibrinogenolysis was obtained by adding Streptokinase (SK, Streptase, Behring Institute, L'Aquila, Italy), at the final concentration of 100 U/ml, to aliquots of FgnS, plasma and heat-defibrinated plasma; to the latter Plasminogen (Kabi) had previously been added at the final concentration of 8 mg%. The plasmin digestion was stopped at different intervals (5, 15, 60 minutes and 16 hours) by means of 500 U/ml of Aprotinin (Richter, Milan, Italy).

Fibrin Monomers (FM) were prepared and stored according to Belitser V.A. et al. (9). For use FM were diluted in PBS albuminated at 10 mg% and this solution was added to FgnS at the v/v proportion 1:10. The Ethanol Gelation (10), the Protamine Sulphate (11) and the FM (BBR) tests were all positive in the final solutions.

Fgn was measured as antigen by means of radial immunodiffusion plates (M-Partigen, Behring Institute) and as clottable protein by means of thrombin polymerization times according to Clauss (12).

FDP were measured with both Thrombo-Wellcotest (Wellcome Italia, Rome, Italy) and the Staphylococcal Clumping test (BBR).

Viscosity was measured by means of a Contraves Low Shear 30 viscometer, at different shear rates (s.r., 0.2; 1.28; 8.1; 94.5 sec. -1). Measurements were made at 37 C, starting from the lowest s.r. to the highest, using the type 1 bob and cup, if the erythrocytes were present in the samples, and the type 2T in the other cases.

The coefficients of variation were:

shear rates	= 0.2	1.28	8.1	94.5	sec-1
FgnS/plasma	= /	5.9	3.4	1.2	%
FgnS/plasma +RBCs	= 4.5	3.1	1.1	0.9	%

Viscosity measurements were carried out on samples of FgnS and plasma before and after fibrinogenolysis, and before and after addition of FM to FgnS. In both cases viscosity measurements were performed before and after addition of fresh washed autologous RBC at 45% haematocrit.

Results were expressed as % variation calculated on the baseline values.

Results

A) Viscosity of FgnS and plasma after SK-degradation.

As shown in fig. 1 the Fgn degradation induced very little changes in the viscosity of plasma. Viscosity of FgnS was slightly increased after early degradation, probably because of the formation of complexes including early FDP.

B) Viscosity of FgnS and plasma after SK-degradation + RBC.

While 5 min degradation (fig. 2) had no effect, a reduction of viscosity was recorded in both RBC suspensions after 15 min. Further degradation gave different results in plasma than in FgnS. In fact the latter showed a further reduction in viscosity after 60 min,

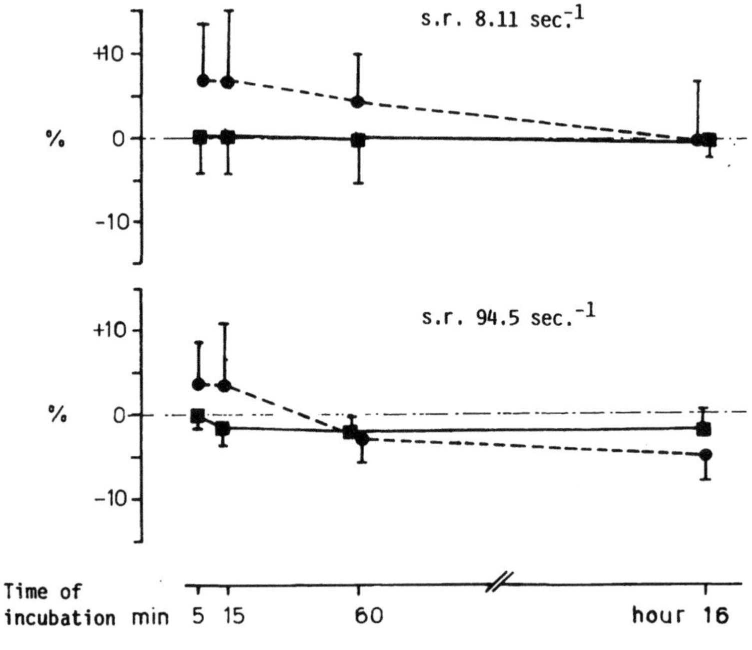

Fig. 1 Viscosity changes (mean +/- Sd of % variations of 6 experiments) of FgnS (-------) and plasma (———) after different times of incubation with Streptokinase. The results obtained with two shear rates are showed.

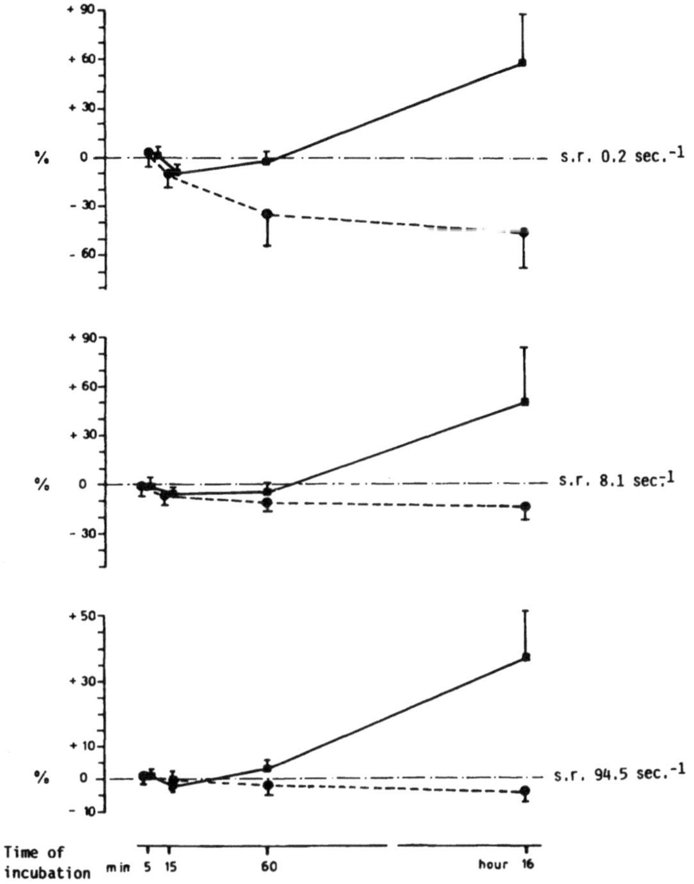

Fig. 2 Viscosity changes (mean+/-SD of % variations of 6 experiments) of FgnS (----) and plasma (——) plus 45% RBC, after different times of incubation with Streptokinase (three shear rates)

much more evident at very low s.r., and remained at the same low level after overnight digestion. The viscosity of plasma plus erythrocytes, on the contrary, returned to the baseline values after 60 min and remarkably and paradoxically increased after overnight digestion, at all the s.r. tested. No different results were obtained using plasma anticoagulated with EDTA-K2 instead CPD.

With the aim of investigating if this phenomenon was due to fibrinogenolysis and/or other proteolytic effects, we treated heat-defi-

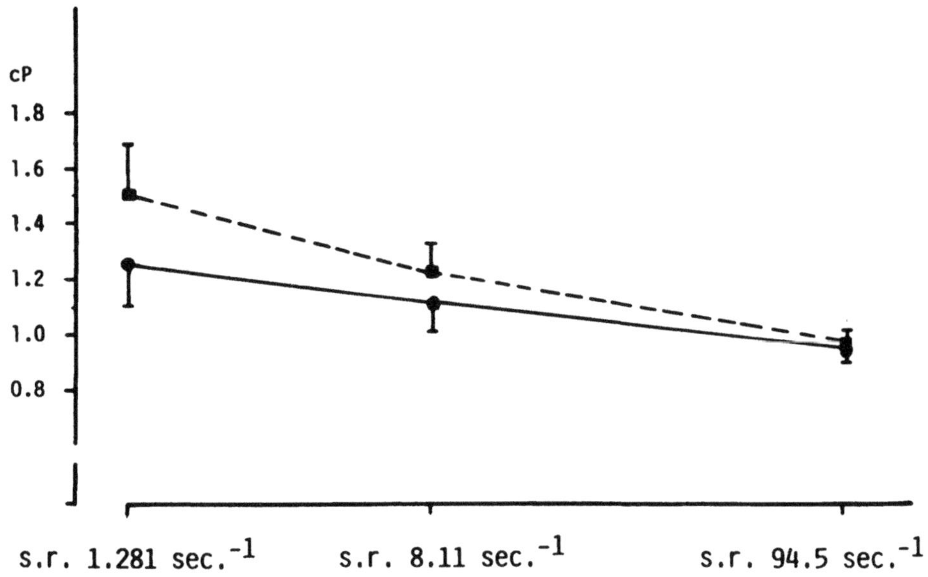

Fig. 3 Viscosity values (mean+/-SD) of FgnS (———) and FgnS plus Fibrin Monomers (-----) at the different shear rates.

brinated plasma with SK overnight and again found an increased viscosity of RBC suspensions in treated plasma, though of a smaller degree than in native plasma (+35+/-32% at 0.2 sec -1 s.r.; +17+/-21% at 8.11 s.r.; +13+/-11% at 94.5 s.r.).

C) Viscosity of FgnS + FM without or with RBC.

The addition of FM to FgnS caused an increase in its viscosity, especially at very low s.r. (+24+/-10% at 1.28 s.r.; +6+/-3% at 8.11 s.r.; +4+/-2% at 94.5 s.r.), thus inducing a clearly non-newtonian rheologic behaviour of FgnS, that was only slightly noticeable in FgnS alone (fig. 3). The addition of FM to a suspension of erythrocytes in FgnS brought about only slight changes in viscosity, and only at the lowest s.r. (+5+/-3% at 0.2 sec -1 s.r.).

Discussion

Blood is a non-newtonian fluid whose viscosity depends on the conditions of shear, increasing greatly with decreasing s.r.. The main determinants of whole blood viscosity are: a) the haematocrit; b) the composition and viscosity of plasma; c) the tendency of red cells to aggregate; c) the deformability of erythrocytes (4). Fgn plays a great role in determining the rheologic properties of blood. In fact it is by far the most important protein influencing plasma viscosity (1,2). Furthermore, elevated Fgn levels, as is also the case with other plasma proteins of larger molecular weight, can overcome the negative zeta potential between erythrocytes, and increase their tendency to form rouleaux thus affecting the erythrocyte sedimentation rate (13) and causing a disproportionate increase in viscosity at low s.r..
Since the Fgn molecule undergoes important changes in size, shape and charge during clotting and lysis, it may be important to study the effects of these changes on blood rheology. Our in vitro study showed that early plasmin degradation products increase the viscosity of FgnS at low s.r., probably because of the formation of complexes. This phenomenon is only evident at low s.r., possibly because camplexes are disrupted at the higher ones. Complete Fgn degradation seemed not to induce significant viscosity changes in absence of RBC, but an effect was evident after addition of erythrocytes. In fact prolonged Fgn digestion (1 and 16 h) caused a sharp reduction in the viscosity of erythocyte suspension, more evident at very low s.r.. This result suggests taht late FDP have less effect on erythrocyte aggregation than does Fgn, and is in accord with both the results of Marsh (14), indicating that fragments D and E differently from Fgn do not accelerate the erythrocyte sedimentation rate, and with those of other Authors (15). The molecular integrity of Fgn seems therefore to be essential for a full effect on RBC aggregation.

We cannot explain the paradoxically increased viscosity values found when RBC were added to long-term SK-treated plasma samples, unless by tentatively attributing this finding to injury to RBC due to small peptides formed during prolonged digestion. Since this effect was also observed in the virtually Fgn free heat-defibrinated plasma but not in FgnS alone, we may speculate that it is probably not merely due to the lysis of Fgn. It should also be noted that different anticoagulants did not affect these results.
Addition of FM to FgnS increased its viscosity only at low s.r. probably through the formation of SFMC that could be disrupted at higher s.r.. Although plasma is generally considered a newtonian fluid (16,17), some recent data showed that its viscosity may become higher at very low s.r. (18). We studied human purified Fgn and also found similar results, probably because of the presence of activated molecules in the Fgn concentrate. The addition of FM furtherly enhanced this non-newtonian rheologic behaviour. Furthermore, our study showed that FM did not exert a significantly greater effect on RBC aggregation than native Fgn. This result is not in accordance with those of other Authors (19) who found a significant correlation between the level of SFMC and the erythrocyte sedimentation rate.

The present study shows that plasmin and thrombin Fgn degradation products have specific rheologic properties that may greatly differ from those of the parent molecule and may be relevant in clinical situations.

References

1. Harkness, J. 1981. Measurement of Plasma Viscosity. In: Clinical Aspects of Blood Viscosity and Cell Deformability. (G.D.O. Lowe, J.C. Barbenel and C.D. Forbes, eds.). Springer-Verlag, Berlin Heidelberg New York. pp 79-87.

2. Chien, S., S. Usami, R.J. Dellenback, M.I. Gregersen. 1970. Shear-dependent interaction of plasma proteins with erythrocytes in blood rheology. Am. J. Physiol. 219 , 143-153.

3. Wells, R.E., T.H. Gawronski, P.J. Cox, R.D. Perera. 1964. Influence of fibrinogen on flow properties of erythrocyte suspension. Am. J. Physiol. 207 , 1035-1040.

4. Dormandy, J.A., E. Hoare, A.M. Khattab, D.E. Arrowsmith, T.L. Dormandy. 1973. Prognostic significance of rheological and biochemical findings in patients with intermittent claudication. Br. Med. J. 4 , 581-583.

5. Pilgeram, L.O. 1974. Abnormalities in clotting and thrombolysis as a risk factor for stroke. Thromb. Diath. Haemorrh. 31 , 245-264.

6. Clayton, J.K., J.A. Anderson, G.P. McNicol. 1976. Preoperative prediction of postoperative deep vein thrombosis. Br. Med. J. 2 , 910-912.

7. Meade, T.W., R. Chakrabarti, A.P. Haines, W.R.S. North, Y. Stirling, S.G. Thompson, M. Brozovic. 1980. Haemostatic function and cardiovascular death; early results of a prospective study. Lancet ii ,1050-1054.

8. Huestis, D.W., J.R. Bove, S. Busch. 1978. Practical Blood Transfusion. 2nd edition. Little, Brown and Company Boston. p 66.

9. Belitser, V.A., T.V. Varetskaja, G.V. Malneva. 1968. Fibrinogen-fibrin interaction. Biochim. Biophys. Acta 154 , 367-375.

10. Breen, F.A. and J.L. Tullis. 1968. Ethanol gelation: A rapid screening test for intravascular coagulation. Ann. Int. Med. 69 , 1197-1206.

11. Seaman, A.J. 1970. The recognition of intravascular clotting: The plasma protamine paracoagulation test. Arch. Intern. Med.

125 ,1016-1021.

12. Clauss, A. 1957. Gerinnungsphysiologische schnellmethode zur bestmmung des fibrinogens. Acta Haematologica 17, 237-246.

13. Fahraeus, R. 1958. The influence of rouleau formation of erythrocytes on the rheology of blood. Acta Med. Scand. 161 , 151-165.

14. Marsh, N.A. 1979. The acelerating effect of fibrinogen and early fibrinogen degradation products on erythrocyte sedimentation. Thrombos. Haemostas. 42 , 757-763.

15. Rampling, M.A. and J.A. Sirs. 1977. Fibrinogen, fibrinogen degradation products and erythrocyte flexibility. Thrombos. Haemostas. 38 , 668-676.

16. Dormandy, J.A. 1980. Blood Viscosity and Red Cell Deformability. In: Methods in Angiology (M. Verstraete ed.) Martinus Nijhoff, The Hague/Boston/London. pp.214-266.

17. Stuart, J. and M.W. Kenny. 1980. Blood rheology. J. Clin. Pathol. 33 , 417-429.

18. Graf, C. and J.P. Barras. 1979. Rheological properties of human blood plasma - A comparison of measurements with three different viscometers. Experientia 35 , 224-225.

19. Lipinski, B., K. Worowski, M. Mysliwiec, R. Farbiszewski. 1969. Erythrocyte sedimentation and soluble fibrin monomer complexes. Thromb. Diath. Haemorrh. 21 , 196-202.

BINDING OF HUMAN FIBRINOGEN TO STREPTOCOCCI AND ITS ROLE IN STREPTOCOCCAL PATHOGENICITY

G.S. Chhatwal and H. Blobel

Institut für Bakteriologie und Immunologie, Justus Liebig-Universität,
Frankfurter Strasse 107, 6300 Giessen, Federal Republic of Germany

Introduction

Several species of gram-positive cocci possess on their surface specific binding sites for fibrinogen (1,2,3). Human fibrinogen interacts with pathogenic staphylococci, causing their clumping (1,4). Besides staphylococci, pathogenic streptococci of various serological groups have the capacity to interact with fibrinogen (5,6,7). The binding sites on group A streptococci which are pathogenic for human beings, have been identified as streptococcal M protein (2). The significance of interactions between fibrinogen and streptococci increased after M protein was shown to be associated with the virulence of group A streptococci (8). M protein inhibits phagocytosis of group A streptococci, thus permitting multiplication of these organisms in the absence of specific antibody (9). Streptococci lacking M protein activate complement via the alternate pathway leading to opsonization and phagocytosis (10,11). It has recently been shown that the interaction of fibrinogen with M protein enhances the resistance of group A streptococci to opsonization by inhibiting the fixation of the third component of complement on the bacterial surface (12). Although most group B, C, G, U and L streptococci lack M protein, they possess surface structures capable of binding fibrinogen (3,13). It is not yet known whether these binding sites also play a role in streptococcal pathogenicity. In the present study we characterized the binding of fibrinogen and its monomer chains to selected cultures of pathogenic streptococci. We also investigated the effects of fibrinogen binding on C3 fixation with streptococcal strains belonging to serological groups A, B, C, G, U and L.

Material and Methods

Streptococci: Of the 47 streptococcal cultures 8 belonged to serological group A, 8 to group B, 14 to group C, 10 to group G, 4 to group U and 3 to group L. Of the 14

Fibrinogen - Fibrin Formation and Fibrinolysis, Vol. 4
© 1986 Walter de Gruyter & Co., Berlin · New York - Printed in Germany.

group C cultures 5 were S.dysgalactiae, 5 S.equi and 4 S.zooepidemicus. Twenty-one cultures of Staphylococcus aureus were included for comparative studies.

Fibrinogen and the monomer chains. Human fibrinogen (Deutsche Kabi, Munich, FRG) was purified by affinity chromatography on gelatine-sepharose followed by gel filtration on Sephacryl S-300. The carboxymethylatet fibrinogen was separated into α, β and γ-chains by high-performance liquid chromatography according to method of Kehl et al. (14).

Binding assay: Fibrinogen as well as monomer chains were radiolabelled with ^{125}I, using the chloramin T method (15). The binding assay was performed with 0.2 μg labelled protein and 2 x 10^8 streptococci in 0.2 ml phosphate buffered saline, pH 7.5 containing 0.05% Tween 20 and 0.1% serum albumin (16).

Quantitation of C3 fixation: The amount of C3 fixed on the surface of streptococci during opsonization was determined by quantitative fluorescent immunoassay (17,18). The streptococci opsonized in normal or inactivated serum (56°C, 30 min) were washed in PBS and suspended in 1:40 PBS-dilution of anti-human-C3-serum conjugated with fluorescein isothiocyanate (Nordic Immunology, Tilburg, Netherlands) for 30 min at room temperature. The streptococci were washed again in PBS and resuspended in 2.5 ml of 0.1 N NaOH for dissocation of the fluorescein. The intensity of fluorescein in the supernatant was measured in a spectrofluorometer with excitation and emmission wavelengths of 485 and 525 nm respectively. The results were expressed as percentages of C3 fixation ranging from 0 (control of bacteria opsonized with buffer alone) to 100% (maximal emission intensity in the series tested) which correlates directly with the amount of C3 bound to the bacteria (18). In inhibition experiments the streptococci were pre-treated with fibrinogen for 1 h at room temperature before incubation with serum for opsonization. The streptococci were trypsinized as described previously (16), in order to determine the effects of trypsinization on C3 fixation.

Results

Binding of fibrinogen and its chains: All 8 group A streptococcal cultures interacted with fibrinogen, 4 of these with high binding activities (mean of 78%). Among 8 group B streptococcal cultures 4 showed moderate (mean 39%) and the others weak or no binding activities. Of the group C cultures S.equi did not interact with fibrinogen

S.dysgalactiae cultures bound fibrinogen weakly and S.zooepidemicus strongly. The streptococcal cultures of group G and U bound fibrinogen strongly and those of group L moderately (fig. 1).

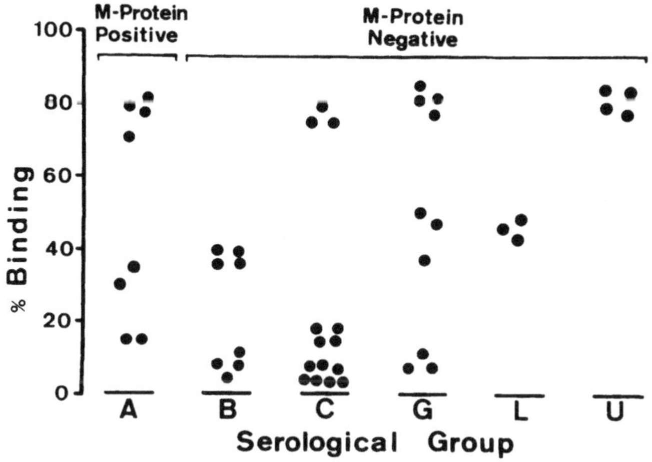

Figure 1: Binding of ^{125}I-labelled fibrinogen to streptococcal cultures belonging to various serological groups. Binding-activity is expressed as percent of total radioactivity bound. 100% was 34,000 cpm. Each point represents a mean of duplicates for 1 streptococcal culture.

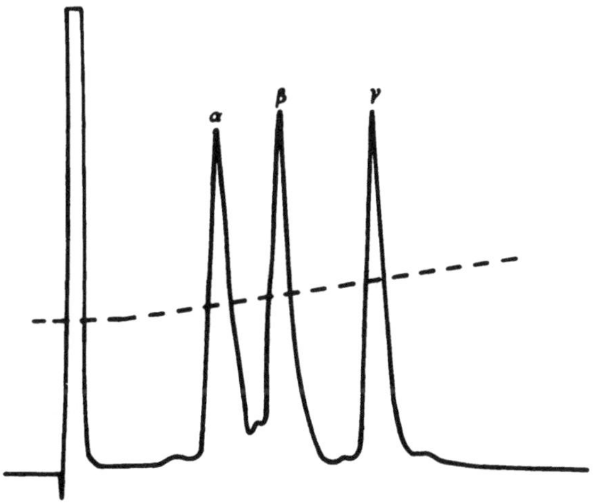

Figure 2: High-performance liquid chromatography of human S-(carboxymethyl) fibrinogen on a Vydac TPRP 10 column using 0.1% trifluoroacetic acid and acetonitrile gradient (36-48%) for elution.

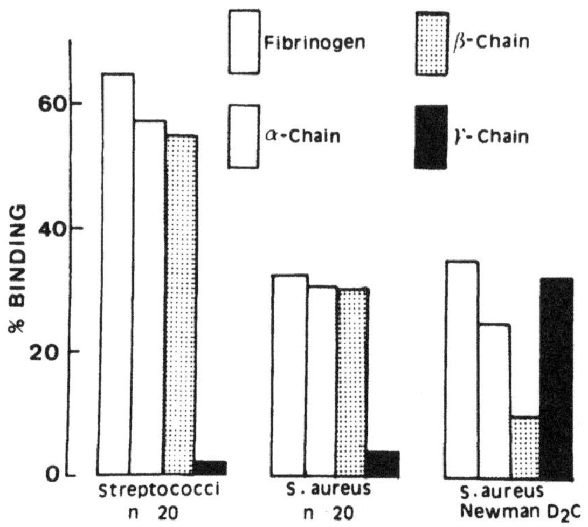

Figure 3: Binding of human fibrinogen and its chains to streptococci of various serological groups and selected cultures of S.aureus.

Human S-(carboxymethyl) fibrinogen could be separated into Aα-, Bβ- and γ-chains by high performance liquid chromatography (fig. 2). Analysis with radiolabelled chains revealed the binding of only α- and β-chains to all streptococcal and staphylococcal cultures tested, but not that of γ-chain. Only S.aureus strain Newman D_2C bound γ-chain (fig. 3).

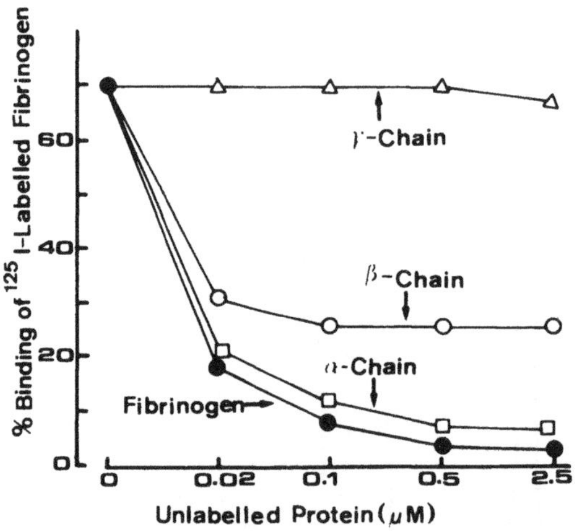

Figure 4: Inhibition of ^{125}I-labelled fibrinogen binding to streptococcal strains 281 A and 290 G by increasing concentrations of unlabelled fibrinogen and its chains. Each point is the means from 2 strains.

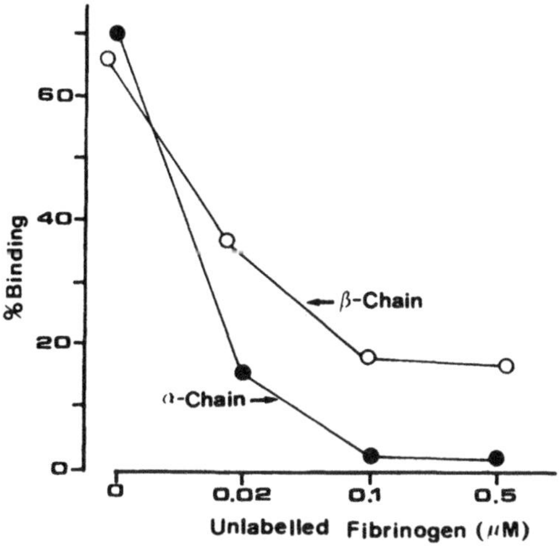

Figure 5: Inhibiton of ^{125}I-labelled α- and β-chains binding to streptococcal strains 281 A and 290 G by increasing concentrations of unlabelled fibrinogen. Each point is the means from 2 strains.

The bindings of fibrinogen and its α- and β-chains to streptococci were saturable and specific. The binding sites had a high sensitivity to trypsin indicating their protein nature. Other plasma proteins such as albumin, IgG, fibronectin, α_2-macroglobulin and haptoglobin (all of which also bound to some streptococci) did not influence the binding of fibrinogen and its chains. The binding of fibrinogen to streptococci could be completely inhibited by α-chain and moderately by β-chain, γ-chain had no influence (fig. 4). Similarly, the bindings of α- and to a large extent that of β-chain to streptococci were inhibited by unlabelled fibrinogen (fig. 5). Detailed analysis of bindings revelaed that both α-chain and whole fibrinogen bound to the same streptococcal sites with similar affinity. The dissociation constant (K_d) for both was in the range of 10^{-10} M. The number of binding sites approximated 19000. Sensitivities towards trypsin (IC_{50}-values) were in the same range for fibrinogen and α-chain. Both could be mutually displaced (table 1).

Table 1: Binding of Fibrinogen and α-Chain to Streptococcal Strain 290 G

Protein	K_d (M)	Binding sites (n)	IC_{50}*		
			Trypsin (μg)	Fibrinogen (nM)	α-chain (nM)
Fibrinogen	1.19×10^{-10}	18500	1.45	18	17
α-chain	1.3×10^{-10}	19140	1.12	20	15

*concentration required for 50% inhibition of binding

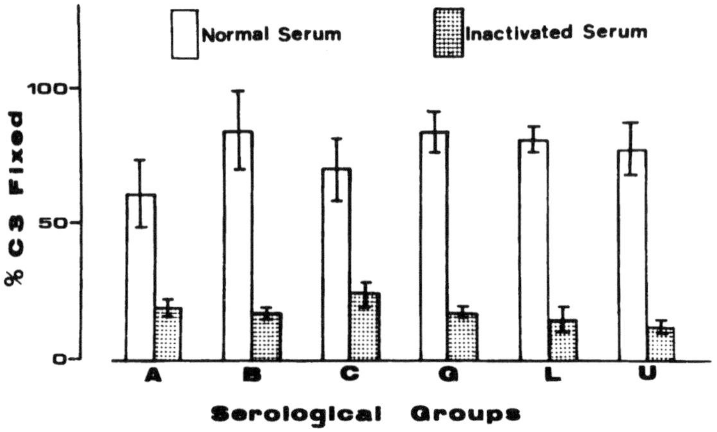

Figure 6: Intensity of C3-specific fluorescence on 4 x 10^8 streptococci after incubation with normal and heat-inactivated serum. The values indicate means and ranges of 8 group A-, 8 group B-, 14 group C-, 10 group G-, 3 group L- and 4 group U- streptococcal cultures.

Influence of fibrinogen binding on C3 fixation: All streptococcal cultures fixed C3 in normal serum with mean values between 69% and 90%. In heated (30 min, 56°C) serum the extent of fixation was much lower (fig. 6). Preincubation of bacteria with fibrinogen inhibited fixation of C3. Inhibition was proportional to the extent of fibrinogen binding. With strongly fibrinogen-positive cultures fixation of C3 was almost completely inhibited. Moderately fibrinogen-positive streptococci showed a less pronounced inhibition of C3 fixation after incubation with fibrinogen. There was no significant inhibition of C3 fixation with fibrinogen-negative cultures (fig. 7). This relationship between the extent of fibrinogen binding and the inhibition of C3 fixation was also observed in S.pyogenes strains with T4 antigens. Treatment of streptococci with trypsin resulted in a complete loss of fibrinogen binding activity, but it did not alter C3 fixation. Thus, trypsin-treated fibrinogen-positive streptococci, even after their incubation with fibrinogen, showed no reduction in C3 fixation (fig. 8). The streptococci with species-specific pathogenicity showed a higher binding affinity for fibrinogen from the susceptible species (table 2). In equimolar concentrations α-chain inhibited C3 fixation much less than whole fibrinogen (fig. 9). This could possibly be explained by the difference of their molecular weight.

Table 2: Binding of Human, Bovine and Equine Fibrinogen to Streptococci with Species-Specific Pathogenicity

Streptococcus Species	Origin	K_d (M)		
		Human Fibrinogen	Bovine Fibrinogen	Equine Fibrinogen
S.pyogenes	Human	2.3×10^{-10}	3.1×10^{-7}	6.1×10^{-6}
S.dysgalactiae	Bovine	1.2×10^{-6}	4.2×10^{-11}	8.2×10^{-6}
S.equi	Equine	2.6×10^{-7}	8.2×10^{-6}	9.6×10^{-9}

Representative of 5 experiments. The values are means of 6 strains from each species.

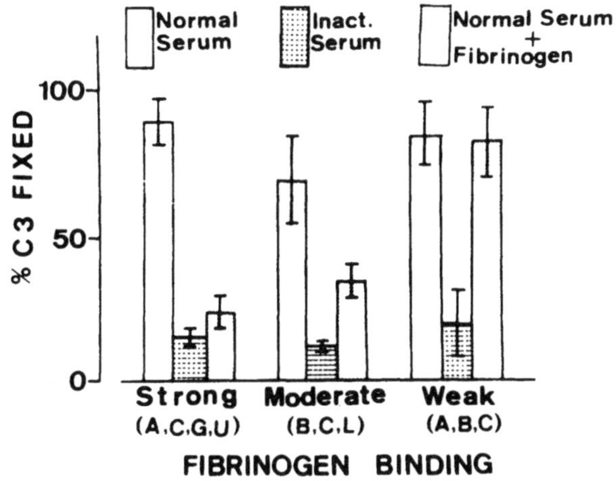

Figure 7: Effects of fibrinogen (100 µg) on fixation of C3 to 4×10^8 streptococci with strong (more than 60%), moderate (20-40%) and weak (less than 10%) fibrinogen binding-activities. The values are means and ranges from selected strains of various serological groups mentioned in parenthesis.

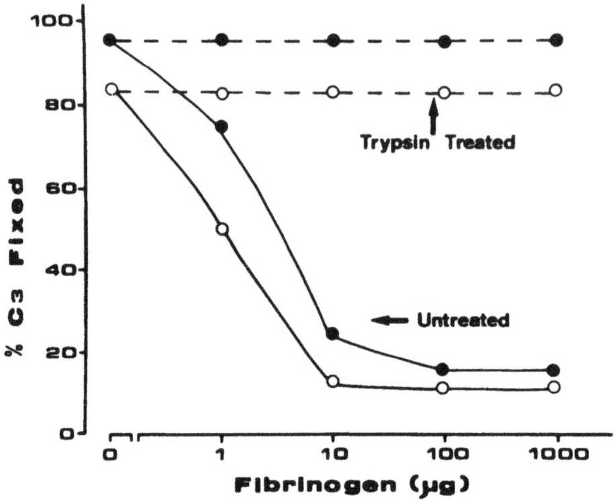

Figure 8: Influence of fibrinogen on C3 fixation to untreated (——) and trypsin-treated (- - - -) streptococcal strains 290 G (●) and K 8 (○).

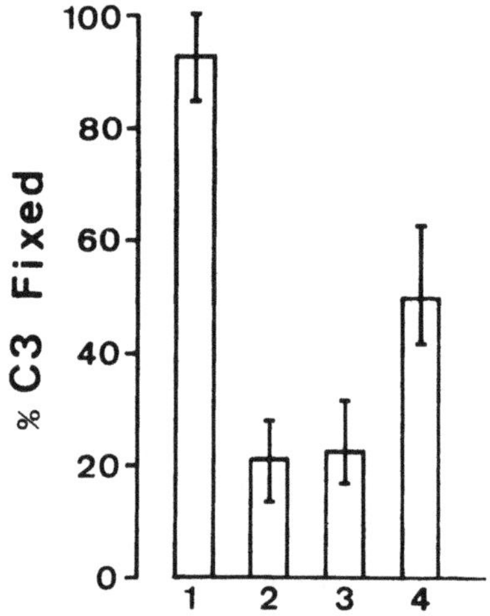

Figure 9: Influence of fibrinogen and its α-chain on C3 fixation to streptococci. The values are means and ranges from 8 fibrinogen-positive cultures belonging to groups A, C and G. 1 = normal serum; 2 = inactivated serum; 3 = serum + fibrinogen; 4 = serum + α-chain.

Discussion

Surface structures of certain streptococci interact specifically with mammalian proteins, leading to unexpected intrusions into common pathways of mammalian reactivities (19). These interactions might play an important role in host-parasite relation. The fibrinogen binding structures of group A streptococci had been identified as M protein (2). In these studies fibrinogen binding sites could be detected on streptococci of serological groups B, C, G, U and L. Monomer chains were used to identify the binding region of the fibrinogen molecule. With S.aureus strain Newman D_2C Hawiger et al. (20) identified the γ-chain as binding region of human fibrinogen. In our studies all streptococcal and staphylococcal strains did not bind the γ-chain of fibrinogen, except strain Newman D_2C. Analysis and kinetics of our studies revealed identical binding sites for fibrinogen and its α-chain.

M protein, located with lipoteichoic acids in the fimbriae of group A streptococci (21,22) appeared to inhibit activation of complement by the alternate pathway and thus delay phagocytosis (10,11). The lack of complement activation could possibly be attributed to an interaction of fibrinogen with M protein (12). M protein, however, has been found only in streptococci of group A and rarely in those of group G (8,23). Most of group B, C, G, L and U streptococci have no M protein, but bind fibrinogen. Thus, it was of interest to study the effects of fibrinogen binding to these strains on streptococcal pathogenicity. Fixation of C3 served as a marker for pathogenicity, since it has been shown to facilitate phagocytosis (18).

Fixation of C3 was observed in all streptococcal test cultures. Inhibition of C3 fixation by fibrinogen, however, occured only in fibrinogen-positive and not in fibrinogen-negative streptococci. The degree of inhibition of C3 fixation was determined by the extent of fibrinogen binding and not by M protein. Treatment of streptococci with trypsin destroyed their capacity to bind fibrinogen, but also the ability of fibrinogen to inhibit C3 fixation. It was noteworthy that streptococci with certain host-specificity showed much higher affinities for fibrinogen of the respective susceptible species. The inhibition of C3 fixation on the bacterial surface by fibrinogen could possibly be explained by a masking effect. The larger fibrinogen molecule, because of their molecular size, blocked much more of the bacterial surface than the smaller α-chain, although both have most likely identical binding sites.

Acknowledgement

This research was supported by a grant from Deutsche Forschungsgemeinschaft, Bonn, FRG. We are grateful to Dr. Agnes Henschen of Max Planck-Institut, Martinsried, for her help in the fractionation of fibrinogen by HPLC.

References

1. Duthie, E.S. 1955. J. Gen. Microbiol. 13, 383.

2. Kantor, F.S. 1965. J. Exp. Med. 121, 848.

3. Kronvall, G., C. Schönbeck, E. Myhre. 1979. Acta Pathol. Microbiol. Scand. (B) 87, 303.

4 Lewis, J.H., J.H. Wilson. 1973. Thromb. Res. 3, 419.

5. Yoshida, K., M. Takahasi, T. Ohtomo, Y. Usui, S. Narikawa. 1979. J. Infect. Dis. 139, 242.

6. Lämmler, C., G.S. Chhatwal, H. Blobel. 1983. Med. Microbiol. Immunol. 172, 149.

7. Chhatwal, G.S., C. Lämmler, H. Blobel. 1984. Med. Microbiol. Immunol. 173, 19.

8. Fox, E.N. 1974. Bact. Rev. 38, 57.

9. Lancefield, R.C. 1962. J. Immunol. 89, 307.

10. Bisno, A.L. 1979. Infect. Immun. 26, 1172.

11. Peterson, P.K., D. Schmeling, P.P. Cleary, B.J. Wilkinson, Y. Kim, P.G. Quie. 1979. J. Infect. Dis. 139, 575.

12. Whitnack, E., E.H. Beachey. 1982. J. Clin. Invest. 69, 1042.

13. Lämmler, C., G.S. Chhatwal, H. Blobel. 1983. Med. Microbiol. Immunol. 172, 191.

14. Kehl, M., F. Lottspeich, A. Henschen. 1982. Hoppe-Seyler's Z. Physiol. Chem. 363, 1501.

15. Hunter, W.H., F.C. Greenwood. 1962. Nature (London) 194, 495.

16. Chhatwal, G.S., H.P. Müller, H. Blobel. 1983. Infect. Immun. 41, 959.

17. Gillis, T.P., J.J. Thompson. 1978. J. Clin. Microbiol. 7, 202.

18. Verbrugh, H.A., V.C. van Dijk, M.E. van Arne, R. Peters, P.K. Peterson, J. Verhoef. 1979. Infect. Immun. 26, 808.

19. Kronvall, G., R.C. Williams. 1969. Ann. Intern. Med. 70, 1043.

20. Hawiger, J., S. Timmons, D.D. Strong, B.A. Cottrell, M. Riley, R.F. Doolittle. 1982. Biochemistry 21, 1407.

21. Swanson, J., K.C. Hsu, E.C. Gotschlich. 1969. J. Exp. Med. 130, 1063.

22. Beachey, E.H., I. Ofek. 1976. J. Exp. Med. 143, 759.

23. Maxted, W.R., E.V. Potter. 1967. J. Gen. Microbiol. 49, 119.

VI. Assays to Fibrin(ogen) Fragments and their Use

DISCRIMINATION BETWEEN FIBRIN AND FIBRINOGEN BY A MONOCLONAL ANTIBODY AGAINST A SYNTHETIC HEXAPEPTIDE REPRESENTING THE AMINO-TERMINUS OF THE ALPHA-CHAIN OF FIBRIN

U. Scheefers-Borchel, G. Müller-Berghaus

Clinical Research Unit for Blood Coagulation and Thrombosis of the Max-Planck-Gesellschaft at the Justus-Liebig-Universität, Giessen, W.-Germany

P. Fuhge, N. Heimburger

Behringwerke AG, Marburg, W.-Germany

Introduction

Blood coagulation is reflected by the transformation of the soluble plasma protein fibrinogen to an insoluble and visible fibrin clot. This final step in the coagulation process is catalysed by thrombin sequentially splitting off one pair of fibrinopeptides A (FPA) and one pair of fibrinopeptides B (FPB) from one fibrinogen molecule (1,2,3). By cleaving off FPA from the A α-chains of fibrinogen, polymerisation sites of the generated fibrin monomer (desAA-fibrin) become available (4,5,6). DesAA-fibrin may polymerise to a clot but can also form soluble intermediates (7,8) which have been identified in the circulating blood with patients (9,10,11) and animals (12,13). We produced a monoclonal antibody against the synthetic hexapeptide Gly-Pro-Arg-Val-Val-Glu representing the amino-terminus of the α-chain of fibrin. This antibody can be used to quantify fibrin in the presence of fibrinogen in blood.

Results

The hexapeptide Gly-Pro-Arg-Val-Val-Glu representing the amino-terminus of the α-chain of fibrin was synthesised using conventional procedures of fragment condensation (14,15). To obtain an optimally exposed position of the hexapeptide, ε-aminocaproic

Fibrinogen - Fibrin Formation and Fibrinolysis, Vol. 4
© 1986 Walter de Gruyter & Co., Berlin · New York - Printed in Germany.

acid was used as a spacer. The purity of the hexapeptide was evaluated by thin layer chromatography, and the racemisation was tested by gas chromatography (16). The racemisation rate of each amino acid was less than 2%. The spacer-coupled hexapeptide was activated with DDC in the presence of hydroxysuccinimide, and then reacted with albumin (17). BALB/c mice were immunised with the carrier bound synthetic hexapeptide. The majority of sera of immunised mice showed a positive immune response against the unconjugated peptide and desAA- and desAABB-fibrin as well, but did not demonstrate an immune response to fibrinogen. Spleens of mice whose sera showed the strongest immune reponse to fibrin and no reponse to fibrinogen were chosen to generate hybridomas. Spleen cells were fused with x63-SP8-653 myeloma cells (a non-producer line, kindly provided by Dr. T. Tamura) using polyethylene glycol (M_r = 3,400) as described by Köhler & Milstein (18). Out of 31 hybridomas 18 clones showed an immune response to desAA-fibrin but not to fibrinogen. Subcloned hybridoma populations (n = 14), whose supernatants showed the strongest anti-fibrin reaction, were chosen for the production of monoclonal antibodies in ascitic fluid of Pristane primed BALB/c mice.

Selection of a fibrin specific antibody

Different purified antibodies obtained were tested by treating human plasma with thrombin or batroxobin, respectively.The concentrations of these enzymes were chosen so low that the plasma did not clot within two minutes. All the monoclonal antibodies showed a positive reaction with plasma treated with thrombin or batroxobin, whereas only a weak reaction was observed with control plasma not treated with these enzymes. The antibody with the highest anti-fibrin response was chosen for all further experiments and is designated anti-fbn 17.

In a purified system, anti-fbn 17 showed the following characteristics. It did not react with fibrinogen and bovine serum albumin (BSA), the carrier protein to which the peptide was coupled, but it reacted with desAA-fibrin with des AABB-fibrin and with the unconjugated fibrin specific hexapeptide (Table 1).

Table 1: Specificity of the monoclonal anti-fibrin antibody 17 tested in a purified system. From: Scheefers-Borchel et al. (19).

Fibrinogen	desAA-Fibrin	desAABB-Fibrin	BSA	Hexapeptide
(A_{414})	(A_{414})	(A_{414})	(A_{414})	(A_{414})
0.061	1.298	0.873	0.05	1.096

Polystyrene microtitre plates were coated with different antigens.Fibrin-specific antibodies were identified by ELISA.

Sensitivity and Specificity in Plasma

The ability of anti-fbn 17 to recognise fibrin in plasma which had been treated with thrombin or batroxobin, respectively, is demonstrated in Figure 1.

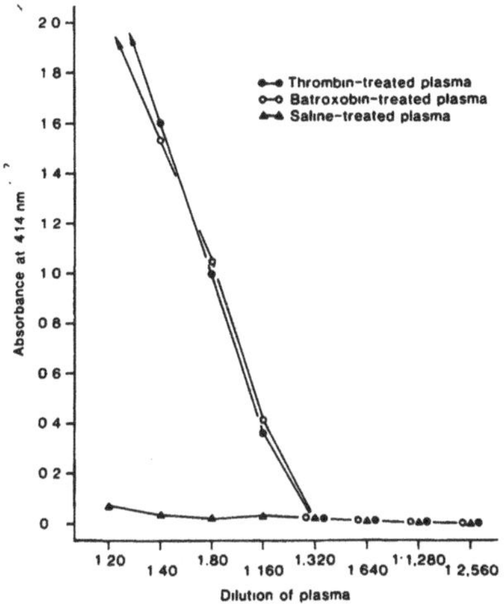

Fig. 1: Detection of fibrin by the monoclonal anti-fibrin antibody (anti-fbn 17) in plasma treated with thrombin (●) or batroxobin (O), respectively, tested by ELISA. To measure the amount of fibrin bound a polyclonal peroxydase-conjugated rabbit anti-fibrinogen antibody was added. Peroxydase activity was assessed by adding hydrogen peroxide and 2.2-azino-di (3-ethylbenzthiazoline sulfonic acid). Control plasma (▲) was treated with isotonic saline. Thrombin or batroxobin was added to plasma at a final concentration of 0.4 U/ml or 0.1 U/ml, respectively. Enzyme-treated plasma was incubated for 2 min or 4 min, respectively. Coagulation was interrupted by adding PBS containing 5 mM EDTA, 2 mM EACA, 200 KIU/ml aprotinin to give a final dilution of 1:20. From: Scheefers-Borchel et al (19).

Fibrin could be measured even in the presence of fibrinogen and in the presence of other plasma components. Fibrinolytic degradation products generated by incubating purified fibrinogen with plasminogen and urokinase did not show any immunoreactivity with anti-fbn 17. Control plasma samples only showed a negligible reaction with anti-fbn 17. This minor reaction indicate small amounts of fibrin present in plasma also under physiological conditions. This observation is in a agreement with findings indicating small amounts of FPA in plasma under physiological conditions.

To test the reactivity of anti-fbn 17, known concentrations of desAA-fibrin in PBS, 3 M urea, were added to plasma, and this mixture was diluted for testing (Fig. 2).

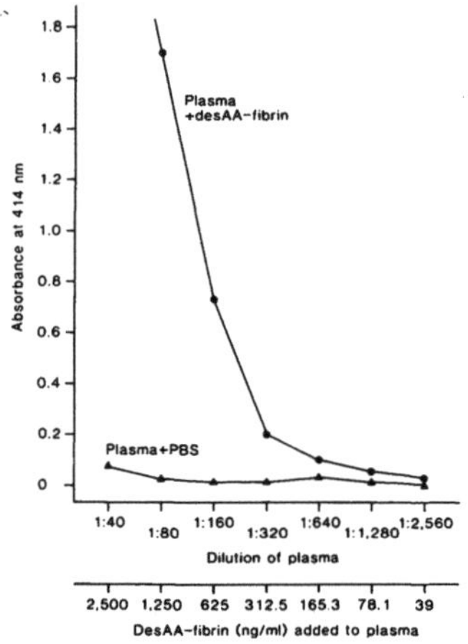

Fig. 2: Detection of purified desAA-fibrin added to plasma (●). In order to test the reactivity of the anti-fbn 17 antiserum towards known concentrations of desAA-fibrin, 20 µl of purified desAA-fibrin containing in PBS, 2.6 M urea were added to 180 µl of anticoagulant plasma to give a final concentration of 100 µg desAA-fibrin/ml. In the control (▲), PBS, 2.6 M urea was added to plasma. Thereafter, the samples were diluted with PBS, 5 mM EDTA, 2 mM EACA, 200 KIU/ml aprotinin, 0.2% Tween 20 and incubated in 96 well microtitre plates coated with anti-fbn 17. The abscissa gives the concentrations of desAA-fibrin contained at different dilutions. From: Scheefers-Borchel et al (19).

When this mixture of fibrin and plasma was further diluted, fibrin could be detected in the presence of fibrinogen concentrations being 20 times higher than those of fibrin up to 78 ng/ml of fibrin.

Determination of Soluble Fibrin in Blood

To determine soluble fibrin in blood, blood was drawn from volunteers and kept in polystyrene test tubes at 37°C without adding any anticoagulants. At different time intervals subsamples were removed and on-going coagulation was interrupted by the addition of an anticoagulant solution. After removing blood cells by centrifugation the obtained plasma was diluted and the presence of fibrin measured by ELISA (Fig. 3).

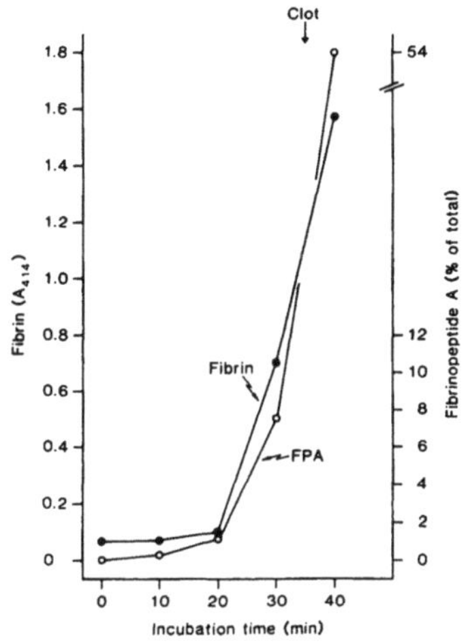

Fig. 3: Increase in fibrin (●) and fibrinopeptide (FPA) (○) concentrations in blood undergoing coagulation. Fibrin generated in blood was determined in diluted plasma samples by ELISA on microtitre plates coated with anti-fbn 17. FPA was measured according to Nossel et al (20) using a commercially available test kit from Mallinckrodt, St. Louis, MO, USA.
From: Scheefers- Borchel et al (19).

Fibrin could not be detected by anti-fbn 17 up to 20 minutes after drawing the blood. At 30 minutes and 40 minutes, a 12-fold and a 30-fold, respectively, increase in fibrin concentration was measured. This increase in fibrin concentration goes in parallel with the increase in FPA concentration. Visible fibrin strands could only be detected in the 40-minute sample. This experiment indicates that soluble fibrin generated in blood in the absence of an anticoagulant can be recognised by the monoclonal antibody anti-fbn 17.

Discussion

The monoclonal antibody used was produced to a synthetic hexapeptide representing the amino-terminus of the human α-chain of fibrin. This antibody was produced to a hexapeptide whose amino-acid sequence is hidden within the fibrinogen molecule and becomes the amino-terminus of the α-chain of fibrin after splitting off the fibrinopeptides A from the fibrinogen molecule. This approach may be a new general strategy to differentiate an activated protein from its unactivated precursor form by means of immunological methods.
The defined epitope of the α-chain of fibrin was selected, as mainly desAA-fibrin and not desAABB-fibrin is found in the circulating blood of patients with on-going intravascular coagulation (21,22). The fibrinopeptide B is assigned to be only cleaved from desAA-fibrin if it has polymerised to a fibrin clot (3). For these reasons an antibody directed to the amino-terminus of the α-chain of desAA-fibrin seems to be the ideal antibody for detecting soluble fibrin. Vice versa the antibody to the β-chain of desAABB-fibrin (23) will not recognise soluble fibrin. The antibody described can be used to measure fibrin in the presence of fibrinogen in blood of patients with intravascular coagulation. The detection and localisation of thrombi using this antibody would be of considerable clinical importance.

Acknowledgement

We thank Andrea Michel for excellent technical assistance and Dr. Teruko Tamura for providing myeloma cells for fusing. This work was supported by the Stiftung Volkswagenwerk, Hannover.

References

1. Bettelheim, F.R. 1956. Biochim.Biophys.Acta 19, 121.

2. Blombäck, B., A. Vestermark. 1958. Ark.Kemi 12, 173.

3. Blombäck, B., B. Hessel, D. Hogg, L. Therkildsen. 1978. Nature 275, 501.

4. Ferry, J.D. 1954. Physiol.Rev. 34, 753.

5. Laurent, T.C., B. Blombäck. 1958. Acta Chem.Scand. 12, 1875.

6. Kudryk, B.J., D. Collen, K.R. Woods, B. Blombäck. 1974. J.Biol.Chem. 249, 3322.

7. Shainoff, J.R., I.H. Page. 1962. J.Exp.Med. 116, 687.

8. Lipinski, B., Z. Wegrzynowicz, A.Z. Budzynski, M. Kopec, Z.S. Latallo, E. Kowalski. 1967. Thromb.Diath.Haemorrh. 17, 65.

9. Godal, H.C., U. Abildgaard. 1966. Scand.J.Haemat. 3, 342.

10. Fletcher, A.P., N. Alkjaersig, J. O'Brien, V.G. Tulevski. 1970. Trans.Assoc.Am.Physicians 83, 159.

11. Matthias, F.R., R. Reinicke, D.L. Heene. 1977. Thromb.Res. 10, 365.

12. Shainoff, J.R., I.H. Page. 1960. Circ. Res. 8, 1013.

13. Thomas, L., R.T. Smith, R. von Korff. 1954. Proc.Soc.Exp. Biol.Med. 86, 813.

14. Wünsch, E. (ed.). 1974. In: Methoden der organischen Chemie Thieme, Stuttgart.

15. Gross, G., J. Meienhofer (eds.). 1979. In: The Peptides 1, Major Methods of Peptide Bond Formation. Academic Press, New York.

16. Frank, H., G.J. Nicholson, E.J. Bayer. 1977. J.Chromatogr.Sci. 15, 174.

17. Weygand, F., D. Hoffmann, E.Z. Wünsch. Naturforschg. 21b, 426.

18. Köhler, G., C. Milstein. 1975. Nature 256, 495.

19. Scheefers-Borchel, U., G. Müller-Berghaus, P. Fuhge, R.Eberle, N. Heimburger. 1985. (Submitted for publication)

20. Nossel, H.L., I. Yudelman, R.E. Canfield, V.P. Butler, K. Spanondis, G.D. Wilner, G.D. Qureshi. 1974. J.Clin. Invest. 54, 43.

21. Kierulf, P., H.C. Godal. 1972. Scand.J.Haemat. 9, 370.

22. Nossel, H.L. 1981. Nature 291, 165.

23. Hui, K.Y., E. Haber, G.R. Matsueda. 1983. Science 222, 1129.

A NEW ENZYME IMMUNOASSAY OF FIBRIN(OGEN) DEGRADATION PRODUCTS IN PLASMA USING A MONOCLONAL ANTIBODY

J. Koopman, F. Haverkate, P. Koppert, W. Nieuwenhuizen, E.J.P. Brommer, W.G.C. van der Werf

Gaubius Institute, Health Research Division TNO, Herenstraat 5d, 2313 AD Leiden, The Netherlands.

Introduction

The determination of fibrinogen/fibrin degradation products (FDP) in serum is a well accepted procedure in the diagnosis of disseminated, and occasionally of local intravascular, coagulation (1). However, assays in serum carry the risk of falsely positive results, if residual fibrinogen in serum reacts with the antiserum used to detect FDP or, if lysis occurs during serum preparation. Falsely negative results can be expected during serum preparation, if particular degradation products, such as fragments X, coagulate or are adsorbed to the clot.

To overcome the disadvantages adherent to the use of serum, we determined FDP in plasma. As polyclonal antisera usually have low titres of the antibodies needed, monoclonal antibodies are required as they combine a high specificity with a high titre and can be produced in large amounts. Monoclonal antibodies reacting with the cross-linked fibrin D dimer fragment, but not with fibrinogen, have been used to determine fibrin degradation products in plasma (2,3). The present study describes an enzyme immunoassay (EIA) of FDP in plasma which is based on the use of monoclonal antibody (no. FDP-14) directed against a neoantigenic determinant (E_{neo}) exposed in fragment E after plasmin digestion of fibrin(ogen), but not in the parent molecule. The detailed characterization of the antibody no. FDP-14 has been described elsewhere (manuscript submitted). The present paper shows that the assay developed is specific for FDP and enables the detection of low levels of FDP in plasma.

Fibrinogen - Fibrin Formation and Fibrinolysis, Vol. 4
© 1986 Walter de Gruyter & Co., Berlin · New York - Printed in Germany.

Methods

Human fibrinogen (4), fibrin monomer (5) fibrinogen fragments X and Y (6,7), and fragment D_{cate} and E (8) were purified as described previously. Tissue-type plasminogen activator was purified from human melanoma cells (9).

Preparation of plasma, defibrinated plasma and serum

Human blood collected in plastic tubes containing 0.11 M sodium citrate solution (1 volume per 9 volumes of blood), was centrifuged at 2300 g for 20 min at 4°C. Plasma obtained was stored at -20°C. Serum was prepared from blood collected in glass tubes containing 1 NIH bovine thrombin per ml blood. After incubation for 2 h at 37°C, the clotted blood was centrifuged at 2300 g for 20 min at room temperature. The serum obtained was stored at -20°C. When plasma and serum were prepared in the presence of inhibitors, the tubes for blood collection contained in addition to citrate 2.0 vol.% of a solution containing 25 KIU trasylol/ml and 25 mg ε-aminocaproic acid (EACA)/ml. In order to prepare defibrinated plasma, we added to plasma 10 vol.% of a solution containing 50 NIH thrombin/ml, 10 KIU Trasylol/ml and 10 mg EACA/ml. The mixture was incubated for 30 min at 37°C and the fibrin clot formed was removed by centrifugation for 5 min at 10,000 g.

Immobilization of IgG from a pool of rabbit antisera against fibrin(ogen) and its plasmin degradation products

Several rabbit polyclonal antisera against human fibrinogen, fibrin monomer, fibrinogen fragments X, Y, D_{cate} and E and fibrin fragment D dimer (8) were pooled. Immunoglobulins (IgG) were isolated from the pool by precipitation with 18% (w/v) sodium sulphate (10). The isolated IgG were immobilized to CH activated Sepharose 4B using the manufacturer's guidelines (Pharmacia, Uppsala, Sweden).

Blood lysate

Whole blood was collected from a healthy volunteer in a plastic tube. After quick mixing with a solution of tissue-type plasminogen activator (final concentration 90 IU/ml) the contents were transferred to a glass tube containing thrombin (final concentration 1 NIH/ml). The tube was incubated at 37°C. After complete lysis (2 h) of the clot formed, Trasylol (final concentration 100 KIU/ml) and 1 vol.% of Diisopropylfluorophosphate (DFP) solution were added. After removal of cells by centrifugation at 2300 g for 20 min at room temperature, the supernantant, here designated as "blood lysate", was collected and stored at -20°C.

Isolation of FDP from blood lysate

One ml of the blood lysate was diluted 4 times with borate buffer and applied to the column of immobilized IgG prepared from a pool of antisera against fibrinogen and its fragments. The column (bed volume 2 ml) was washed successively with 100 ml of borate buffer, pH 7.4, with 20 ml of this buffer containing 0.5 M NaCl, and with 20 ml of ten-fold diluted borate buffer. FDP were eluted with 0.01 M NaOH, and the FDP solution obtained was immediately neutralized with 0.1 M HCl. After dialysis against distilled water and lyophilization, the FDP preparation was dissolved in 0.15 M NaCl (1,3 mg FDP/ml), and stored at -20°C.

Monoclonal Antibody

FDP from blood lysate were injected into mice. After a number of fusion experiments, a hybridoma cell line that secretes an antibody (No. FDP-14) reacting specifically with fragment E, but not with fibrin(ogen), was established. The antibody was purified by adsorption to Protein A Sepharose and subsequent elution according to Ey et al. (11). The selection and characterization are described in detail elsewhere.

Rabbit anti FDP conjugate

IgG were purified from the pool of rabbit antisera against fibrin(ogen) and its degradation products, using caprylic acid (12). The purified IgG were conjugated with Horse Radish Peroxidase (HPO) using SPDP as a bifunctional reagent (13), essentially as described by Pharmacia, Stockholm, Sweden.

FDP enzyme immunoassay

Coating of microtiter plates was achieved by adding 120 µl of a PBS (phosphate buffered saline, pH 7.4) solution containing 3 µg purified monoclonal antibodies (no. FDP 14) per ml to each well.

After incubation for at least 16 h at 4°C, the plates were washed three times immediately before use with PBS containing 0.05% Tween 20. From normal plasma or serum samples, serial dilutions were made starting with a two-fold dilution with PBS containing 0,2% Tween 20, further dilutions were made by diluting with PBS containing 0.1% Tween 20. From patients' samples a dilution series was made in PBS containing 0.1% Tween 20, starting with a 20-fold dilution. For routine analyses of patients' samples only 4 dilutions were made i.e. 1:20, 1:100, 1:500 and 1:2500. 100 µl of the sample to be tested was added to the plate. After incubation for 30 min at room temperature, the plate was washed three times with PBS containing 0.05% Tween 20. 100 µl anti-FDP conjugate diluted 1:500 with PBS containing 0.1% Tween 20 was added to each well of the plate. The plate was incubated for 30 min at room temperature and washed four times with PBS containing 0.05% Tween 20. Then 200 µl of a solution containing the HPO substrate hydrogen peroxide and TMB (14) were added to each well of the plate. After conversion of the substrate the reaction was stopped by adding 50 µl 2 M sulphuric acid which caused a color change from blue to yellow. The absorbance at 450 nm was read with a Titertek Multiscan (Flow Laboratories, Irvine, UK).
A_{450} values of the blanks of PBS containing 0.1% Tween 20, and treated similarly to the samples, ranged from 0.075 to 0.150. A calibration curve was made using a serial dilution of blood lysate (containing 2 mg FDP/ml) in PBS containing 0.1% Tween 20, starting with a 1000-fold dilution. The FDP concentration of the sample, after correction for the blank value, was read from the calibration curve. FDP values in plasma below 0.25 µg/ml were considered as normal.

Results

Specificity of the FDP Enzyme Immunoassay

To investigate the specificity of the EIA, we determined dose--response curves of fibrinogen, fibrin, blood lysate, and purified fibrinogen degradation products. The assay (Fig. 1) responds to low concentrations of lysate, and fibrinogen fragments X, Y, and E, but not or only slightly to fibrinogen, fibrin, or fragment D. Concentrations of fibrin monomers higher than 10 µg/ml could not be used due to polymerization of fibrin monomer. The optimum response of fragment E was lower than that of lysate, fragments X, and Y. The EIA is specific for a neoantigenic determinant in fragments X, Y and E (E_{neo}) which is exposed after plasmin digestion, but not present in the parent molecule.

Dose-response curves of blood lysate diluted in buffer and diluted in buffer containing 5% normal pooled plasma did not differ, which indicates that a large excess of fibrinogen (at a dilution of $1:10^5$ the ratio (w/w) fibrinogen/FDP amounts to 5000:1) does not disturb the determination of FDP in the EIA.

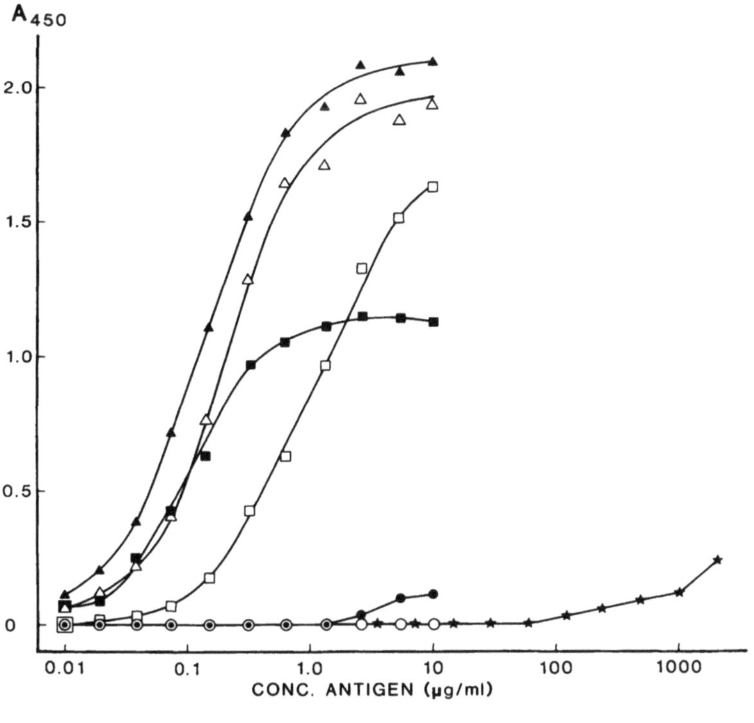

Fig. 1.

Semi-logarithmic dose-response curves obtained in the enzyme immunoassay (EIA) of blood lysate (▲), fibrinogen (*), fibrin monomer (●), fibrinogen fragment X (□), Y (△), D_{cate} (o), and E (■).

Expression of results

Comparison of responses of sample and reference material is allowed only when the straight parts of their semilogarithmic dose-response curves run parallel. Fig. 2 shows that the curves of plasma taken from 3 patients with disseminated intravascular coagulation, having widely differing FDP concentrations, run parallel with the reference curve. Furthermore, other patients' plasmas tested exhibited parallel curves.

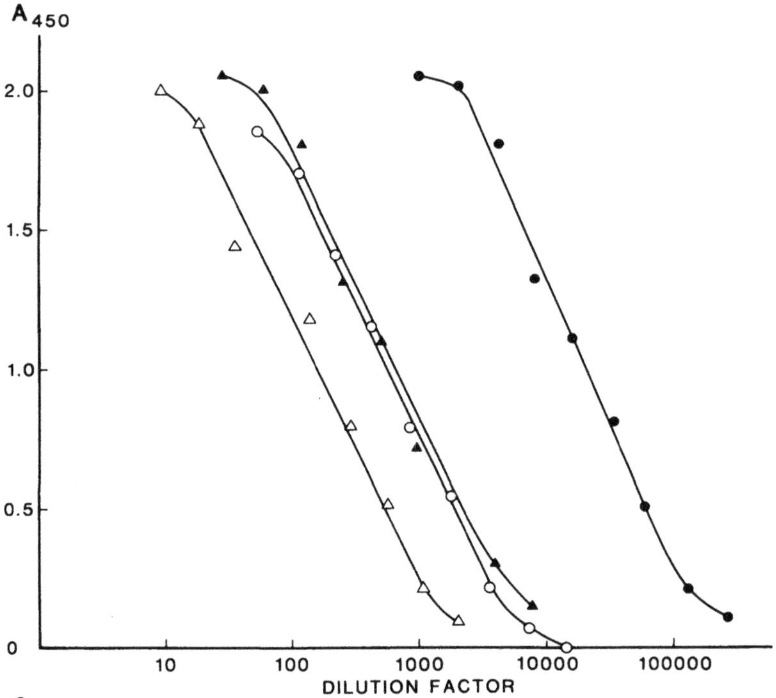

Fig. 2.
Dose-response curves obtained in the EIA of plasmas of patients (△,▲,o) with different FDP levels, as compared with the calibration curve (Blood Lysate) (●).

Normal values

FDP values of 8 normal individuals were determined in plasma and serum prepared both with and without the protease inhibitors Trasylol and EACA (Table 1). Values below 60 ng/ml might be less accurate as the corresponding response is not located on the straight part of the dose-response curve.

FDP values in patients' plasmas

a. Disseminated Intravascular Coagulation (DIC). Out of 28 plasma samples collected from 18 patients suspected of having DIC, 26 samples showed increased FDP levels in the EIA ranging from 0.6 to 137 µg/ml. Two samples had values below 0.25 µg/ml, defined here as "normal".

In order to investigate whether FDP in the patients' plasma can be captured in the clot during coagulation, we compared FDP values by the EIA in plasma and in plasma defibrinated by addition of thrombin. In 8 of the plasmas of the 28 patients studied (Table 2), we found a considerable decrease of FDP after defibrination, indicating loss of FDP with removal of the clot.

b. Thrombolytic therapy. We studied 4 patients who were admitted for acute myocardial infarction and treated within 4 hours with intracoronary streptokinase, 4000 U/minute for one hour. Blood samples were collected as soon as the patient arrived at the recovery room, i.e. about 2 h after the beginning of the therapy, and at various time intervals up to 20 h. FDP-levels were below 0.25 µg/ml on admission, but very high, ranging from 117 to 372 µg/ml, after thrombolytic therapy. The FDP disappeared from the patient's plasma with a half-time of approximately 5 h.

Table 1. FDP values (ng/ml) determined by the EIA in plasma and serum of 8 normal individuals. Blood was collected in the presence (+) and absence (-) of the inhibitors Trasylol and EACA.

	Plasma		Serum	
subject.no.	+	-	+	-
1	30	43	180	1100
2	32	48	44	1300
3	52	64	74	2400
4	42	52	48	400
5	46	58	50	1000
6	28	36	62	900
7	80	90	150	6800
8	40	40	32	60

Table 2. FDP values (µg/ml) of patients with suspected disseminated intravascular coagulation.

	Plasma	Defibrinated Plasma
1	2,1	1,1
2	137	27
3	5,6	2,0
4	0,8	0,25
5	0,6	0,25
6	2,3	1,0
7	1,0	0,25
8	2,0	1,0

Discussion

The choice of the immunogen i.e. a whole mixture of fibrin degradation products isolated from blood lysate, was based on the premise that such products may have a better chance of eliciting antibodies against FDP in the blood of patients than products prepared from purified fibrinogen. The hybridoma cell line selected produces antibodies which react specifically with a neoantigenic determinant in fragment E, exposed after plasmin digestion, but not in the parent fibrinogen molecule.

In conventional FDP assays, proteolytic activity during serum preparation should be suppressed by adding inhibitors such as Trasylol, EDTA, and EACA (15). Accordingly, serum of normal individuals prepared without inhibitors, showed highly elevated FDP values in our EIA of FDP (Table 1), whereas their serum prepared with inhibitors had values near those of their plasma. In normal plasma (Table 1) no significant differences were found between samples with and without inhibitors. In FDP assays, suppression of proteolytic activity is, therefore, more important in serum than in plasma. Even in serum prepared with inhibitors from 3 normal individuals (no. 1,6,7, Table 1), the FDP values were higher than those of their plasma prepared without inhibitors (Table 1). On the other hand, FDP formation might occur during preparation of plasma from patients with high proteolytic activity. We, therefore, advise to add inhibitors, also when using plasma samples.

The higher FDP values in normal serum (with inhibitors) as compared with those in plasma (no. 1,6,7 in Table I) indicate the risk of falsely positive results when using serum. The loss of FDP with removal of clots formed in patient's plasma (Table II) indicates the risk of falsely negative results when using serum.

Normal FDP values in plasma amounted to 30-90 ng/ml. It is not known whether these values should be ascribed to the occurrence of E_{neo} determinants in normal plasma, or to interference by non-specific factors.

The assay is sensitive to plasmin-induced split products of both fibrin and fibrinogen. After thrombolytic therapy for acute myocardial infarction, fibrinogen degradation can be expected. In DIC mainly fibrin degradation products will be found. Since our test detects split products of both fibrinogen and fibrin, it can be used in both cases and has, therefore, a wide field of application.

In conclusion, the quantitative assay developed has a low detection limit, and can be applied in plasma. It is a useful diagnostic tool in a wide variety of clinical diseases, and can be used to follow thrombolytic therapy.

Acknowledgements

We are indebted to Drs. J. Engbers and J. Stibbe for providing us with patients' samples.

References

1. Bick, R.L. 1982. The clinical significance of fibrinogen degradation products. Semin. Thromb. Haemostas. 8, 302-330.

2. Rylatt, D.B., A.S. Blake, L.E. Cottis, D.A. Massingham, W.A. Fletcher, P.P. Masci, A.N. Whitaker, M. Elms, I. Bunce, A.J. Webber, D. Wyatt and P.G. Bundesen. 1983. An immunoassay for human D dimer using monoclonal antibodies. Thromb. Res. 31, 767-778.

3. Soria, J., C. Soria, C. Boucheix, M. Mirshahi, J.Y. Perrot, A. Bernadou, M. Samama and Rosenfeld C.S. 1983. Monoclonal

antibodies that react preferentially with fibrinogen degradation products or with crosslinked fibrin split products. Ann. New York Acad. Sci. 408, 665-666.

4. Van Ruijven-Vermeer, I.A.M. and W. Nieuwenhuizen. 1978. Purification of rat fibrinogen and its constituent chains. Biochem. J. 169, 653-658.

5. Haverkate, F. and G. Timan G. 1976. In: Progress in Chemical Fibrinolysis and Thrombolysis, Vol 2, Davidson JF, Samama MM, and Desnoyers PC, eds. Raven Press, New York, pp. 67-71.

6. Nieuwenhuizen, W. and M. Gravesen. 1981. Anticoagulant and calcium-binding properties of high molecular weight derivatives of human fibrinogen produced by plasmin (fragments X). Biochim. Biophys. Acta 668, 81-88.

7. Nieuwenhuizen, W., M. Voskuilen and J. Hermans. 1982. Anticoagulant and calcium-binding properties of high-molecular weight derivatives of human fibrinogen (plasmin fragments Y). Biochim. Biophys. Acta 708, 313-316.

8. Van Ruijven-Vermeer, I.A.M., W. Nieuwenhuizen, F. Haverkate and G. Timan. 1979. A novel method for the rapid purification of human and rat fibrin (ogen) degradation products in high yields. Hoppe-Seyler's Z. Physiol. Chem. 360, 633-637.

9. Rijken, D.C., G. Wijngaards, M. Zaal de Jong and J. Welbergen. 1979. Purification and partial characterization of plasminogen activator from human uterine tissue. Biochim. Biophys. Acta 580, 140-153.

10. Keckwick, R.A. 1940. The serum proteins in multiple myelomatosis. Biochem. J. 34, 1248-1257.

11. Ey, P.L., S.J. Prowse and C.R. Jenkin. 1978. Isolation of pure IgG1, IgG2a, and IgG2b immunoglobulins from mouse serum using protein A-Sepharose. Immunochem. 15, 429-436.

12. Steinbuch, M., R. Audran. 1969. The isolation of IgG from mammalian sera with the aid of caprylic acid. Arch. Biochem. Biophys. 134, 279-284.

13. Carlsson, J., H. Drevin and R. Axen. 1978. Protein thiolation and reversible protein-protein conjugation. Biochem. J. 173, 723-737.

14. Bos, E.S., A.A. Van der Doelen, N. Van Rooy and A.H.W.M. Schuurs. 1981. 3,3',5,5'-Tetramethyl benzidine as an Ames test negative chromogen for horse-radish peroxidase in enzyme immunoassay. J. Immunoassay 2, 187-204.

15. Donati, M.B. 1975. Assays for fibrinogen-fibrin degradation products in biological fluids: some methodological aspects. Thromb. Diath. Haemorrh. 34, 652-660.

FIBRIN(OGEN) DEGRADATION PRODUCTS. DETERMINATION USING A MONOCLONAL ANTI D NEO ANTIBODY. ADVANTAGES IN CLINICAL INVESTIGATION.

M.Mirshahi, J.Soria, C.Soria, J.Y.Perrot, A.Bernadou, C.Boucheix.

Services des Pr Bernadou, Fabiani et Samama, Hotel DIEU, Paris.

Services des Pr Caen et Rousselet, Hopital Lariboisière, Paris.

Fibrin(ogen) degradation products (FDP) were determined in plasma, using an anti D neo monoclonal antibody (McAb) called F2C5, either by a latex agglutination assay or by an immunoenzymological procedure, depending on the pathological case to be tested.

Material and Methods.

Fibrin degradation products (FbDP) were obtained according to Gaffney (1). Fragment D was isolated according to Nilhen (2) Anti D neo McAb (F2C5) was obtained and characterized as previously described (3)(4)(5). This Mc Ab was tested by both a direct immunoenzymological assay and a competitive inhibition binding assay . It did not react with fibrinogen (Fg) or its early degradation products or with fibrin monomers, but reacted with FbDP and fragment D. Furthermore, it has been demonstrated that the reactivity of this McAb F2C5 against FbDP is 10 times greater than that observed with fragment D.

Fibrinogen - Fibrin Formation and Fibrinolysis, Vol. 4
© 1986 Walter de Gruyter & Co., Berlin · New York - Printed in Germany.

- Ig from ascitic fluids of mice injected with the F2C5 clone was isolated by DEAE trisacryl gel chromatography according to Corthier et al (6).

-Latex agglutination assay (for high levels of FDP) :
Latex particles (0.3 μ diameter- Rhone Poulenc) were coated with F2C5 -Ig according to Singer (7).
20 μl of the latex suspension was added to 50 μl of diluted plasma onto a glass plate, and the mixture stirred with a glass rod until forming a ring of 2 cm diameter. The lowest dilution of plasma (in 0.15 M saline buffer containing 0.1 M glycine, pH 8.2) that induced agglutination of the F2C5- latex particles after 6 min. gentle rocking of the plate was determined.

-Immunoenzymological procedure (for lower levels of FDP) :
This method involves the binding of FDP onto plates coated with F2C5- Ig. Then, in a second step, FDP bound to the plate are revealed using peroxidase labelled polyclonal anti D-Ig.
Experiments were performed using a 96 well microtitration plate (Dynatech M 26 B). The protocol was similar to that described by WHITAKER (8), except that the detection of FbDP bound to the plates was performed by adding a peroxidase labeled polyclonal anti D Ig, and that immune peroxidase bound to the wells was determined using orthophenylene diamine and pehydrol as described by WOLTERS et al (9).

Cases reports
26 cases of intravascular coagulation (D.I.C.) were examined.

These were characterized by a decreased platelet count, decrease in factor V, the presence of soluble complexes detected by the test of LARGO et al using FS Prest (Stago Laboratories). FDP in serum was measured using latex particles coated with both F2C5 McAb and polyclonal Ig Anti D + anti E (Spli prest-Stago Laboratories)

1 patient under SK therapy was examined: at the moment of the biological determination, the fibrinogen level dropped to 36 mg/ 100 ml.

Results

a) Sensitivity of the techniques.

- An agglutination of F2C5 - coated latex particles is induced by 7 µg/ml of fragment D and 1 µg/ml of FbDP expressed in terms of the fragment D.
- Using the immunoenzymological procedure, there is a linear dose- response curve between the logarithm of the FbDP concentration (from 1.5 to 200 ng/ml) and the amount of immuneperoxidase bound to the coated polystyrene, expressed as units of optical density at 492 nm.

b) Results in Clinical Investigation :

1°) Latex agglutination assay:

For the diagnosis of disseminated intravascular coagulation

(DIC) , the latex procedure was used because it is very convenient for urgent measurements and is sufficiently sensitive.

Among the 25 patients tested,

- in 19 cases, a good correlation (r = 0.93) was observed between FDP levels determined in plasma using F2C5- coated latex particles and FDP levels determined in serum using both F2C5 and polyclonal Ig anti D + anti E coated latex particles.
- in 3 cases, however, the FDP level was within the upper limit of the normal range when determined in serum, whatever F2C5 or polyclonal anti D + anti E was used, but was 2 or 3 times higher than normal when determined in plasma using F2C5.
- in 3 other cases, when the patients were under heparin therapy, the FDP level was found to be higher in serum when using the polyclonal Ig-coated latex particles than when using F2C5 whether serum or the corresponding plasma was used. However, using polyclonal IG anti D + anti E, FDP levels in serum dropped to the same value than that found using F2C5 , when serum was allowed to remain for a further hour at 37°C with another thrombin addition (10 U/ml final concentration).

For patients with hyperfibrinolysis (euglobulin lysis time less than 30 min), the levels of plasma FDP were within the normal range.

In one patient under SK therapy, although fibrinogen levels dropped from 200 mg/100 ml to 38 mg/100 ml, no increase in fragment D was seen using F2C5 coated latex particles. In this patient, immunoelectrophoresis showed that the fibrinogen was degraded into early degradation products.

- 2°) Immunoenzymological assay.

Because of the increased sensitivity of this test, it was carried out in order to detect a thrombotic disorder. Normal values of FDP was less than 100 ng/ml expressed in terms of the fragment D.

Discussion

Immunoassay of FDP determined using a D neo McAb presents several advantages

Concerning the diagnosis of DIC, we have used the latex agglutination assay because this test is very convenient and very rapid to perform in urgent cases.

This test was directly applicable in plasma , therefore

1°) it is not time consumming because it avoids the need to prepare serum totally depleted of fibrinogen which takes at least 2 hours.

2°) it avoids an overestimation of FDP due to the presence of non- clottable fibrinogen (patients under heparin therapy for example)

3°) it avoids underestimation of FDP due to the fact that in some patients, FbDP may remain occluded in the fibrin clot formed during serum preparation.

4°) The McAb used did not discriminate totally between fragment

D and FbDP. This does not seem to be of importance even in cases of dramatic hyperfibrinolysis or in patients under SK therapy, since no increase in fragment D was found in such patients.

This is due to the fact that in plasma, hyperfibrinogenolysis is always limited to the early stages of degradation because of the presence of alpha 2 anti- plasmin and of the low affinity of plasminogen for tissue plasminogen activator in the absence of fibrin.

Because of its high sensitivity,the immunoenzymological assay seems promising for the diagnosis of thrombotic disorder.

References

1 - GAFFNEY, P.J., JOE, F., MAHMOUD, M. 1975. Thromb.Res.7, 89.

2 - NILHEN, J.E. 1967. Thromb. Diath. Haemorrh. 18, 89.

3 - BOUCHEIX,C., MIRSHAHI, M., SORIA, J., SORIA, C., PERROT, J.Y., BERNADOU, A., ROSENFELD, C. 1982 . In : Protides of the Biological fluids (Peeters H. ed) Pergamon Press, p.399.

4 - SORIA, J., SORIA, C., MIRSHAHI, M.,BOUCHEIX, C.,

PERROT, J.Y., BERNADOU, A., SAMAMA, M. 1983. In: Fibrinogen. Structure. Functional aspects. Metabolism. (HAVERKATE F., HENSCHEN A., NIEUWENHUIZEN W.,STRAUB P. ed.) Walter de Gruyter , p.227.

5 - MIRSHAHI, M., SORIA, J., SORIA, C., BOUCHEIX, C., PERROT, J.Y., NIEUWENHUIZEN , W., BERNADOU, A., SAMAMA, M., ROSENFELD ,C. 1983. Thromb.Haemost.,50, 301.

6 - CORTHIER, G., BOSCHETTI, E., CHARLEY-POULAIN, J. 1984. J.Immunol.Methods 66, 75.

7 - SINGER, J.M., PLOTZ, C.M. 1956. Amer. J. Med. 21, 888.

8 - WHITAKER, A.N., ELMS, M.J., MASCI, P.P., BUNDESEN, P.G., RYLATT, D.B., WEBER, A.J., BUNCE, I.H. 1984. J.Clin.Path. 37, 882.

9 - WOLTERS, G., KUIJPERS, L., KACAKI, J., SCHUURS, A. 1976. J.Clin.Path. 28, 873.

A MONOCLONAL ANTIBODY, SPECIFIC FOR HUMAN FIBRINOGEN AND FIBRINOPEPTIDE A-CONTAINING FRAGMENTS. ITS APPLICATION IN AN ENZYME-IMMUNOASSAY FOR FIBRINOGEN DEGRADATION PRODUCTS, SUITABLE FOR USE IN PLASMA.

P.W. Koppert, C.M.G. Huijsmans, F. Haverkate, J. Engbers, E.J.P. Brommer, W. Nieuwenhuizen*

TNO Gaubius Institute for Cardiovascular Research, Herenstraat 5d, 2313 AD Leiden, The Netherlands

*To whom all correspondence should be addressed

Introduction

One of the goals of our present research is to develop monoclonal antibodies to be used in specific enzyme immunoassays for the determination of fibrin(ogen) degradation products in plasma or blood. Most existing assays for degradation products are based on polyclonal antibodies, which cross-react with fibrinogen. As a consequence these assays must be performed on serum. The use of serum, however, can cause falsely positive (e.g. by incomplete clotting or by lysis of fibrin during serum preparation) or falsely negative results (e.g. because some fibrin(ogen) degradation products become associated with the clot).

We used two different immunogens to develop degradation product-specific monoclonal antibodies.

- A mixture of fibrin degradation products, isolated from a lysate of a whole blood clot (J. Koopman et al., elsewhere in this volume). This approach yielded a monoclonal antibody, specifically reactive with degradation products both of fibrin (designated as XDP) and of fibrinogen (designated as FDP), and not with fibrinogen or fibrin. This monoclonal antibody (FDP-14) is used as capture antibody in an enzyme-immunoassay (EIA) for the total of FDP + XDP directly in human plasma or blood, without the need of serum preparation.
- Purified fibrinogen fragment Y. During the latter work we observed an interesting clone, which produces an antibody, specifically reactive with normal human fibrinogen,

Fibrinogen - Fibrin Formation and Fibrinolysis, Vol. 4
© 1986 Walter de Gruyter & Co., Berlin · New York - Printed in Germany.

fibrinopeptide A-containing fragments and not with free fibrinopeptide A.

This paper describes the development and characterization of this monoclonal antibody, and its application (in combination with FDP-14) in an assay for fibrinogen degradation products directly in plasma, without interference by free fibrinopeptide A.

Materials and Methods

Fibrinogens and fibrin monomer

Fibrinogens of man (normal and genetic variants), rat, cat, pig and cow were purified as described before (1).

Fibrinogen Milan II is an abnormal fibrinogen with decreased thrombin-binding and a slow thrombin-catalyzed fibrinopeptide A (and B) release (2).

Fibrinogen Metz (a gift of drs J. and C. Soria, Hôtel Dieu, Paris, France) is a homozygous fibrinogen variant in which arginine at position A α 16 (= the thrombin/arvin cleavage site) is replaced by cystein (3).

From fibrinogen Amsterdam (patient referred to us by Dr. H.L. Haak) only one of the two fibrinopeptides A can be released (3; and F. Haverkate, in press).

Fibrinogen Kassel (from Dr. H. Janzarik, Klinikum der Justus-Liebig Universität, Giessen, FRG) has a prolonged thrombin time but the molecular defect is not known at present.

Fibrin monomer was prepared as described by Haverkate (3a).

Human fibrinogen Aα, Bβ and γ chains were separated by reduction and carboxymethylation of fibrinogen and purified as described by Doolittle and coworkers (4).

Plasmin-generated fibrin(ogen) degradation products

Fragment X was prepared and purified as described before (5), Y as in (6), and D_{cate}, D_{EGTA} and E as in (7).

Cyanogen bromide (CNBr) fragments of fibrin(ogen)

The amino-terminal disulphide knots (NDSK) of fibrinogen and fibrin were prepared and purified as described by Blombäck et al. (8) and Olexa et al. (9), respectively.

Fragment FCB-2 (10,11) (also known as HO1-DSK (12)), its Aα chain remnant (= Aα 148-207), and fragment FCB-3 (11) were purified as described before (10).

Fragment Aα 1-51 was prepared either by reduction and carboxymethylation of the NDSK of fibrinogen (NDSK-fbg) or by CNBr treatment of purified Aα chain.

(Partial) purification was in both cases achieved by gel filtration on Sephadex G50 in 50% acetic acid. Aα 1-51 containing

Table 1. Summary of the chain (remnant) composition of fibrin(ogen)-derived fragments. The figures indicate the numbers of amino acids.

	Amino acid stretches derived from			
product	Aα chain	Bβ chain	γ chain	references
Fibrinogen	$(1-610)_2$	$(1-461)_2$	$(1-410)_2$	(11)
Fibrin monomer	$(17-610)_2$	$(15-461)_2$	$(1-410)_2$	(11)
X	$(1-208)_2$	$(1-461)_2$	$(1-410)_2$	(14,15)
Y	1-208/1-78	1-461/54-122	1-410/1-58	(14,15)
D_{cate}	111-197	134-461	86-410	(16)
D_{EGTA}	111-197	134-461	86-303	(16)
E	$(1-78)_2$	$(54-122)_2$	$(1-58)_2$	(17)
NDSK (fbg)	$(1-51)_2$	$(1-118)_2$	$(1-78)_2$	(8)
NDSK (fb)	$(17-51)_2$	$(15-118)_2$	$(1-78)_2$	(8)
FCB-2	148-207	191-224 225-242 243-305	95-265	(10-12)
FCB-3	241-476	-	-	(11)
Fibrinopeptide A	1-16	-	-	(18)
Fibrinopeptide B	-	1-14	-	(18)

fractions were identified by end group analysis (13) (alanine and some aspartic acid) and molecular weight determinations by SDS-PAGE.

Table 1 summarizes the chain (remnant) composition of the fibrin-(ogen)-derived fragments, used in this study.

Immunization scheme

Purified fibrinogen fragment Y (25 µg) in Freunds complete adjuvant (Difco) was injected intraperitoneally in female Balb/c mice (Centraal Proefdierenbedrijf TNO, Zeist, The Netherlands); then at 3 weeks intervals with 25 µg fragment Y in incomplete Freunds adjuvant. An intravenous injection of 25 µg fragment Y in PBS was given three days before fusion (see below).

Fusion

The immunized mice were killed in ether vapour, and spleen cells were harvested. 8.10^7 spleen cells were fused with 2.10^7 nonproducing myeloma P3 x 63 Ag 8653 cells in the presence of 40% polyethyleneglycol 4000 (Baker), essentially as described by Köhler and Milstein (19).

The cell suspension was diluted and divided over 96-wells microtiter plates (Costar). Media of growing cells were screened for antibody production as described below.

Cell lines producing reactive antibodies were subcloned twice by limiting dilution (0.5 cells per well) as described in (20).

Screening procedure (ELISA)

Screening was performed by a procedure analogous to that originally described by Engvall and Perlman (21) on plates, coated with fibrinogen, fibrin monomers or fragment Y, and using a rabbit--anti-mouse immunoglobulin coupled with urease (Sanbio) for visualisation. In some cases such as the cross-reactivity assay (see below) a horse radish peroxidase conjugate was used in combination with 5-aminosalicylic acid (0.8 mg/ml) and hydrogen peroxide (0.005%).

Cross-reactivity assay (CRA) according to Soria et al. (22)

In this assay a dilution of a solution of monoclonal antibody is chosen, which gives 80% of the maximum response in the assay described under the heading Screening procedure on fragment Y-coated plates. The antibody solution at this dilution is preincubated (16 hrs, 4°C) with different concentrations of fibrin(ogen) fragments (0-200 μg/ml) to be tested for cross-reactivity with fragment Y and then applied to a fragment Y-coated plate. A concentration-dependent decrease of response from 80% downward is indicative for cross-reactivity.

Purification of the monoclonal antibody and subclass assessment

After dialysis for 16 hrs at 4°C against 0.015 M Tris.HCl, pH 7.0, the antibody-containing solutions were applied to a DE-52 cellulose column (Whatman) equilibrated with the same buffer. Elution of immunoreactive material was performed with 0.15 M Tris.HCl, pH 7.0. This material was dialyzed against 0.1 M NH_4HCO_3, freeze-dried, dissolved in PBS/Tween and applied to a Sephacryl S-200 column (Pharmacia) in 0.1 M $NaHCO_3$, pH 7.5. Material eluting near the void volume of this column was immunoreactive. Purity was checked by immunoelectrophoresis as described by Radl (23). Antisera against mouse α, μ, δ, ε, γ and κ and λ chains were gifts from Dr. Radl (Institute for Experimental Gerontology TNO, Rijswijk, the Netherlands).

Influence on thrombin and arvin clotting times

This assay was performed, essentially as described before (24). Increasing amounts of monoclonal antibody (pretreated with 10^{-4} M DFP) were added to a constant amount of fibrinogen (0.1 ml, 2 mg/ml in PBS pH 7.4) and incubated for 2.5 hrs in the presence of 4 KIU of aprotinin. A monoclonal antibody raised against tissue--type plasminogen activator and not reactive with fibrinogen was used as a control. In another control experiment human fibrinogen was replaced by rat fibrinogen.

Fibrinopeptide release

The thrombin-catalyzed fibrinopeptide release with time before and after treatment with DFP-treated monoclonal antibody was performed according to Kehl et al. (25) with an LKB 2152 HPLC apparatus equipped with a CP-Spher C18 reversed phase column (Chrompack).

Results

A. Characterization of the monoclonal antibody

All of the 172 wells, initially filled with the fusion mixture, showed cell growth upon visual inspection after 3 weeks. The media of the cells in only 2 wells were immunoreactive in ELISA with fibrinogen and fragment Y, and not with fibrin monomers. The cells in these 2 wells were cloned and gave 9 stable clones. When one of these clones was recloned by limiting dilution (0.5 cells/well), 30% of the wells showed cell growth. The media in all wells with hybridoma growth immunoreacted with fibrinogen, fragment Y and not with fibrin monomers. This clone is, up till now, stable in culture for over 18 months. It has been injected also into the peritoneal cavity of pristane-primed Balb/c mice for ascites production. It has been productive for more than 9 months (15 passages). The monoclonal antibody, described in this paper, will be designated as Mab-Y18. Both the results of the subclass assessment and the elution position of Sephacryl S-200 during purification (see section materials and methods) showed that Mab-Y18 is of the IgM, κ type.

Table 2. Immunoreactivity of Mab-Y18 with fibrinogen and fibrin (ogen)-derived fragments.

Antigen	response in ELISA	Antigen	response in ELISA
FCB-2	-	fpA	-
FCB-3	-	fpB	-
Aα 148-207	-	X (fbg)	+++
NDSK (fbg)	+++	Y (fbg)	+++
NDSK (fb)	-	D_{cate}, D_{EGTA}	-
Aα chain	+++	E_3 (fb)	-
Bβ chain	+	fibrinogen	+++
γ chain	-	fibrin monomers	-

- = no reaction;

+ = less than 3 times the blank response (O.D.);

+++ = more than 10 times the blank response (O.D.).

The blank response is generally around 0.15 in this assay.

Table 2 shows the immunoreactivity of Mab-Y18 with fibrinogen and 15 fibrinogen-derived proteins and peptides, as observed in the ELISA system.

Fibrinogen and its fibrinopeptide-containing fragments react with Mab-Y18. It is remarkable that both the fibrinogen Aα- and Bβ-chain give a positive result in the ELISA. Free fibrinopeptides A (fpA) and B (fpB) are not reactive.

The affinity of Mab-Y18 for fragment Y is difficult to assess, since fragment Y is a plasmin-generated product, the structure of which varies from preparation to preparation. Fibrinogen and its Aα-chain are much better defined and therefore we have estimated the affinity of Mab-Y18 for these two proteins from cross-reactivity assays. K_d values for intact fibrinogen and its Aα-chain do not differ significantly. They are 6×10^{-9} M and 2×10^{-9} M, respectively.

Table 3. Cross-reactivity of different derivatives of fibrinogen with fragment Y adsorbed to plastic plates, both before and after treatment with thrombin or arvin.

Antigen tested for	Cross-reactivity of the antigen		
cross-reactivity	non-treated	thrombin-treated	arvin-treated
normal human fibrinogen	+++	-	-
fragment Y (fbg)	+++	-	-
A α chain	+++	-	-
B β chain	++	-	-
γ chain	-	-	-
A α 1-51[1)]	+++	-	-
fpA	-	-	-
fpB	-	-	-

- = no cross-reaction;
+++ = 50% inhibition with 10^{-8} M or less;
++ = 50% inhibition with approximately 10^{-7} M;
+ = more than 10^{-6} M required for 50% inhibition.
1) Either prepared from NDSK (fbg) or from Aα-chain (see section Materials and Methods).

The results of the CRA's with different antigens, before and after treatment with thrombin or arvin, are summarized in Table 3. These results confirm and extend those of Table 2.
Fibrinogen and fibrinopeptide A-containing fibrinogen fragments in solution compete with adsorbed fragment Y. Furthermore these fragments loose their reactivity with Mab-Y18 upon treatment with thrombin or arvin. The Bβ-chain preparation shows cross-reactivity, although less than the Aα-chain. However, this cross-reactivity of the Bβ-chain is lost upon treatment with either thrombin or arvin. As arvin can only cleave off fpA, these results show clearly, that the Bβ-chain preparation is contaminated with Aα-chain. This was confirmed with HPLC experiments, where we could show that fpA was released from this Bβ-chain preparation by thrombin or arvin (results not shown). The Bβ-chain preparation showed, however, only one band on SDS-PAGE and therefore it is conceivable that it contains partly degraded Aα-chains with the same molecular weight as intact Bβ-chains.
Information as to the epitope of Mab-Y18 can be obtained by studying the cross-reactivities of fibrinogens of other species and those of genetically abnormal human fibrinogens. The results of such experiments are summarized in the Tables 4 and 5.

Table 4. Mab-Y18 cross-reactivities of fibrinogens from different species with fragment Y. Sequences of the fibrinopeptide A are given for comparison.

Fibrinogenspecies	Cross-reactivity	Sequence fpA[1)]
normal human	+++	ADSG-EGDFLAEGGGVR
pig	-	AEVQDKGEFLAEGGGVR
rat	-	ADTGTTSEFIEAGGDIR
cat	-	GDVQ-EGEFIAEGGGVR
cow	-	EDGSDPP-SGDFLTEGGGVR

1) from reference (18).

Table 5. Mab-Y18 cross-reactivities of some genetically abnormal human fibrinogens (before and after exhaustive treatment with thrombin and arvin) with fragment Y of normal human fibrinogen.

Abnormal fibrinogen	Cross-reactivity of fibrinogen		
	non-treated	thrombin-treated	arvin-treated
Milan II	+++	-	-
Metz	+/-	+/-	+/-
Amsterdam	+++	++	+
Kassel	+++	-	-
Normal	+++	-	-

- = no cross-reactivity;
+++ = 50% inhibition at 10^{-8} M (see text under cross-reactivity assay);
++ = 50% inhibition at approximately 10^{-7} M;
\+ = 50% inhibition at 10^{-6} M;
+/- = inhibition observed; too much fibrinogen needed to reach 50% inhibition in cross-reactivity assay (see text).

The results in Table 4 show the specificity of Mab-Y18 for human fibrinogen. None of the other fibrinogen species tested exhibits any cross-reactivity with human fragment Y. The results in Table 5 point to a possible involvement of Aα 16, since fibrinogen Metz (A α 16 arginine replaced by cysteine (3)) cross-reacts only slightly. The (normal) fpA's of fibrinogen Milan II are released at a slow rate probably as a result of a decreased thrombin binding (2). If this decreased thrombin binding is caused by mutations of amino acids outside fpA, these mutations do not destroy the immunoreactivity between Mab-Y18 and fibrinogen Milan II.

Only one fpA per molecule of fibrinogen Amsterdam (heterozygous) can be released by thrombin or arvin (6). The defect in fibrinogen Amsterdam is not known in detail, but our results suggest that the defect has no effect on the immunoreactivity with

Mab-Y18. This seems to be true also for the 50% of the molecules which are abnormal, since cross-reactivity is maintained even after thrombin or arvin treatment, when the normal fibrinogen molecules loose their fpA's. The defect in fibrinogen Kassel is not known at present, but the results in Table 5 may be explained, by the assumption that its immunoreactivity with Mab-Y18 is normal and that all fpA can be cleaved off by thrombin and arvin. An alternative explanation at this stage would be that fibrinogen Kassel is heterozygous and that the population of abnormal molecules has no reactivity at all with Mab-Y18.

Fig. 1 shows the effect of Mab-Y18 on the thrombin and arvin clotting times of normal human fibrinogen. A strong concentration-dependent effect of Mab-Y18 is seen both for the thrombin and for the arvin clotting times.

A monoclonal antibody directed against tissue-type plasminogen activator, used as a control, has no effect on the clotting times (Fig. 1). As expected from the lack of immunoreactivity of Mab-Y18 with rat fibrinogen (Table 4), Mab-Y18 had no effect on the thrombin and arvin (latter not shown) clotting times of rat plasma (Fig. 1, curve C).

Fibrinopeptide A release by thrombin from normal human fibrinogen after incubation with Mab-Y18, as measured by HPLC, was decreased, whereas fpB release was normal. After 90 minutes incubation with thrombin or arvin only about 1 mole of fpA per mole of Mab-Y18 treated fibrinogen had been released, whereas after the same incubation period the release of fpA from the same fibrinogen with anti-tissue-type plasminogen activator was 2 moles fpA per mole of fibrinogen. After 24 hours 2 moles of fpA had been released from Mab-Y18 treated fibrinogen. The rates of release of the different forms of fibrinopeptides of normal human fibrinogen i.e. of fibrinopeptides A, AP (phosphoserine at Aα 3) and AY (lacking Aα 1) were inhibited to the same extent.

B. <u>The application of Mab-Y18 in an EIA for FDP in plasma</u>

The details of the EIA for FDP's will be described elsewhere. Suffice it to explain here the principle of the assay. The first step of the EIA is the same as that of the FDP + XDP assay, described elsewhere in the volume (J. Koopman et al.) i.e. plasma is pipetted into the wells of an FDP-14 coated microtiter plate.

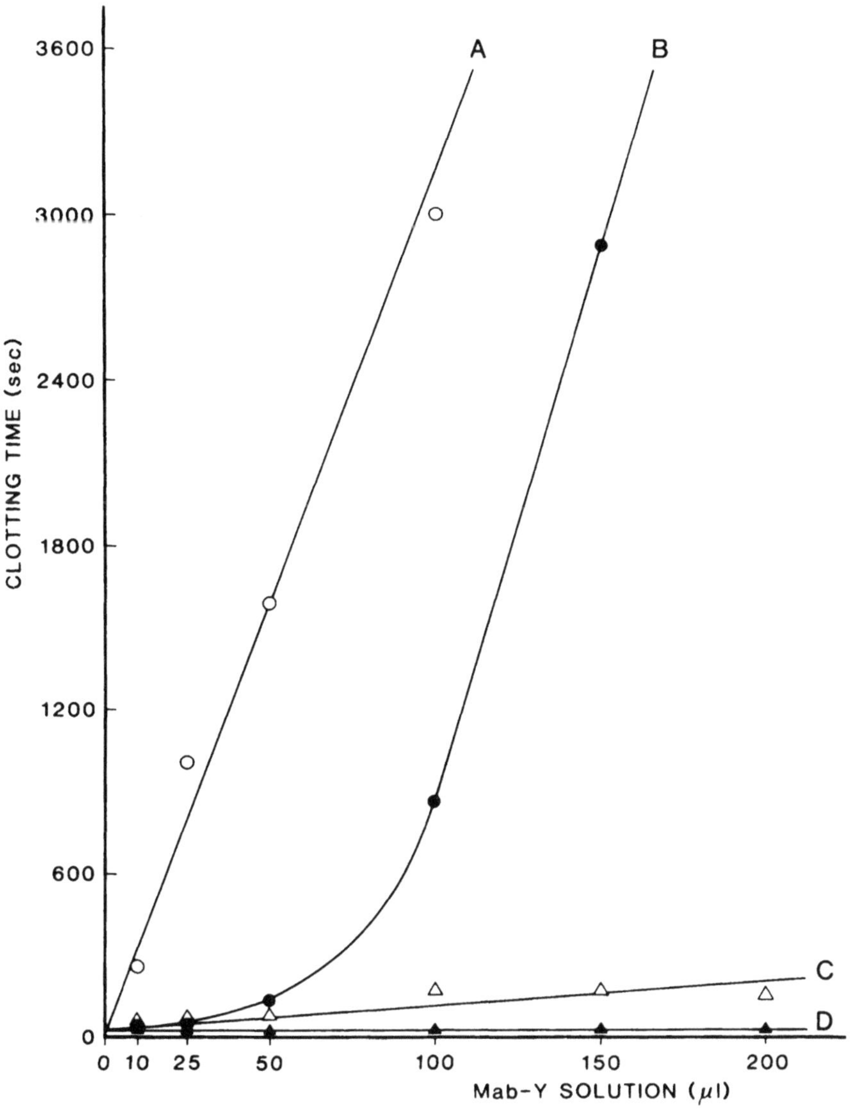

Figure 1
<u>Influence of Mab-Y18 on thrombin and arvin clotting times.</u>
Curve A: dependence of arvin clotting time (human fibrinogen) upon Mab-Y18 concentration.
Curve B: the same for thrombin.
Curve C: thrombin time of rat fibrinogen.
Curve D: thrombin time of normal human fibrinogen in the presence of an anti tissue-type plasminogen activator monoclonal antibody.
(Details in the text).

This step is the selection for FDP + XDP. In the second step a conjugate of horse-radish peroxidase with Mab-Y18 is used, which selectively reacts with FDP's (containing fibrinopeptide A). A schematic depiction of the EIA is shown in Fig. 2.

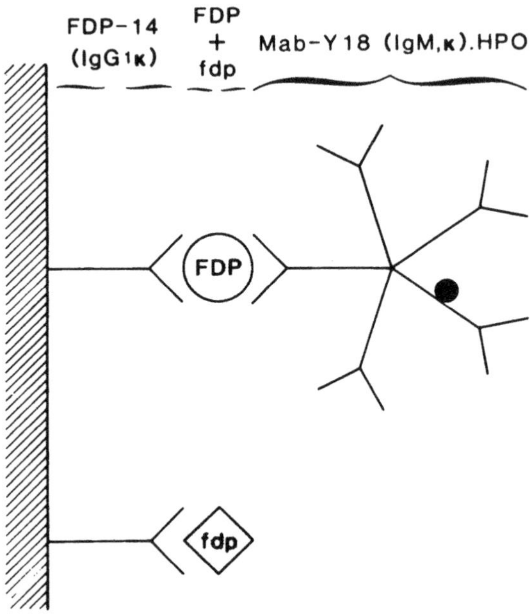

Figure 2
Schematic representation of the two-step EIA for FDP's.

Substrate solutions and measurements are the same as those described for the FDP + XDP assay by Koopman et al. This EIA for FDP's can be performed on plasma or even on whole blood. Back--ground values are very low i.e., lower than 0.1. The assay is specific for FDP's, since XDP's, fibrin monomers and fibrinogen gave no response in the EIA, but fibrinogen fragments X, Y and E gave strong responses. We have applied the FDP EIA to plasma samples taken at different times from patients undergoing streptokinase therapy for acute myocardial infarction. A typical result is shown in Fig. 3, where the results of the FDP + XDP assay and the present FDP have been plotted in a semilogarithmic way.

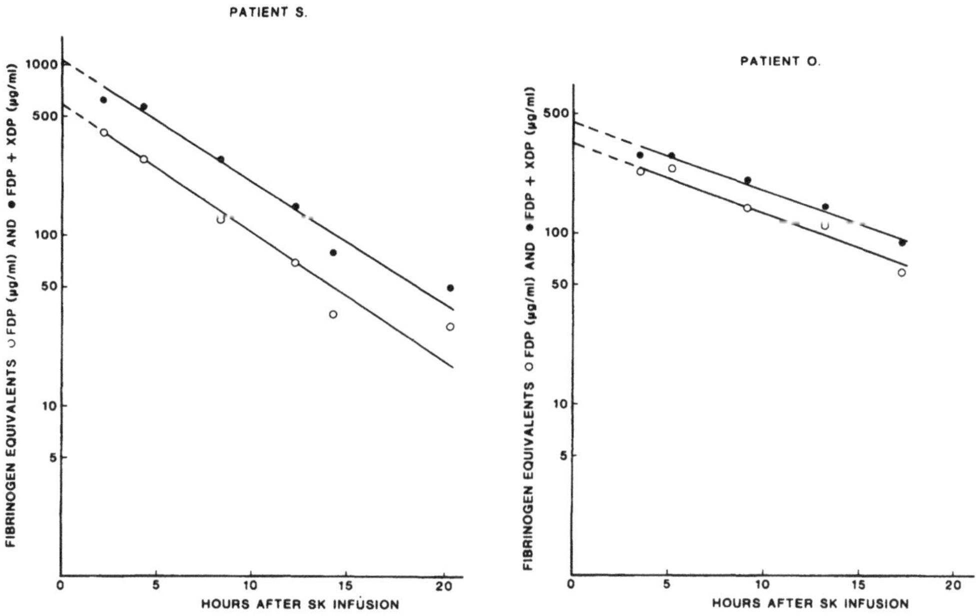

Figure 3
Time-dependent decrease of FDP's and (FDP + XDP) in blood of two patients, SK treated for acute myocardial infarction.

As can be seen both FDP + XDP and FDP levels show a normal clearance profile with a $T\frac{1}{2}$ of 5 to 6 hours. Patients with acute myocardial infarction not treated with streptokinase did not have measurable levels of FDP (or FDP + XDP).

Discussion

The monoclonal antibody (Mab-Y18), characterized in this study, reacts specifically with fibrinopeptide A-containing derivatives of normal human fibrinogen as is clearly shown by the results in Tables 2 and 3. It is surprising that Mab-Y18 also exhibits some reactivity with purified Bβ-chain. This could indicate that Aα- and Bβ-chains have similar epitopes. However, as shown in Table 2, the explanation is much more trivial. As our Bβ -chain preparation loses its reactivity with Mab-Y18 upon treatment with arvin and as we could demonstrate (by HPLC) that fibrinopeptide A is released from the Bβ-chain preparation, we conclude that our Bβ-chain preparation contains some partially degraded Aα-chain. Since the preparation showed only one homogeneous band upon SDS-PAGE, this means that this partly degraded Aα-chain has the same molecular weight as the Bβ-chain and was therefore not recognized.

Since it is our experience and that of others (22) that some monoclonal antibodies interacts with some antigens only when the latter are adsorbed e.g. to the plastic wall of a microtiter plate and not with the antigens in solution, we decided to introduce CRA as described by Soria et al. (22). We found that Mab-Y18 does not discriminate between adsorbed antigens and antigens in solution (compare tables 2 and 3).

Free fibrinopeptides A are not recognized by Mab-Y18. Furthermore fibrinopeptide A-containing fibrinogen derivatives loose their reactivity with Mab-Y18 upon release of fibrinopeptide Aα by thrombin or arvin (Table 3). This could indicate that fibrinopeptide A does not comprise the full Mab-Y18 epitope, but is rather an essential part of it. As judged from the strong cross--reactivity of Aα 1-51 (Table 3), the rest of the epitope would be localized, in that case, between Aα 17 and 51. An alternative possibility is, that fibrinopeptide A comprises the full Mab-Y18 epitope but that the extra carboxyl group on Aα 16 in free fibrinopeptide A has an adverse effect on the complex formation between Mab-Y18 and fibrinopeptide A.

Comparison of the reactivities of fibrinogens of other mammalian species with Mab-Y18 shows the high specificity of Mab-Y18 for human fibrinogen (Table 4). Even porcine fibrinogen, which has a fibrinopeptide A in which residues Aα 9-16 are identical with human fibrinopeptide A does not react with Mab-Y18, indicating that residues Aα 1-8 play an essential role in the Mab-Y18 epitope. Since we have found (not shown) that the release of other forms of fibrinopeptide A i.e. AP (phosphoserine at Aα 3) and AY (lacking Aα 1) is inhibited to the same extent as that of fibrinopeptide A, it is conceivable that residues Aα 2 and 4-8 play a crucial role in the Mab-Y18 epitope, and that Aα 1 and 3 are less essential.

As indicated above, it seems that arginine A 16 (i.e. the thrombin/arvin cleavage site) is crucial for the recognition by Mab-Y18. This is further supported by our results obtained with fibrinogen Metz; in this homozygous dysfibrinogen arginine A 16 is replaced by cysteine. This single mutation destroys the interaction with Mab-Y18 completely.

As shown in Fig. 1, Mab-Y18 prolongs the thrombin and arvin times of human plasma, by different profiles i.e. at low Mab-Y18 concentrations the increase in arvin clotting times is much stronger than that of the thrombin clotting time. This may be due to the fact that thrombin can cleave off both fibrinopeptides A and B. Mab-Y18 inhibits fibrinopeptide A release but does not affect the fibrinopeptide B release thus favouring the formation of des BB-fibrin by thrombin. Des BB-fibrin forms weak clots (26).

We have been able to set up a specific EIA for FDP in plasma or whole blood, which is not disturbed by fibrinogen, fibrin or XDP's. The examples of patients undergoing streptokinase therapy clearly demonstrate the great potential of this EIA to monitor FDP levels during therapy since the EIA time to result is only 45 minutes.

References

1. Van Ruijven-Vermeer, I.A.M. and W. Nieuwenhuizen. 1978. Purification of rat fibrinogen and its constituent chains. Biochem. J. 169, 653-658.

2. Haverkate, F., P.M. Mannucci, A. d'Angelo, C. Kluft, J. Koopman, W. Nieuwenhuizen, R.M. Bertina, A. Henschen and M. Kehl. 1983. An abnormal fibrinogen (Milan II) with a defective thrombin binding and thrombin clotting time, but with normal reptilase and arvin times. Thromb. Haemostas. 50, 1061, (abstr).

3a. Haverkate, F. and G. Timan. 1976. Preparation of highly purified bovine fibrin plates. In: Progress in Chemical Fibrinolysis and Thrombolysis, Vol. 2 (J.F. Davidson, M.M. Samama and P.C. Desnoyers, eds.) Raven Press, New York. pp. 67-71.

3. Henschen, A., M. Kehl, C. Southan, F. Lottspeich and D. Georgopoulos. 1983. In: Fibrinogen - Structure, Functional Aspects, Metabolism, Vol. 2 (F. Haverkate, A. Henschen, W. Nieuwenhuizen and P.W. Straub, eds.) Walter de Gruyter, Berlin-New York. pp. 125-144.

4. Doolittle, R.F., K.G. Cassman, B.A. Cottrell, S.J. Friezner, J.T. Hucko and T. Takagi. 1977. Amino acid sequence studies on the ³chain of human fibrinogen. Characterization of 11 cyanogen bromide fragments. Biochemistry 16, 1703-1709.

5. Nieuwenhuizen, W. and M. Gravesen M. 1981. Anticoagulant and calcium-binding properties of high molecular weight derivatives of human fibrinogen, produced by plasmin (fragments X). Biochim. Biophys. Acta 668, 81-88.

6. Nieuwenhuizen, W., M. Voskuilen and J. Hermans. 1982. Anticoagulant and calcium-binding properties of high molecular weight derivatives of human fibrinogen (plasmin fragments Y). Biochim. Biophys. Acta 708, 313-316.

7. Van Ruijven-Vermeer, I.A.M., W. Nieuwenhuizen, F. Haverkate and T. Timan T. 1979. A novel method for the rapid purification of human and rat fibrin(ogen) degradation products. Hoppe-Seyler's Z. physiol. Chem. 360, 633-637.

8. Blombäck, B., M. Blombäck, A. Henschen, B. Hessel, S. Iwanaga and K.R. Woods. 1968. N-terminal disulphide knot of human fibrinogen. Nature 218, 130-134.

9. Olexa, S.A. and A.Z. Budzynski. 1979. Binding phenomena of isolated unique plasmic degradation products of human cross--linked fibrin. J. Biol. Chem. 254, 4925-4932.

10. Nieuwenhuizen, W., J.H. Verheijen, A. Vermond and Chang GTG. 1983. Plasminogen activation by tissue activator is accelerated in the presence of fibrin (ogen) cyanogen bromide fragment FCB-2. Biochim. Biophys. Acta 755, 531-533.

11. Henschen, A. 1981. Fibrinogen - Blutgerinnungsfaktor I. Biochemische Aspekte. Haemostaseologie 1, 49-61.

12. Gårdlund, B., B. Hessel, G. Marguerie, G. Murano and B. Blombäck B. 1977. Primary structure of human fibrinogen. Characterization of disulfide-containing cyanogen-bromide fragments. Eur. J. Biochem. 77, 595-610.

13. Gray, W.R. 1967. Dansyl chloride procedure. Meth. Enzymol. 11, 139-151.

14. Graeff, H. and R. Hafter. 1982. Detection and relevance of crosslinked fibrin derivatives in blood. Seminars in Thromb. & Hemostas. 8, 57-86.

15. Takagi, T. and R.F. Doolittle. 1975. Amino acid sequence studies on plasmin-derived fragments of human fibrinogen: Amino-terminal sequences of intermediate and terminal fragments. Biochemistry 14, 940-946.

16. Nieuwenhuizen, W. and F. Haverkate. 1983. Calcium-binding regions in fibrinogen. Ann. N.Y. Acad. Sci. 408, 92-96.

17. Olexa, S.A., A.Z. Budzynski, R.F. Doolittle, B.A. Cottrell and T.C. Greene TC. 1981. Structure of fragment E species from human cross-linked fibrin. Biochemistry 20, 6139-6145.

18. Dayhoff, M.O. 1972. Atlas of Protein Sequence and Structure. 5, D87-D97.

19. Köhler, G. and C. Milstein C. 1975. Continuous cultures of fused cells secreting antibody of predefined specificity. Nature 256, 495-497.

20. McKearn, T.J. 1980. In: Monoclonal Antibodies. Hybridomas; a new dimension in biological analyses. (R.H. Kennett, T.J. McKearn and K.B. Bechtol, eds.) Plenum Press, New York 1980, pp. 374

21. Engvall, E. and P. Perlman. 1972. Enzyme-linked immuno sorbent assay. III. Quantitation of specific antibodies by labelled anti-immunoglobulin in antigen coated tubes. J. Immunol. 109, 129-135.

22. Soria, J., C. Soria, C. Boucheix, M. Mirshahi, J.Y. Perrot, A. Bernadou and M. Samama. 1983. In: Fibrinogen - Structure, Functional Aspects, Metabolism, Vol. 2 (F. Haverkate, A. Henschen, W. Nieuwenhuizen and P.A. Straub, eds.) Walter de Gruyter, Berlin-New York. pp. 227-233.

23. Radl, J. 1981. In: Immunological techniques applied to aging research. (W.H. Adler and A.A. Nordin, eds.) CRC Press Inc., Boca Raton, Fla, USA, pp. 122-139.

24. Haverkate, F., G. Timan and W. Nieuwenhuizen W. 1979. Anti-clotting properties of fragments D from human fibrinogen and fibrin. Eur. J. Clin. Invest. 9, 253-255.

25. Kehl, M., F. Lottspeich and A. Henschen. 1981. Analysis of human fibrinopeptides by HPLC. Hoppe-Seyler's Z. physiol. Chem. 362, 1661-1664.

26. Shainoff, J.R. and B.N. Dardik. 1979. Fibrinopeptide B and aggregation of fibrinogen. Science 204, 200-202.

A MONOCLONAL ANTIBODY AGAINST THE CNBR-PEPTIDE F-CB3 OF THE Aα-CHAIN OF HUMAN FIBRINOGEN

R. Gollwitzer, G. E. Kulbe, D. Gabrijelčič
Max-Planck-Institut für Biochemie, D-8033 Martinsried, FRG

R. P. Linke
Institut für Immunologie der Universität München, D-8000 München, FRG

Introduction

F-CB3 (Aα 241-476) is the largest single chain cyanogen bromide peptide of fibrinogen (1). It is contained in the highly exposed carboxy-terminal two third of the Aα-chain, not integrated in the D-domain but located on the surface of the molecule (1) as a "free swimming appendage" (2). Because of its location outside the three-domainal structure, this part of the molecule is easily and early cleaved off by several proteases including plasmin (3,4). Several potential plasmic cleavage sites are close to the amino- and carboxy-terminal end of the peptide (5). One cleavage site, residues 424/425, is contained in the peptide (6). The very early plasminolysis or proteolysis of fibrinogen and fibrin is correlated to an increase of α-chain peptides also in vivo. A radioimmunoassay for F-CB3 was developed by us earlier (7). Elevated serum levels of F-CB3 related antigen were demonstrated in patients with various haemorhagic disorders (8,9).

In this paper we report on the production and characterization of monoclonal antibodies produced against F-CB3.

Results and Discussion

Four to six months old Balb/c Han male mice were immunized with peptide F-CB3. The serum was tested for anti-F-CB3 antibody activity before cell fusion of the spleen cells with murine

Fibrinogen - Fibrin Formation and Fibrinolysis, Vol. 4
© 1986 Walter de Gruyter & Co., Berlin · New York - Printed in Germany.

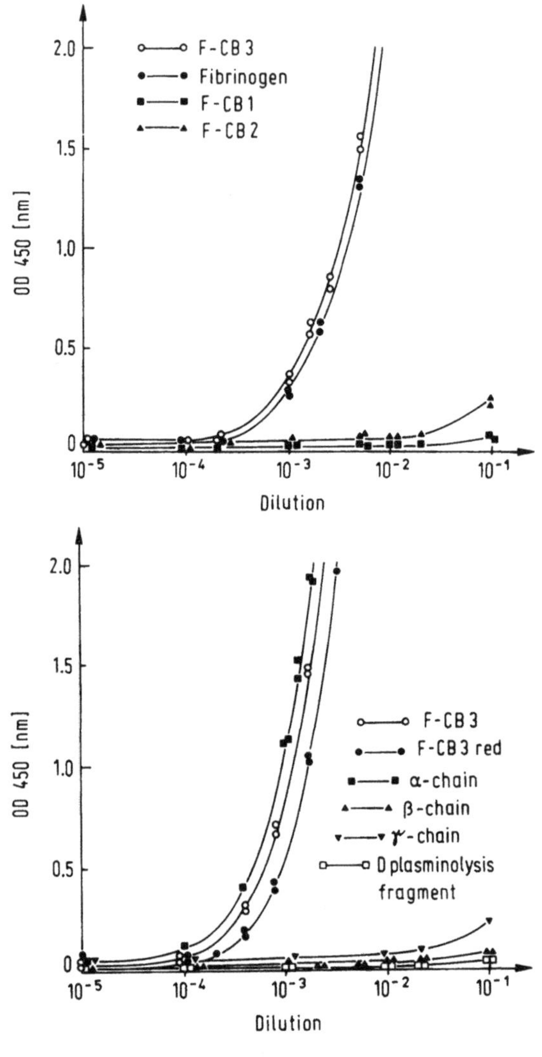

Fig. 1. Enzyme-immunoassay with supernatant of cell line 125. The wells of the microtiter plates were coated with fibrinogen, F-CB1, F-CB2, F-CB3 unreduced and reduced, the isolated α-, β- and γ-chain and with plasminolysis fragment D, resp., using a concentration of 5 µg/ml. Bound antibody was detected by reaction with goat anti-mouse IgG (bridge antibody) and a murine monoclonal peroxydase-anti-peroxydase complex (11). 3,3',5,5' tetra-methyl-benzidine (TMB)(Miles) was used as colorimetric substrate. The titration curve of fibrinogen was corrected by a factor of 7,according to the fact that the dimeric molecule contains two F-CB3 peptides and according to the difference in molecular weight:F-CB3: 23878, fibrinogen: 340000,assuming equal coating with the protein and the peptide.

P3x63-Ag8.653 myeloma cells was performed. 23 of 800 primary culture supernatants reacted with the antigen. These 28 cell lines were expanded and cloned. Finally, 5 stable cell lines secreting antibodies against F-CB3 were used for further studies.

The isotype of the F-CB3 binding immunoglobulins was characterized by immunodiffusion using antisera specific for murine Ig-subclasses and immunoglobulin light chains. One of the antibodies, mc 125, was identified as $IgG_1\kappa$, the four other ones (mc 124, 126, 127, 128) were found to be IgMκ. Isolation of the pure immunoglobulins was performed by stepwise pH-gradient elution of the culture supernatants from protein A-Sepharose (10). Only antibodies from one cell line (mc 125) bound to protein A and could subsequently be eluted at pH 6.5 to 6.

The specificity of mc 125 was tested against a panel of antigens, including the isolated α-, β- and γ-chain, the cyanogen bromide

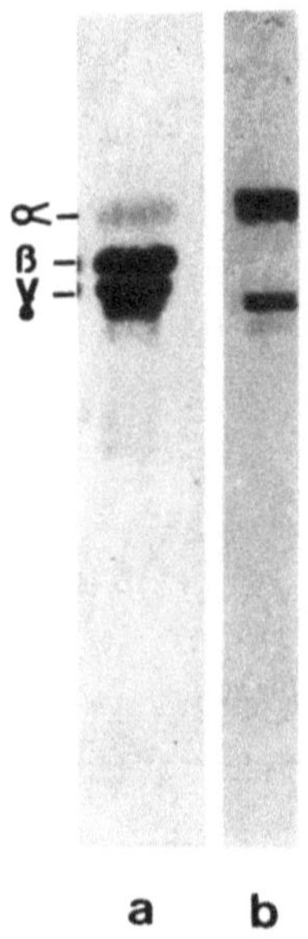

Fig. 2. Immunoblot reaction of mc 125 with reduced fibrinogen. After reduction and separation on 15% SDS PAGE and after electrophoretic transfer to nitrocellulose, the bands were either colored with amido black 10 B (lane a), or incubated with mc 125 (2 μg/ml) and goat anti-mouse IgG-peroxidase--conjugate. Antigen -antibody complexes were detected with a substrate containing catechol and 1,4-phenylenediamine in cacodylate buffer (12) (lane b).

peptides F-CB1 (N-terminal disulfide knot) and F-CB2 (the multichain peptide containing the second disulfide knot), plasminolysis fragment D and native human and bovine fibrinogen. As demonstrated by micro-ELISA (Fig.1), mc 125 reacts strongly with F-CB3, with the α-chain and with human fibrinogen. No reaction can be observed with any of the other antigens: F-CB1, F-CB2, β- or γ-chain and plasminolysis fragment D. The finding that mc 125 reacts equally well with the unreduced and the reduced form of the peptide, but does not bind to bovine F-CB3 (not shown) may indicate a nonconformational antigenic determinant.

The specificity of the purified antibody was also checked by Western blotting. Reduced fibrinogen incubated with mc 125 revealed two bands on nitrocellulose: one in α-chain position, as expected, the other one slightly lower than γ-chain position (Fig.2). Isolated β- and γ-chains did not react with the antibody (not shown). Therefore we assume that the band migrating slightly ahead of γ is a degraded α-chain fragment with a molecular weight around 47 kD.

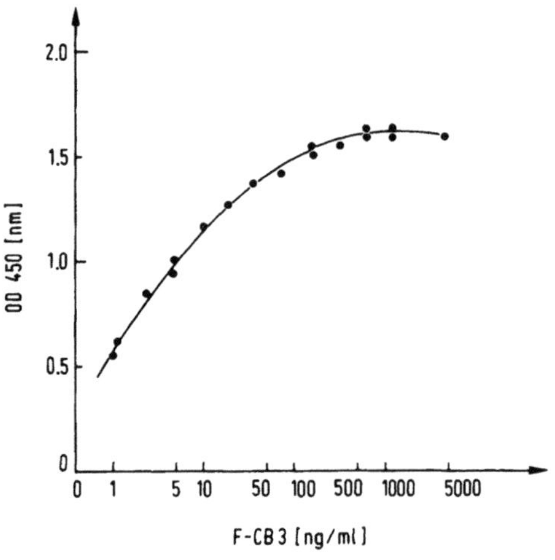

Fig. 3. Standard curve of F-CB3, measured in double sandwich micro-ELISA.
Coating with first antibody, immunoselective rabbit anti-F-CB3 (concentration 1,1 μg/ml). Second antibody, purified mc 125 (concentration 2 μg/ml). The amount of bound second antibody was detected by reaction with goat anti-mouse IgG coupled to peroxidase (Dianova). TMB was used as chromogen.

This indicates a cleavage of the α-chain between residues 424 and 425, i.e. in the last quarter of the sequence of F-CB3. From this finding it can be deduced that the antigenic determinant should be located before this cleavage site. This assumption is consistent with our finding that the antibody reacted only at very high concentrations with the earliest X-fragments, while no reaction with late X (MW 220 kD), Y, D or E could be observed.

In addition, a double sandwich micro-ELISA was developed in order to quantitate F-CB3 in sera of patients with various thrombo-embolic disorders. Our present standard curve is shown in Fig. 3. The assay allows to measure F-CB3 concentrations in the range of 1 - 100 ng/ml. This result suggests, that the monoclonal anti-F-CB3, mc 125, might prove useful in the diagnosis of early proteolysis and plasminolysis in the sera of patients.

Acknowledgement

We would like to express our gratitute to Miss J. Tüpel for expert technical assistance. This research was supported by the Sonderforschungsbereich der Deutschen Forschungsgemeinschaft 0207, Teilbereich A 1 and C 6. One of us (D.G. from the institute "Jožef Stefan", Ljubljana, Yugoslavia) was supported by a training grant from I.A.E.A., Vienna.

References

1. Gollwitzer, R., R. Timpl. 1975. FEBS LETTERS 58, 269-272.

2. Doolittle, R.F.. 1977. Horizons Biochem. Biophys. 3, 164-191.

3. Hessel, B.. 1975. Thromb. Res. 7, 75-87.

4. Gollwitzer, R., W. Bode. 1980. Haematologica 65, 528-534.

5. Furlan, M.. 1978. In: Fibrinolysis: Current fundamental and clinical concepts (P.J. Gaffney and S. Balkuv-Ulutin, eds.). Academic Press London, New York, San Francisco, p. 97-108.

6. Strong, D.D., K.W.K. Watt, B.A. Cottrell, R.F. Doolittle. 1979. Biochemistry 18, 5399-5404.

7. Gollwitzer, R., R. Hafter, R. Timpl, H. Graeff. 1977. Thromb. Res. 11, 859-868.

8. Schramm, W., K.H. Duswald, R. Gollwitzer. 1982. In: Hämostase, Thrombophilie und Arteriosklerose (J. van de Loo, F. Asbeck eds.). F.K. Schattauer Verlag, Stuttgart, New York, p. 160-169.

9. Hafter, R., W. Klaubert, R. Gollwitzer, R. von Hugo, H. Graeff. 1984. Thromb. Res. 35, 53-64.

10. Ey P.L., S.J. Prowse, C.R. Jenkin. 1978. Immunochemistry 15, 429-436.

11. Linke, R.P.. 1984. J. Histochem. Cytochem. 32, 322-328.

12. Dziadek, M., H. Richter, M. Schachner, R. Timpl. 1983. FEBS LETTERS 155, 321-325.

CLINICAL ASPECTS OF FIBRIN FORMATION AND FIBRINOLYSIS MEASURED WITH MONOCLONAL ANTIBODIES AGAINST D-DIMER

R. Hafter, R. Schröck, R. von Hugo und H. Graeff
Frauenklinik der Technischen Universität, D-8000 München

Introduction

D dimer and related crosslinked fibrin derivatives were measured in plasma of normal subjects and in patients with thromboembolic disorders and malignant diseases in an ELISA technique with specific monoclonal antibodies (MAb) developed by Rylatt and colleagues (1, 2, 3). The assay does not detect fibrinogen nor its degradation products (X, Y, D, E) and can therefore be employed on diluted plasma samples. Proof of crosslinked fibrin derivatives in plasma samples of patients was first documented in 1979 (4).

Materials and Methods

Monoclonal antibodies (MAb) were a gift of MAbCO, Springwood, Australia. The test was performed on 96 well micro-titer plates (Dynatech Immulon Cat N^{O} 655061) in a two way sandwich technique essentially according to EIA protocol (MAbCO) under use of a monospecific MAb (DD-3B6/22) as capture Ab and a panspecific MAb conjugated to horse radish peroxidase (DD-4D2 HRP) as tag Ab.

Plasma samples were diluted 1:5 (or higher if necessary) with PBS/Tween/BSA (phosphate buffered saline, pH 7.4/0.2 % Tween/2 % bovine serum albumine).
D dimer standard provided by MAbCO was diluted with the same diluent to concentrations (100 ng to 1000 ng/ml) to assess the standard curves. o-Tolidine dihydrochloride (Sigma T6269) was used as a substrate. Absorbance was recorded at 450 nm with the microtiter plate photometer Titertek Multiskan (Flow Lab.). Further details of the test are described elsewhere (1, 2, 3, 5).

Plasma samples: Blood was collected by clean venipuncture in the presence of anticoagulant (1:10), containing 0.13 mol/l sodium citrate, 0.06 mol/l TES (N-tris(hydroxymethyl)methyl-2-aminoethanesulfonic acid), 0.05 mol/l EDTA (disodium salt), and 2000 KIU/ml aprotinin (Trasylol, Bayer), adjusted to pH 7.4. Plasma was obtained by centrifugation (10 min 300 g, then 5 min 5000 g).

Fibrinogen - Fibrin Formation and Fibrinolysis, Vol. 4
© 1986 Walter de Gruyter & Co., Berlin · New York - Printed in Germany.

Samples were stored at -20^{0} C.

Cancer antigen 125 (CA 125) was measured by RIA (Diagnostic Kit, Centocor, Inc., Malvern, Pa.) according to manufacturer's instructions.

Results and Discussion

Fig. 1 shows a binding curve of D dimer standards with its typical sigmoidal shape, when plotted semilogarithmically. Measurements can be read in the range from 10 to 1000 ng DD/ml. In the flat part of the curve, that is in the range from 10 to 100 ng DD/ml, they are, however, rather unreliable. This becomes evident if serial dilutions of plasma samples are measured. If (for instance) the absorbance of a sample from an undiluted plasma sample is below 0.1, further dilutions (1:2, 1:4, 1:8 etc.) will not change the absorbance proportionally to the rate of dilution.

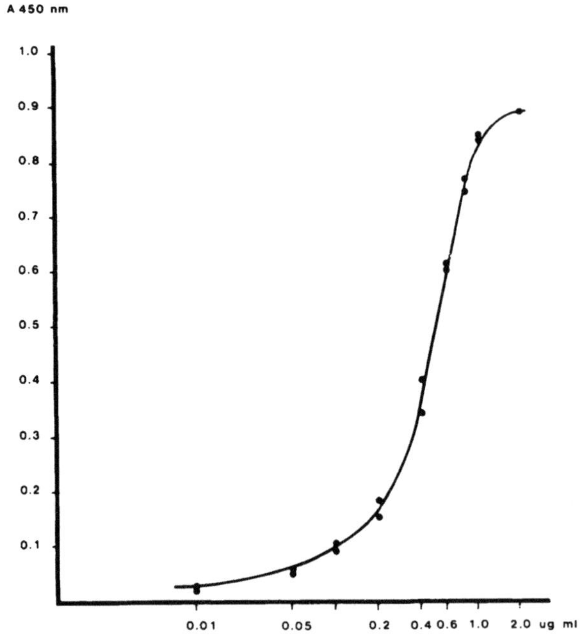

Fig. 1

D dimer standard curve. 0.01 to 2.0 µg DD/ml. Semilogarithmic plot. ELISA method with monoclonal antibodies.

The test is recommended (from MAbCO protocol) to be used on plasma dilutions of 1:5. We used 1:5 dilutions throughout this study except from samples with D dimer concentrations > 2000 ng/ml where we used dilutions of 1:10 or more. But we were aware that under the described conditions, which refer to healthy subjects, normal values might be overestimated.

To establish the reliability criteria of the D-dimer test we determined the coefficient of variation (CV) which was 4.9 % in the intraassay precision (DD range in plasma 45 - 488 ng/ml) and 12.3 % or 15.1 % in the interassay precision, dependent on the DD concentration range (Table 1).

The recovery test (Table 2) revealed 100 % recovery when 100 ng DD was added to 1 ml plasma samples and 84 % or 73 % recovery when 200 or 400 ng DD were added to the same 1 ml plasma samples. Corresponding results were achieved when DD prepared in our laboratory was used instead of the MAbCO standard.

Table 1

Coefficient of Variation (CV) at D-Dimer Measurement by ELISA

	DD ng/ml	N	CV %	Range of CV %
Intraassay precision	45 - 488	10x10	4.9	3.1 - 7.0
Interassay precision	45 - 118	5x10	12.3	9.6 -15.4
	184 - 488	5x10	15.1	12.3 -18.4

Table 2

Recovery Test : Human D-Dimer added to identical Plasma Samples

Added ng/ml	Found ng/ml	N assays	Recovery %
0	223 ± 30	3x6	
100	323 ± 15	3x6	100
200	391 ± 33	3x6	84
400	513 ± 23	3x6	73

Furthermore, we compared D dimer measurements in plasma and serum. In serum samples prepared with thrombin from citrated plasma in the presence of Trasylol we found mostly somewhat lower values of DD (Table 3, left side) than in the original plasma samples, while in serum samples prepared in the absence of Trasylol higher values of DD were found (Table 3, right side).

Table 3

D-Dimer Concentrations in Plasma and Serum (ng/ml)

N°	Plasma	Serum	Deviation %	N°	Plasma	Serum	Deviation %
1	255	280	+ 9.8	7	525	632	+20.4
2	495	446	-10.1	8	575	803	+39.6
3	575	385	-33.1	9	750	979	+30.5
4	750	704	- 6.2	10	890	1109	+24.3
5	775	715	- 7.8	11	1485	2409	+62.2
6	1560	1512	- 3.1	12	1540	2403	+59.0

Serum prepared from plasma samples with thrombin (o.1 ml/ml plasma; 3 IU) in presence (N° 1 - 6) of aprotinin (200 KIU/ml plasma) and (N° 7 - 12) in absence of aprotinin

These findings seem to indicate, on one hand, that part of the crosslinked fibrin derivatives is adsorbed to or occluded into the fibrin clot when fibrinogen is clotted with thrombin in vitro. On the other hand, when Trasylol is absent during clotting a greater part of D dimer and related compounds is released by fibrinolysis from crosslinked fibrin. Whitaker (3) and Gaffney (6) reported similar observations. Whitaker (3) suggested that higher plasma values might also be explainable as some part of still clottable crosslinked fibrin derivatives.

The following chapter deals with clinical findings.

To evaluate the D-dimer test in respect to its sensitivity towards thromboembolic episodes we measured D-dimer in six young non pregnant patients with apparatively diagnosed deep vein thrombosis (DVT) in absence of any other interfering disease. The mean D-dimer concentration found (808 ∓ 430 ng/ml) was significantly higher compared with a control group (n = 20) of similar age (168 ∓ 67 ng/ml). In one patient with additional pulmonary embolism a D-dimer concentration of 4950 ng/ml was measured (Table 4). Fibrinogen and fibrinopeptide A (FPA) were found elevated in these patients, too, and AT III was decreased.

Table 4

Thromboembolic Disease in Young Non Pregnant Patients
(Mean ± SD)

	N	Age Years	DD ng/ml	Fbg mg/ml	FPA ng/ml	AT III %
DVT	6	29 ± 9	808 ± 430	4.01 ± 1.7	25 ± 8	71 ± 12
PE	1	18	4950	4.46	40	53
Controls	20	25 ± 4	168 ± 87	1.99 ± 0.2	10 ± 5	95 ± 16
p DVT/Contr.			<0.001	<0.0005	<0.005	<0.005

Since thromboembolic episodes more often occur during gestation and in childbed in which already a hypercoagulable state is observed with rise of soluble fibrin monomer complexes (SFMC) (7, 8), it was of interest to measure D-dimer also in healthy women during gestation and puerperium in order to obtain comparable base-line values. Measurements on a small group of 23 healthy pregnant and on 8 puerperal women revealed a distinctive increase in D-dimer dependent on duration of pregnancy. Highest values of about 600 ng DD/ml were noted between third trimenon and delivery, compared to 168 ng/ml in matched controls. A further marked increase up to 2500 ng/ml was observed in the puerperium (mean 1525 ∓ 630) (Table 5).

DD levels in puerperium turned out to be even higher than those of young non pregnant patients with DVT. Noteworthy in this connection is that no relevant changes of AT III levels were observed. The increase of FPA was also smaller than expected, for which the shorter half-life of FPA might be responsible.

Table 5

Uncomplicated Pregnancy and Childbed
(Mean ± SD)

	Weeks	N	Age Years	DD ng/ml	Fbg mg/ml	FPA ng/ml	AT III %
Gestation	9 - 19	9	30 ± 6	248 ± 70	2.78 ± 0.6	13 ± 3	94 ± 16
	20 - 29	5	30 ± 4	330 ± 84	3.62 ± 0.5	19 ± 6	88 ± 3
	30 - 40	9	28 ± 4	586 ± 57	3.30 ± 0.2	23 ± 6	81 ± 11
Childbed		8	31 ± 3	1525 ± 630	4.78 ± 0.9	25 ± 3	89 ± 13
Controls	–	20	25 ± 4	168 ± 87	1.99 ± 0.2	10 ± 5	95 ± 16

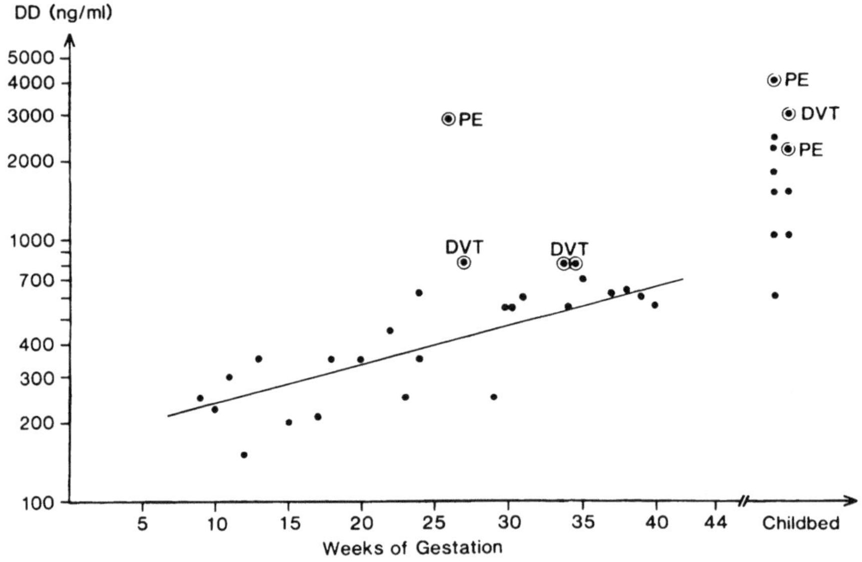

Fig. 2: Concentrations of D-dimer in 31 healthy females (see Table 5) and in seven females with deep vein thrombosis (DVT) and pulmonary embolism (PE) during gestation and childbed

Out of seven patients who suffered DVT with and without pulmonary embolism (PE) during pregnancy and childbed, DD concentrations were distinctively elevated in four, in comparison to women with uncomplicated gestation (Fig. 2).

As a second possibility to test hypercoagulability as an interfering factor for the specificity of D dimer release in thrombotic disease the postoperative phase was investigated (Table 6).

Table 6

Postoperative Phase (Mean ± SD)

	N	Age Years	DD ng/ml	Fbg mg/ml	FPA ng/ml	AT III %
Patients	9	44 ± 10	1280 ± 580	4.06 ± 0.7	29.9 ± 5.0	80 ± 14
Controls	20	25 ± 4	168 ± 87	1.99 ± 0.2	10.3 ± 4.5	95 ± 16
Controls	20	44 ± 19	197 ± 52	–	–	–

For this purpose plasma samples were investigated from the first and second postoperative day from patients operated electively because of benign gynecological disorders. The average age of these nine patients was 44 ∓ 10 years, the mean D dimer concentration 1280 ∓ 580 ng/ml. In a matched control group mean D-dimer concentration was 197 ∓ 52 ng/ml. Similar to the situation in childbed the changes in FPA and AT III were less marked.

Another interfering disease for detecting thromboembolic episodes by DD measurement is malignancy. In a previous paper (5) we have reported about D dimer concentrations in patients with gynecological malignant diseases. Especially in patients with epithelial ovarian cancer we found a strong correlation between concentrations of D dimer and tumor associated antigen CA 125 on one hand, and clinically staged tumor situation (tumor activity) on the other hand (5). Measurement of CA 125 by RIA is hitherto the most specific and sensitive method available to monitor the response of treatment in epithelial ovarian cancer (9).

In eight from nine preoperative patients (Fig. 3) in whom tumor marker concentration was normal (< 65 U/ml) D dimer concentration was also low (< 400 ng/ml). In sixteen patients (from sixteen) with pathological values of CA 125 (> 65 U/ml) D dimer concentrations were > 400 ng/ml. The tumor situations (expressed in activities A_1, A_2, A_3) in all patients except one, correlated to D dimer and CA 125 concentrations (Fig. 3). A_1 refers to a non-detectable tumor although a recurrence is suspected, A_2 to a tumor in stabilized phase or undergoing remission, A_3 to a tumor in progression with spreading local or distant metastases.

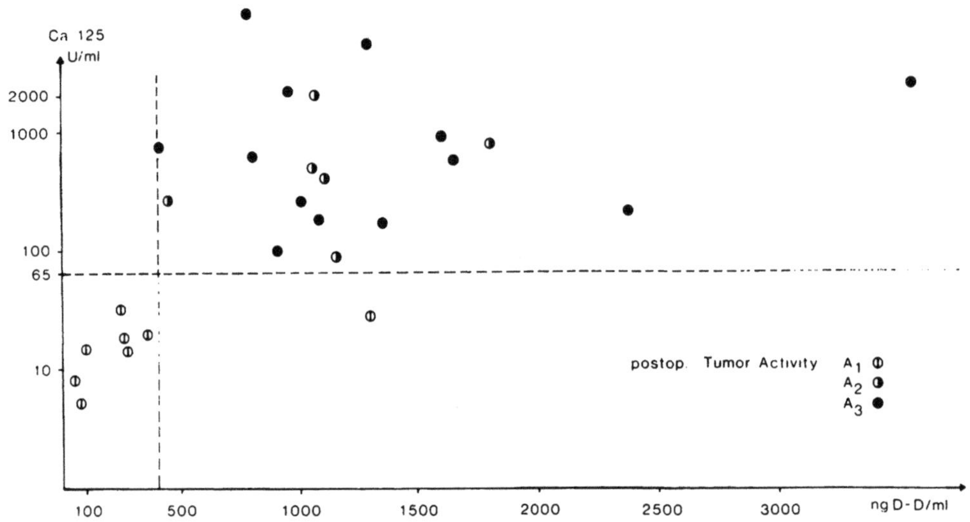

Fig. 3: Concentrations of tumor associated antigen CA 125 and D-dimer in plasma of 27 patients with ovarian cancer (FIGO II - IV) of different tumor situations: A_1 ↓, A_2 ◑, A_3 ●

The good correlation of CA 125 and D dimer to the clinical situation was also observed in some single patients in whom under therapy a parallel behaviour of CA 125, D-dimer and the tumor situation was assessed. One case of a patient with ovarian cancer (FIGO III) under therapy over a period of more than eight months is shown in Fig. 4. The close parallel course in DD and CA 125 concentrations is only once divergent (between Sept 28 and Oct 9) when the patient suffered from an episode of DVT which was phlebographically confirmed a few days later.

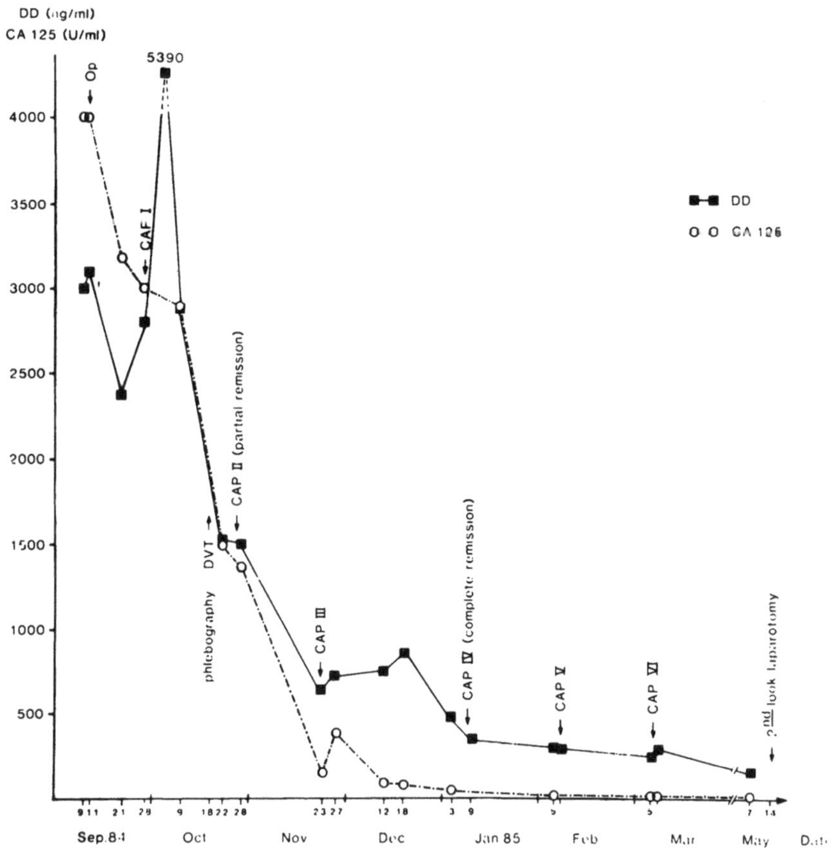

Fig. 4: Course of CA 125 and D dimer concentrations in a patient with epithelial ovarian cancer (FIGO III) undergoing tumorreductive surgery and six cycles of chemotherapy (CAP I - VI).
CAP = Cyclophosphamide + Adriamycin + Cisplatin

In conclusion, the above findings confirm that thromboembolic episodes are recognizable with high sensitivity by D-dimer test, although the specificity of the test is somewhat lowered during pregnancy, puerperium and in the postoperative phase, as well as in malignant diseases, caused by D-dimer increase under these conditions.

Acknowledgements

This study was supported by the Deutsche Forschungsgemeinschaft (Sonderforschungsbereich 0207, München). The technical assistance of Mrs. E. Sedlaczek and Mrs. M. Schulte-Jahn is gratefully acknowledged. We are thankful to MAbCO, Australia, for supplying us with the monoclonal antibodies for the D-dimer test.

References

1. Rylatt, D.B., A.S. Blake, L.E. Cottis, D.A. Massingham, W.A. Fletcher, P.P. Masci, A.N. Whitaker, M.J. Elms, I.H. Bunce, A.J. Webber, D. Wyatt, P.G. Bundesen. 1983. Thromb. Res. 31, 767 - 778.

2. Elms, M.J., I.H. Bunce, P.G. Bundesen, D.B. Rylatt, A.J. Webber, P.P. Masci, A.N. Whitaker. 1983. Thromb. Haemostas. 50 (2), 591 - 594.

3. Whitaker, A.N., M.J. Elms, P.P. Masci, P.G. Bundesen, D.B. Rylatt, A.J. Webber, I.H. Bunce. 1984. J. Clin. Pathol. 37, 882 - 887.

4. Graeff, H., R. Hafter, L. Bachmann. 1979. Thromb. Res. 16, 313 - 328.

5. Hafter, R., R. Schröck, R. von Hugo, H. Graeff. 1985. Scand. J. clin. Lab. Invest. (in press).

6. Gaffney, P.J., M.J. Perry. Assay methods for fibrinogen and fibrin degradation products (FDP). Presented at First International Postgraduate Course, Fibrinolysis in Clinical Medicine, Venice 1984.

7. Hafter, R., T. Schneebauer, K. Tafel, E. Ernst, H. Graeff. 1975. Geburtsh. u. Frauenheilk. 35, 518 - 525.

8. Graeff, H., A. Wiedemann, R. von Hugo, R. Hafter. 1976. Am. J. Obstet. Gynecol. 124, 21 - 24.

9. Bast, R.C., T.L. Klug, E.S. John, E. Jenison, J.M. Niloff, H. Lazarus, R.S. Berkowitz, T. Leavitt, C.T. Griffiths, L. Parker, V.R. Zuranoski, R.C. Knapp.1983. New Engl. J. Med. 309, 883 - 887.

FIBRINOGEN DERIVATIVES IN ACUTE STROKE

J.T. Douglas, G.D.O. Lowe, C.D. Forbes

University Department of Medicine, Royal Infirmary, Glasgow, U.K., G31 2ER

I. Knight, D.A. Lane

Department of Haematology, Charing Cross Hospital Medical School, Hammersmith, London

M.J. Perry, P.J. Gaffney

National Institute for Biological Standards and Control, Holly Hill, Hampstead, London, NW3 6RB

Introduction

This study reports preliminary findings on the activation products of platelets, coagulation and fibrinolysis in patients with acute stroke. Activation of blood coagulation and fibrinolysis generates thrombin which cleaves fibrinopeptide (FPA) and plasmin which cleaves Bβ 15-42 containing fragments from fibrin (ogen). Later lytic fragments include fragment E (FgE) and high molecular weight cross-linked fibrin degradation products commonly referred to as X-oligomers (X-L FDP). Activation of platelets results in the release of betathromboglobulin (BTG) from platelet α - granules.

Around 80% of strokes are thromboembolic in origin (1) and their onset and further progression are thought to be the result of the formation of intravascular thrombi and/or embolization. Such thrombi are formed by the interaction of platelets and fibrin.

In this study we have determined BTG, fibrinogen, FPA, plasminogen activator, Bβ 15-24, serum fibrin(ogen) degradation products (FDP), serum fragment E (FgE) and X-L FDP in patients with acute stroke, and have related them to controls, changes in the first 10 days and their prognostic value for death.

Fibrinogen - Fibrin Formation and Fibrinolysis, Vol. 4
© 1986 Walter de Gruyter & Co., Berlin · New York - Printed in Germany.

MATERIALS AND METHODS

Venous blood samples were collected by careful venepuncture without stasis. Plasma BTG was determined by radioimmunoassay (Amersham kit) as described previously (2). FPA and Bβ15-42 were measured by the IMCO radioimmunoassay kits as previously described (3).

Blood for fibrinogen, plasminogen activator and X-L FDP was anti-coagulated with 0.11M trisodism citrate (9:1, V:V). Plasminogen activator was measured by the lysis area of the euglobulin fraction on fibrin plates and fibrinogen by the Dade fibrometer as previously described (4). Blood for FgE antigen and FDP concentration was collected into trypsin inhibitor (final concentration 1800 NF units/ml) and thrombin (10 NIH Units/ml) and allowed to clot at room temperature for 1 hour. Serum was obtained by centrifugation and stored at -20°C. FgE antigen was measured by radioimmunoassay as described previously (5). Serum FDP were measured using the conventional Wellcome FDP kit (Wellcome Diagnostics). Plasma concentrations of X-L FDP were measured using a monoclonal antibody technique as described previously (6).

Blood was obtained from 15 control patients undergoing elective surgery for non malignant disease and 39 patients with acute stroke as defined by the sudden onset of focal neurological symptoms of presumed vascular origin, excluding primary sub-arachnoid haemorrhage. Patients with acute stroke were sampled within 24 hours following admission and subsequently on days 5 and 10.

Results

Betathromboglobulin (Fig 1)

When compared to the control group (24.3 ± 2.1 ng/ml, mean ± SEM) significantly increased levels of plasma BTG were observed in patients on days 1 (52.9 ± 4.8 ng/ml, $P < 0.001$), 5 (50.9 ± 10.3 ng/ml, $p < 0.01$) and 10 (65.5 ± 12.2 ng/ml, $p < 0.01$) after stroke. On day 1, BTG levels were significantly higher in the stroke patients who died (61.2 ± 5.6 ng/ml) when compared to the level in patients who survived (44.6 ± 3.9 ng/ml, $p < 0.02$).

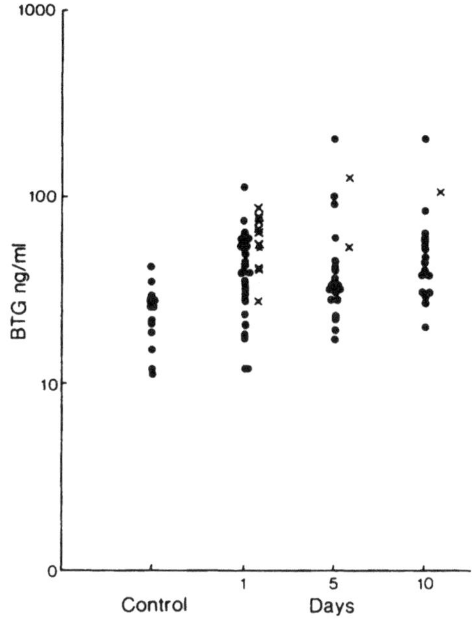

Fig 1. Plasma BTG in controls, patients on day 1,5 and 10 after acute stroke●represents controls and patients who survived. X represents patients who died.

Fibrinogen (Fig 2)

Significantly increased fibrinogen levels were found, when compared to controls (3.2 ± 0.2 g/l), in patients on days 1 (4 ± 0.2 g/L, $p < 0.05$), 5 (4.3 ± 0.3 g/L, $p < 0.05$) and 10 (4.2 ± 0.3 g/L, $p < 0.05$) after stroke. There was no significant difference on day 1 between the fibrinogen levels of the stroke patients who died (4.6 ± 0.4 g/L) and the patients who survived (3.8 ± 0.2 g/L).

Fibrinopeptide A (Fig 3)
Significantly increased FPA levels were found, when compared to controls (3.0 ± 0.4 pmol/ml), in patients on days 1 (9.6 ± 2.2 p mol/ml, $p < 0.05$), 5 (9.6 ± 2.7 p mol/ml, $p < 0.05$) and 10 (6.1 ±

1.1 p mol/ml, $p < 0.05$) after stroke. On day 1, FPA levels were significantly higher in the stroke patients who died (median, 6 p mol/l when compared to the levels in patients who survived (median, 2.6 p mol/ml, $p < 0.002$).

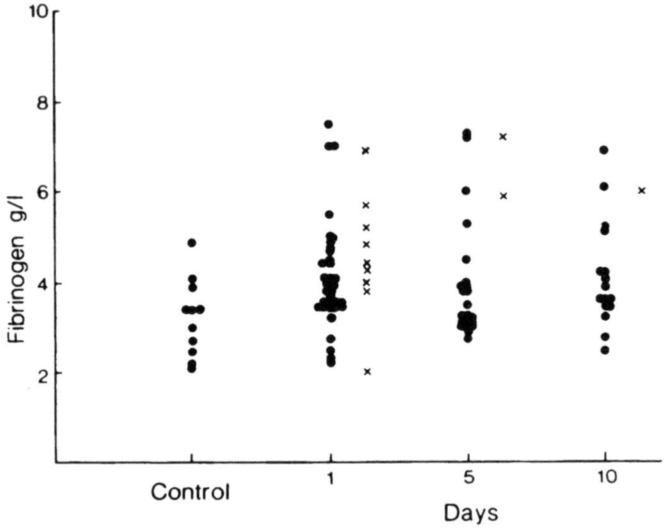

Fig 2. Plasma fibrinogen in controls, patients on days 1, 5 and 10 after stroke.

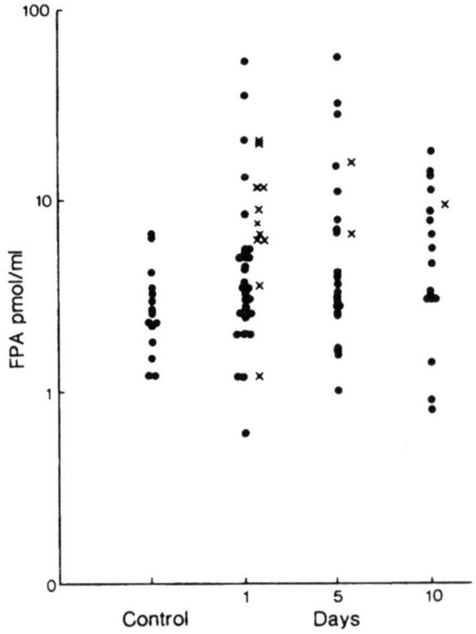

Fig 3. Plasma FPA in controls, patients on days 1, 5 and 10 after stroke.

Plasminogen Activator (Fig 4)

Significantly increased plasminogen activator levels were found, when compared to controls (70.3 ± 4.2 mm^2), in patient on days 1 (85.7 ± 4.6 mm^2, $p < 0.05$), 5 (84.5 ± 4.7 mm^2, $p < 0.05$) and 10 (96.1 ± 6.2 mm^2, $p < 0.05$) after stroke. On day 1, while not significant there appears to be a trend towards lower plasminogen activator levels in stroke patients who died (78.2 ± 8.8 mm^2) when compared to patients who survived (85.9 ± 4.9 mm^2).

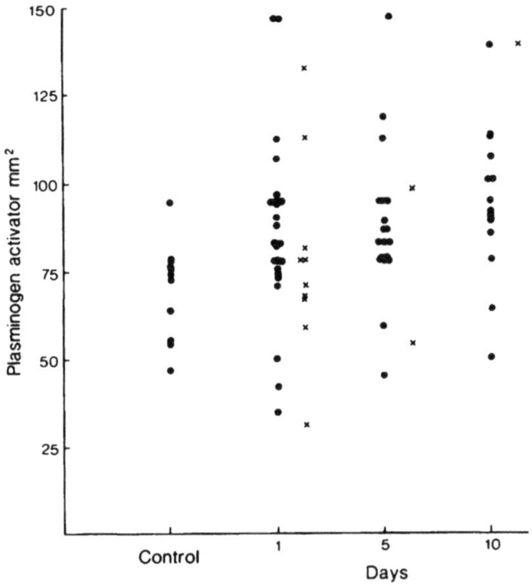

Fig 4. Plasma plasminogen activator in controls, patients on days 1, 5 and 10 after stroke.

Bβ15-42 (Fig 5)

Similar Bβ15-42 levels were observed in the control patients (3.5 ± 0.7 p mol/ml) and stroke patients on days 1 (3.6 ± 0.3 p mol/ml) 5 (3.9 ± 0.5 p mol/ml) and 10 (3.7 ± 0.5 p mol/ml). However, on day 1, the mean Bβ15-42 level in the stroke patients who died (5.3 ± 0.4 p mol/ml) was significantly higher than the mean Bβ15-42 level in the patients who survived (2.9 ± 0.3 p mol/ml, $p < 0.001$). The mean Bβ15-42 level measured in stroke patients on day 5 (3.9 ± 0.5 p mol/ml) was significantly higher than the mean level measured in the same stroke patients on day 1 (3 ± 0.3 p mol/ml).

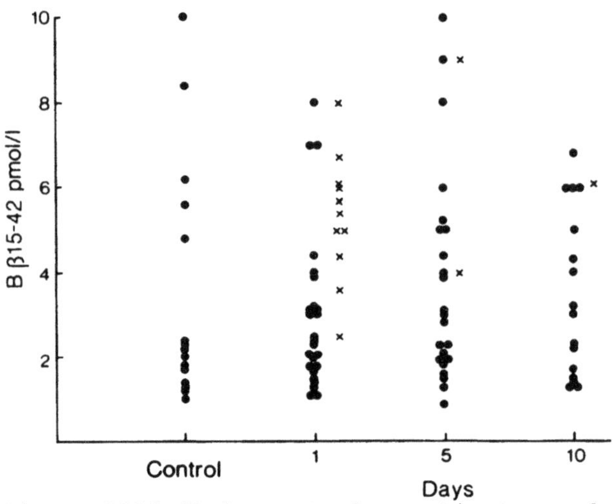

Fig 5. Plasma Bβ15-42 in controls, patients on days 1, 5 and 10 after stroke.

FDP (Fig 6)

Similar FDP levels were obtained in the stroke patients on days 1 (3.2 ± 0.2 µg/ml), 5 (3.5 ± 0.3 µg/ml) and 10 (3.6 ± 0.5 µg/ml) after stroke when compared to the control range for this assay (1.5 - 5 µg/ml). On day 1 the mean FDP level in the stroke patients who died (4.5 ± 0.5 µg/ml) was significantly higher than the mean level in patients who survived (2.8 ± 0.2 µg/ml, $p < 0.01$). The mean FDP level measured in stroke patients on day 5 (3.6 ± 0.4 µg/ml) was significantly higher than the mean level measured in the stroke patients on day 1 (2.9 ± 0.2 µg/ml, $p < 0.01$).

Fragment E (Fig 7)

Greatly elevated FgE levels were obtained in the stroke patients on days 1 (356 ± 55 ng/ml), 5 (393 ± 74 ng/ml) and 10 (426 ± 111 ng/ml) when compared to the control range for this assay (10-80 ng/ml). On day 1 the mean FgE level in patients who died (643 ± 143 ng/ml) was significantly higher than the mean FgE level in the patients who survived (245 ± 36 ng/ml, $p < 0.002$).

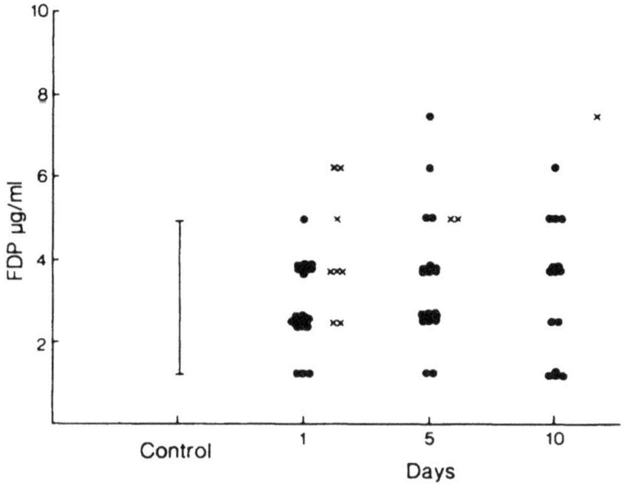

Fig 6. Serum FDP in control range, patients on days 1, 5 and 10 after stroke.

X-L FDP (Fig 8)

Greatly elevated X-L FDP levels were obtained in the stroke patients on days 1 (502 ± 251 ng/ml), 5 (413 ± 163 ng/ml) and 10 (816 ± 312 ng/ml) when compared to the control range for this assay 0-200 ng/ml). On day 1, while not significant, higher X-L FDP levels were observed in stroke patients who died (median, 215 ng/ml) when compared to the levels in patients who survived (median, 81 ng/ml).

Discussion

These results which demonstrated increased FPA, BB15-42 and BTG levels in patients with acute stroke, confirm activation of coagulation, fibrinolysis and platelets in acute stroke. Our finding of increased BTG levels verifies previous reports (7-9) but disputes a previous study which did not find increased BTG levels in acute stroke (10). These previous studies did not

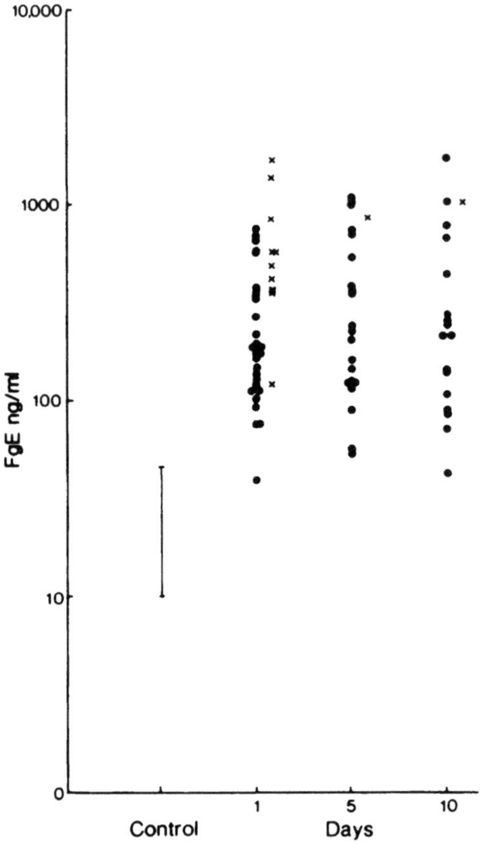

Fig 7. Serum FgE in control range, patients on days 1, 5 and 10 after stroke.

relate FPA, Bβ15-42 or BTG to death versus survival. In our study all 3 parameters were significantly increased on the day following stroke in patients who later died when compared to patients who survived. It may be that these parameters may be related to the size of the thrombus or infarct. At the present time their relation to specificity for infarctcannot be assessed as CT scans have only been performed in approximately 50% of patients. To date only 3 patients had intracranial haemorrhages, therefore larger numbers are required to determine if these parameters differentiate haemorrhages and infarts. This study also showed increased FgE, FDP and X-L FDP levels in patients with acute stroke,

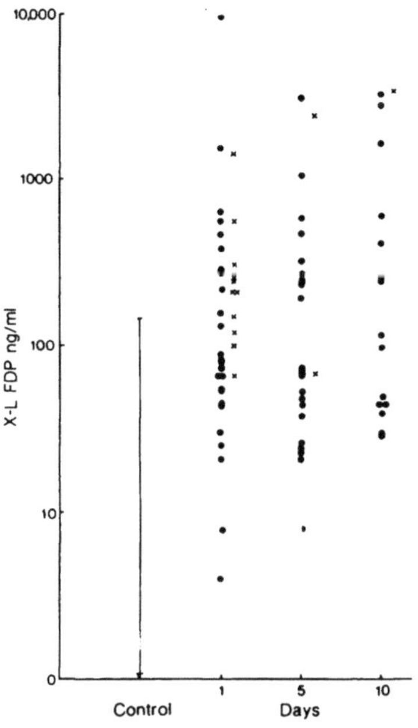

Fig 8. Plasma X-L FDP in control range, patients on days 1, 5 and 10 after stroke.

Although it has been reported previously that FgE levels were increased in stroke patients who progressed (10), our study showed increased FDP and FgE levels on day 1 in patients who died when compared to patients who survived. Interestingly, the conventional Wellcome FDP kit appears to be as good a predictive index of death as the more complicated FgE and X-L FDP assays. In this study we report the first measurement of X-L FDP in acute stroke, which as expected showed increased levels in patients on days 1, 5 and 10 after acute stroke.

This study also showed a decreased plasminogen activator level on day 1 in patients who died when compared to patients who survived and although not significant it may suggest a decreased fibrinolytic response to thrombus formation in such patients. However, BB 15-42 levels were higher in patients who died, hence plasmin generation was ongoing despite lower activator levels. We plan to expand the study to include 100 patients, whom we will follow up for 1 year in order to determine the relationship of the parameters measured in our preliminary study to:

- infarct/haemorrhage on CT scan
- predictors of death or recurrence of stroke
- predictors of functional recovery.

References

1. Allen, C.M.C. 1983. Quart. J. Med. 52, 515-523.

2. Douglas, J.T., G.D.O. Lowe, C.D. Forbes, C.R.M. Prentice. 1983. Thromb. Haemostas. 50, 541-542.

3. Douglas, J.T., S.L. Blamey, G.D.O. Lowe, D.C. Carter, C.D. Forbes. 1985. Thromb. Haemostas. 53, 235-238.

4. Blamey, S.L., B.M. McArdle, P. Burns, G.D.O. Lowe, C.D. Forbes, D.C. Carter, C.R.M. Prentice. 1984. Thromb. Haemostas, 51, 71-74.

5. Gordon, Y.B., J.J. Martin, J. Landon, T. Chard. 1975. Br. J. Haematol, 29, 109-118.

6. Perry, M.J. 1984. VIII International congress on thrombosis. Istanbul, 134.

7. Hoogendijk,E.M.G., C.S.P. Jenkins, E.M. Van Wyk, J. Vos, J.W. Ten Cate. 1979. Thromb. Haemostas. 64, 512-522.

8. Matsuda, T., T. Sekik, M. Ogaware, T. Minra, M. Yokarchi, M. Murokami. 1979. Thromb. Haemostas. 42, 288.

9. Lane, D.A., S. Wolff, H. Ireland, M. Gawel, M. Foadi. 1983. Br. J. Haematol. 53, 655-658.

10. De Boer, A.C., A.G.G. Turpie, R.W. Butt, R.J. Duke, R.F. Bloch, E. Genton. 1982. Br J. Haematol, 50, 327-334.

VII. Fibrin(ogen) and Disease Pathology

TRIGGERING OF THE EXTRINSIC BLOOD COAGULATION SYSTEM

Hans Prydz

Research Institute for Internal Medicine, University of Oslo, Rikshospitalet, Oslo, Norway.

Introduction

Tissue thromboplastin (tissue factor, factor III) is the most potent trigger of blood coagulation known. Recent years have seen an increasing awareness of the role of the extrinsic clotting system (i.e. thromboplastin and factor VII) in various clinical syndromes related to inflammation, immune responses, disseminated intravascular coagulation, transplant rejection etc. It is reasonable to assume that also processes leading to extravascular fibrin deposits in many cases are triggered by the synthesis or release (e.g. by trauma) of thromboplastin.

I shall briefly review the biochemistry, physiology and cell biology of this extrinsic clotting pathway. For a more extensive review and literature list see Prydz (1).

Biochemistry of Thromboplastin and Factor VII

Thromboplastin (tissue factor, factor III) consists of a single-chain integral membrane glycoprotein (apoprotein III) of apparent M_r around 50 kD (about 48-52 kD when isolated from human brain (2,3) 43-45 kD from bovine brain (4). This protein has no procoagulant triggering activity alone, but regains its activity in the presence of certain phospholipids (2,5). The apoprotein was first purified by Bjørklid et al. (2) but the yield of our method was too low to permit any protein chemistry, and even today very little is known about the biochemistry of the apoprotein. This is

Fibrinogen - Fibrin Formation and Fibrinolysis, Vol. 4
© 1986 Walter de Gruyter & Co., Berlin · New York - Printed in Germany.

partly due to its hydrophobicity which makes the presence of detergents mandatory at all steps during the purification. Since the protein alone is inactive as a procoagulant and has no other known function which can be monitored, recombination with phospholipids and removal of the detergent are necessary to be able to follow the activity throughout the purification procedure. For the human apoprotein III a molar ratio of protein:phospholipid of about 1:80-1:100 seemed to give an optimal thromboplastin activity (3). This result is in good accordance with more recent determinations of the molar ratios of other protein-phospholipid interactions.

A bovine preparation has been reported to require a weight ratio of 1:450 (protein to phospholipid), corresponding to a molar ratio of about 1:30,000 (4) and the activity remained unaltered at ratios twice higher. This very high value for the apparent phospholipid requirement of bovine apoprotein may be due to unrecognized losses of phospholipids in the dialysis part of reconstitution experiments.

The nature of the phospolipids necessary for reconstitution of the procoagulant activity of the apoprotein has not been entirely clarified. Nemerson (6,7) and Pitlick and Nemerson (8) reported that PE was the most active, followed by PC, and that PS was inactive. Mixtures of phospholipids were more effective. Lysolecithin was inactive. Wijngaards et al. (9) and Bjørklid and Storm (3) investigated systematically binary and (the latter authors) ternary phospholipid mixtures and reported that negatively charged phospholipids (PS or PG) in mixtures with PC and or PE were the most effective. Nemerson (6) demonstrated a requirement for unsaturated phospholipids, later confirmed by other groups (9).

Human factor VII is a vitamin K-dependent single-chain plasma glycoprotein of M_r 45-48,000 (10,11). Its primary structure is incompletely known but will probably be deduced shortly from the cloning of cDNA in which several laboratories are involved. One reason for the lack of structural information about factor VII is its very low level in plasma, about 0.5 µg/ml (12). Factor VII is mainly produced in the parenchymal liver cells (13) and also in monocytes (14). Its half-life in plasma is very short (4-6 h). Like other clotting factors in plasma, factor VII is a proenzyme and must be activated to a serine protease for its role in coagulation.

Physiology and Triggering of the Extrinsic Coagulation Pathway

Thromboplastin triggers blood coagulation by forming a Ca^{2+}-dependent stoichiometric complex with factor VII which undergoes a conformational change exposing its active site. Factor VII is thereby transformed from a zymogen to an active enzyme. This alters the sensitivity of human factor VII to serine protease inhibitors, from the very low sensitivity of the zymogen to the more normal sensitivity for a serine protease shown by factor VII in complex with thromboplastin. The factor VII-thromboplastin complex is the most potent trigger of coagulation yet known. Purified and reconstituted human thromboplastin can clot normal human plasma in 12-15 s. Human plasma contains a still ill-defined inhibitor most likely of the thromboplastin-VII complex, which may turn out to be very important.

Østerud and Rapaport (15) produced clear evidence that the reaction product of thromboplastin and factor VII activated factor IX in a human system. Activated factor IX itself as well as factor Xa and thrombin failed to activate factor IX, but the thromboplastin/factor VII reaction product replaced the normal factor IX band in SDS-PAG electrophoresis by bands corresponding to the heavy and light chain of activated factor IX. The capability of the extrinsic trigger to activate the intrinsic system was thus firmly established. Similar results have later been reported by other laboratories using bovine reagents.

Østerud and Rapaport (16) showed that this activation of factor IX by thromboplastin and factor VII was of the same order of potency as activation of factor IX by factor XI. Fitting in very well with these observations is the competitive inhibition of factor X activation by factor IX and vice versa. This inhibitory effect has been observed in several types of experiments (17,18) and Jesty and Silverberg (19) have determined the respective K_i values in a bovine system.

Further evidence that activation of IX by thromboplastin and VII is important for normal haemostasis is provided by an interesting patient reported by Bertina et al. (20). Their patient had a factor X deficiency which was demonstrable when straightforward extrinsic activation by thromboplastin and factor VII was studied, but no defect was seen in the activation of factor X by factor IXa alone or by factor IXa and factor VIII. This patient had no bleeding complications suggesting that the normal haemostasis was caused via activation of factor IX by thromboplastin and VII.

In addition to this "classical" activation of factor VII by formation of the thromboplastin-Ca^{2+}-factor VII complex, there are two other ways by which factor VII can be activated:

1. Factor VII from human and bovine sources can undergo a proteolytic nick, giving rise to a two-chain disulphide-linked molecule with 30-100 fold increased activity in a thromboplastin-triggered test system (11). Factor IXa, factor Xa and factor XIIa activate factor VII in this way. There is some evidence that purified two-chain factor VII in the presence of Ca^{2+} and phospholipids can activate factor X.

2. Factor VII activity is high in plasma from pregnant women (21) and from some men at risk for cardiovascular diseases (22). In both cases we have shown that this is due to the presence of factor VII-phospholipid complexes in plasma (23,24). When present in such complexes the specific activity of factor VII can increase 3-4 fold. The complexes do not contain detectable thromboplastin, and they do not consistently shorten the recalcification time of citrated plasma. They are very sensitive to purified phospholipase C (23,24) which breaks down phospholipids to diglycerides. In preliminary gel filtration experiments the apparent size of the complexes suggests that they consist of one factor VII molecule and 20-25 phospholipid molecules. The presence of human factor VII in these phospho-

lipid complex(es) alters its conformation as evidenced by an increased sensitivity for DFP inhibition of its active site serine.

Cell Biology of Thromboplastin

Thromboplastin is of widespread occurrence in the mammalian organism. Especially rich sources are brain, lung, thyroid gland, intraperitoneal and bone marrow fat, and placenta. The liver is a rather poor source. As far as we know today, thromboplastins from these various sources all cross-react with neutralizing antibodies, both polyclonal (3) and monoclonal (25), but whether they are identical in every aspect of their structure is obviously unknown, since no structural information is available.

There is, however, more information available about the cell biology of thromboplastin. Apparently, certain cells in vitro (and their tissue equivalents) synthesize apoprotein III constitutively. Such cells are fibroblasts, glioma cells and placental trophoblasts. Other cells, which normally do not synthesize apoprotein III, can be induced to do so by a number of agents like immune complexes, endotoxins, lymphokines. Such cells are monocytes, macrophages and endothelial cells. Finally, there are cells (lymphocytes, granulocytes, platelets) in which so far no thromboplastin synthesis has been demonstrated in spite of the use of several inducers.

When present, thromboplastin is normally cell-bound and not in contact with plasma. Triggering of coagulation requires such contact. This can be brought about either by tissue injury (surgical or otherwise) or by induction of synthesis of the thromboplastin apoprotein in cells not normally making it. As mentioned, such cells are monocytes and macrophages and at least certain kinds of endothelial cells (human umbilical cord and bovine aorta). The thromboplastin synthesized becomes to a large extent available on the cell surface, so that the intact cells may serve as procoagulant foci. This is of proven or suggested clinical importance in various fields of human medicine (26-29). A third possible way of contact between thromboplastin and plasma is release of thromboplastin from the cellular surface by shedding of plasma membrane vesicles from various cell types (30). Such vesicles are sedimentable in the ultracentrifuge and they can be detected both in vitro and in vivo (in ascites fluid). Shedding of sedimentable vesicles from macrophages and from monocytes activated with phorbol ester has been observed. In the latter case the vesicles contained high thromboplastin activity (31).

Our knowledge about the regulation of thromboplastin (i.e. apoprotein III) synthesis is fragmentary. In inducible cells the increase in thromboplastin activity obviously depends on protein and RNA synthesis. When inducible cells are submitted to PPD (purified protein derivative of Mycobacterium bovis BCG) or endotoxin, the procoagulant activity starts to rise after about 30 min. Most inducers of thromboplastin synthesis interact with the plasma membrane and therefore depend on a second messenger system to induce gene expression. Knowledge of such systems might allow therapeutic or prophylactic intervention in cases of disseminated intravascular coagulation caused by increased thromboplastin expression. A case in point may be meningococcal septicaemia (29). Several of the commonly explored second messenger systems are involved in inducing and/or modulating thromboplastin synthesis and expression, apparently in a concerted action. The systems involved include cyclic AMP, intracellular Ca^{2+} and transmethylation reactions. Increased intracellular levels of cAMP reduce markedly the thromboplastin synthesis triggered by immune complexes and by PPD. There is also a good inhibitory effect on induction by endotoxin and PHA, but less of an effect on TPA or A 23187 induction (32). DbcAMP, forskolin, methylisobutylxanthine and PGE_2, all agents that increase intracellular cAMP via different mechanisms, even inhibited apparent constitutive apoprotein III producers like trophoblasts.

Cellular cooperation, sometimes mediated through soluble extracellular substances, are also important regulators for the thromboplastin response. Lymphocytes influence the response of monocytes to various exogenous inducers of apoprotein III synthesis, but it is still a matter of debate whether lymphocyte/monocyte cooperation is necessary for the response or only enhances and sustains it (33,34). In the case of endothelial cells it appears that both platelets and lymphocytes (and lymphocyte-conditioned medium) have a strong enhancing effect on the thromboplastin response (35,36) but there is no doubt that endothelial cells (human umbilical vein as well as bovine aorta) alone can be induced to make thromboplastin.

Other soluble exogenous substances are also involved. Østerud and Eskeland (37) have produced evidence for the importance of complement in the endotoxin-induced thromboplastin response, although some of their results do not agree with those of others. Complement factor C3b itself appears to be a potent inducer (38). Smariga and Maynard (39) have purified a platelet protein that stimulates thromboplastin synthesis in fibroblasts. Exogenous Ca^{2+} is necessary for a maximum thromboplastin response to TPA and a sine qua non for the response to the ionophore A 23187 in monocytes (Lyberg, unpublished). We have furthermore shown a marked enhancing effect of cyclosporine A on monocyte thromboplastin synthesis (40).

Depending on inducer and cell type the procoagulant activity peaks after 3-4 h (in the case of endotoxin or PPD) and up to 16-20 h when antigen-antibody complexes or phorbol tumor promotors are used as inducers. Subsequently, the procoagulant activity declines, even in the continual presence of the inducing agent, with an apparent half-life which varies from a few hours to about ten. The decline of thromboplastin activity in monocytes is slower in the presence of cyclosporine A or lymphocytes at ratios of 1-10 lymphocytes per monocyte.

Conclusion

There is no reason any longer to uphold the strict separation between the extrinsic and the intrinsic pathways of blood coagulation. Thromboplastin-factor VII complexes and possibly other truly activated forms of factor VII can activate factor IX in the intrinsic cascade as well as factor X in the final common path of the clotting mechanism.

With regard to the role of thromboplastin in various disorders of local or disseminated intravascular coagulation and in the general inflammatory reaction it is likely that we have only seen the top of the iceberg. Induction of procoagulant activity of thromboplastin or thromboplastin complex types is probably part of a general cellular response to a number of agents exogenous to the cell and may play a role in the pathogenesis of atherosclerosis, rheumatoid arthritis, delayed hypersensitivity and other immunopathological, infectious or degenerative conditions where thrombin formation or fibrin deposition are involved.

Acknowledgement

Torill Halvorsen kindly prepared the manuscript. Work in the author's laboratory was supported by grants from the Norwegian Research Council on Science and the Humanities, the Norwegian Research Council on Cardiovascular Diseases, the Laerdal Foundation for Acute Medicine and the Association of the Norwegian Life Insurance Companies.

References

1. Prydz, H. 1984. Triggering of the extrinsic blood coagulation system. In: Blood Coagulation and Haemostasis: A practical guide (J.M. Thomson, ed.) Churchill Livingstone, Edinburgh, p.

2. Bjorklid, E., Storm, E. and Prydz, H. 1973. The protein component of human brain thromboplastin. Biochem. Biophys. Res. Comm. 55, 969-976.

3. Bjorklid, E. and Storm, E. 1977. Purification and some properties of the protein component of tissue thromboplastin from human brain. Biochem. J. 165, 89-96.

4. Bach, R., Nemerson, Y. and Konigsberg, W. 1981. Purification and characterization of bovine tissue factor. J. Biol. Chem. 256, 824-831.

5. Deutsch, E., Irsigler, K. and Lomoschitz, H. 1964. Studien uber Gewebthromboplastin. 1. Reinigung, chemische Charakterisierung und Trennung in einen Eiweiss- und Lipoidanteil. Thromb. Diathes. Haemorrh. 12, 12-34.

6. Nemerson, Y. 1968. The phospholipid requirement of tissue factor in blood coagulation. J. Clin. Invest. 47, 72-80.

7. Nemerson, Y. 1969. Characteristics and lipid requirements of coagulant proteins extracted from lung and brain: the specificity of the protein component of tissue factor. J. Clin. Invest. 48, 322-331.

8. Pitlick, F.A. and Nemerson, Y. 1970. Binding of protein component of tissue factor to phospholipids. Biochemistry 9, 5105-5113.

9. Wijngaards, G., van Deenen, L.L. and Hemker, H.C. 1977. Reconstitution and lipid requirements of porcine tissue thromboplastin. Biochim. Biophys. Acta 488, 161-171.

10. Gladhaug, A. and Prydz, H. 1970. Purification of the coagulation factors VII and X from human serum. Some properties of factor VII. Biochim. Biophys. Acta 215, 105-111.

11. Broze, G.J. and Majerus, P.W. 1980. Purification and properties of human coagulation factor VII. J. Biol. Chem. 255, 1242-1247.

12. Fair,D.S. 1983. Quantitation of factor VII in the plasma of normal and warfarin-treated individuals by radioimmunoassay. Blood 62, 784-791.

13. Prydz, H. 1964. Studies on proconvertin (factor VII) V. Biosynthesis in suspension cultures of rat liver cells. Scand. J. Clin. Lab. Invest. 16, 540-548.

14. Fair, D.S., Tsao, B., Curtiss, L. and Edgington, T. 1983. Monocytes can be induced by lipopolysaccharide stimulated T cells to express factor VII activity. Thromb. Haemostas. 50 (1), abstr. 532.

15. Østerud, B. and Rapaport, S.I, 1977 Activation of factor IX by the reaction product of tissue factor and factor VII: additional pathway for initiating blood coagulation. Proc. Nat. Acad. Sci. 74, 5260-5264.

16. Østerud, B. and Rapaport, S.I. 1980. Activation of ^{125}I-factor IX and ^{125}I-factor X: effect of tissue factor and factor VII, factor X_a and thrombin. Scand. J. Haematol. 24, 213-226.

17. Ørstavik, K.H., Laake, K. 1978. Antiserum against factor IX shortens the bovine thromboplastin coagulation time of human plasma. Thromb. Res. 12, 455-465.

18. Østerud, B., Kasper, C.K., Lavine, K.K., Prodanos, C. and Rapaport, S.I. 1981. Purification and properties of an abnormal blood coagulation factor IX (factor IX_{bm})/kinetics of its inhibition of factor X activation by factor VII and bovine tissue factor. Thromb. Haemostas. 45, 55-59.

19. Jesty, J. and Silverberg, S.A. 1979. Kinetics of the tissue factor- dependent activation of coagulation factors IX and X in a bovine plasma system. J. Biol. Chem. 254, 12337-12345.

20. Bertina, R.M., Alderkamp, G.J.H. and Nooy, E. de. 1981. A variant of factor X that is defective only in extrinsic coagulation. Thromb. Haemostas. 46 (1), abstr. 259.

21. Alexander, B., Meyer, L., Kenny, J., Goldstein, R., Gurewich, V. and Grinspoon, L. 1956. Blood coagulation in pregnancy: proconvertin and prothrombin, and the hypercoagulable state. N. Eng. J. Med. 254, 358-363.

22. Meade,T.W., North, W.R.S., Chakrabarti, R., Stirling, Y., Haines, A.P., Thompson, S.G. and Brozovic, M. 1980. Haemostatic function and cardiovascular death: Early results of a prospective study. Lancet I, 1050-1054.

23. Dalaker, K. and Prydz, H. 1984. The coagulation factor VII in pregnancy. Br. J. Haematol. 56, 233-241.

24. Dalaker, K., Hjermann, I. and Prydz, H. 1985. A novel form of factor VII in plasma from men at risk for cardiovascular disease. Br. J. Haematol., in press.

25. Johnsen, U.L.H., Leoni, P., Nustad, K. and Prydz, H. Monoclonal antibodies against human brain thromboplastin. Development of test systems and characterization of the antibodies. Thromb. Haemostas., in press.

26. Van Ginkel, C.J.W., Thörig, L., Thompson, J., Oh, J.I.H. and van Aken, W.G. 1979. Enhancement of generation of monocyte tissue thromboplastin by bacterial phagocytosis: Possible pathway for fibrin formation on infected vegetations in bacterial endocarditis. Infect. Immunol. 25, 388-395.

27. Miller, C.L., Graziano, C., Lim, R.C. and Chin, M. 1981. Generation of tissue factor by patient monocytes: correlation to thromboembolic complications. Thromb. Haemostas. 46, 489-495.

28. Lyberg, T., Prydz, H., Baklien, K. and Hoyeraal, H.M. 1982. Effect of immune complex-containing sera from patients with rheumatic diseases on thromboplastin activity of monocytes. Thromb. Res. 25, 193-202.

29. Østerud, B. and Flægstad, T. 1983. Increased tissue thromboplastin activity in monocytes of patients with meningococcal infection related to an unfavourable prognosis. Thromb. Haemostas. 49, 5-7.

30. Dvorak, H.F., Van DeWater, L., Bitzer, A.M., Dvorak, A.M., Anderson, D., Harvey, V.S, Bach, R., Davis, G.D., DeWolf, W. and Carvalho, A.C.A. 1983. Procoagulant activity associated with plasma membrane vesicles shed by cultured tumor cells. Cancer Res. 43, 4334-4342.

31. Hetland, Ø., Brovold, A.-B., Holme, R., Gaudernack, G. and Prydz, H. 1985. Thromboplastin (tissue factor) in plasma membranes of human monocytes. Biochem. J. in press.

32. Lyberg, T. 1983. Effect of cyclic AMP and cyclic GMP on thromboplastin (factor III) synthesis in human monocytes in vitro. Thromb. Haemostas. 50, 804-809.

33. Edgington, T.S. 1983. Recognition coupled responses of the monocyte: Activation of coagulation pathways. Nouv. Rev. Fr. d'Hematol. 25, 1-6.

34. Lyberg, T. and Prydz, H. 1983. The role of cellular co-operation in thromboplastin synthesis. Nouv. Rev. Fr. d'Hématol. 25, 291-293.

35. Johnsen, U.L.H., Lyberg, T., Galdal, K.S. and Prydz, H. 1983. Platelets stimulate thromboplastin synthesis in human endothelial cells. Thromb. Haemostas. 49, 69-72.

36. Lyberg, T., Galdal, K.S, Evensen, S.A. and Prydz, H. 1983. Cellular cooperation in endothelial cell thromboplastin synthesis. Br. J. Haematol. 53, 85-95.

37. Østerud, B. and Eskeland, T. 1982. The mandatory role of complement in the endotoxin-induced synthesis of tissue thromboplastin in blood monocytes. FEBS Lett. 149, 75-79.

38. Prydz, H. Allison, A.C. and Schorlemmer, H.-V. 1977. Further link between the complement and the coagulation system. Nature 270, 173.

39. Smariga, P.E. and Maynard, J.R. 1982. Purification of a platelet protein which stimulates fibrinolytic inhibition and tissue factor in human fibroblasts. J. Biol. Chem. 25, 11960-11965.

40. Carlsen, E., Mallet, A.M. and Prydz, H. 1985. Effect of cyclosporine A on thromboplastin activity in mononuclear blood cells and monocytes in vitro. Clin. Exp. Immunol. In press.

EXTRAVASCULAR FIBRIN FORMATION AND FIBRINOLYSIS IN A MODEL OF INFLAMMATION ACCOMPANYING CELLULAR HYPERSENSITIVITY

R.F. Peters, M.K. Jasani, M.F. Tweed
CIBA-GEIGY Pharmaceuticals, Horsham, West Sussex RH12 4AB, U.K.

I. Knight, D.A. Lane
Charing Cross and Westminster Medical School, London, U.K.

Introduction

Extravascular (e-v) fibrin deposition at the inflammatory site is a characteristic feature of cellular hypersensitivity responses. This has been demonstrated in a number of animal models (1, 2, 3), in allergic contact dermatitis (4) and in delayed skin reactions (5, 4) in man. It is also a consistent feature of chronic inflammatory diseases such as rheumatoid arthritis (6,7) and of graft rejection (8,9).

Lymphocyte infiltration into the inflammatory site is also characteristic of these responses (10, 11, 2, 12) and previous studies in these laboratories have shown that e-v fibrin deposition in rejecting allografts involves a role for T-lymphocytes (13, 14).

It is well known that both tissue plasminogen activator (tPA) and plasminogen (Plg) bind to fibrin in an ordered and sequential manner and that fibrinolysis is regulated by specific molecular interactions between them (15). However, it is not known whether such mechanisms operate *in vivo* to control the lysis of e-v fibrin deposits.

This manuscript describes the use of a foot-pad inflammation model of cellular hypersensitivity to Mycobacterium tuberculosis in the rat to investigate e-v fibrin formation, its relationship to T-lymphocytes and the possible involvement of plasminogen and tPA in the processes of e-v fibrin removal.

Fibrinogen - Fibrin Formation and Fibrinolysis, Vol. 4
© 1986 Walter de Gruyter & Co., Berlin · New York - Printed in Germany.

Methods

Rats were immunised by an injection, in the scruff, of M.tuberculosis suspended in liquid paraffin B.P.. Six days later the animals were challenged with a further injection into the right hind paw (16). The formation of e-v fibrin deposits was detected microscopically and formation and removal quantified using ^{125}I-human fibrinogen B.P. (16). Exudation was measured using ^{131}I-human serum albumin B.P. (17). The accumulation of intravenously administered Plg and tPA was investigated using ^{125}I-Plg (5 μi) and ^{125}I-mtPA (5 μCi). The activity and molecular size of plasminogen activators was studied using SDS polyacrylamide-gel electrophoresis of potassium thiocyanate extracts of inflamed tissue (18) followed by fibrin autography (19).

Results and Discussion

Extravascular fibrin formation and removal

Histological study of inflamed tissue revealed that e-v fibrin deposits were present by 16 h post-challenge and persisted up to at least 72 h. The deposits were present throughout the connective tissue and around infiltrating mononuclear cells and were similar in appearance to those seen during the rejection of rabbit skin allografts (9). Quantification of fibrin deposition in the inflamed paw using ^{125}I-fibrinogen (Fig 1a) demonstrated that it reached a maximum at 24 h post-challenge and that this fibrin was then removed, falling by 80% between 24 h and 96 h. Measurement of further fibrin formation beyond 24 h post-challenge (Fig. 1a) indicated that fibrin formation continued in amounts sufficient to compensate for that removed. Thus e-v fibrin levels persisted at the 24 h level as a result of continuous turnover. This was accompanied by similar persistence of oedema (Fig. 1b). This situation can be likened to that in rheumatoid arthritis in which extensive, persistent e-v fibrin deposits are seen in inflamed joints (7, 20).

Lymphocyte involvement

To investigate a possible link between lymphocytes infiltrating the inflammatory site and local e-v fibrin formation during the cellular hypersensitivity response, animals were treated with cyclosporin A (CsA), which has been shown to inhibit T-cell mediated responses in vivo (21), or were

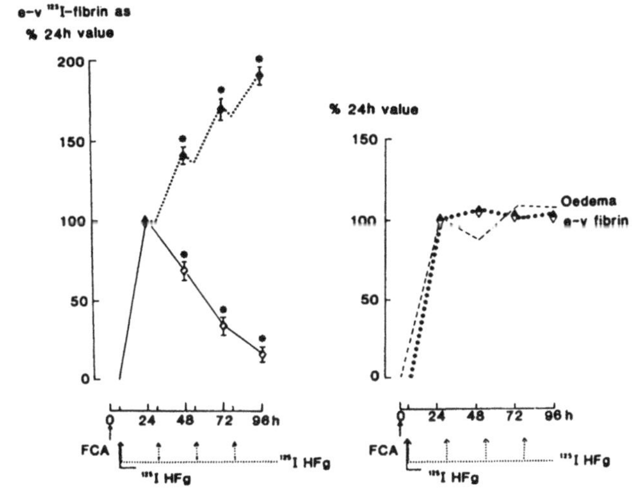

Fig. 1a: Formation of e-v ^{125}I-fibrin at 24 h and its subsequent removal (——) were measured following administration (i.v.) of ^{125}I-HFg at 6 h post-challenge. The continuous formation of e-v ^{125}I-fibrin beyond 24 h (·····) was measured over 18 h periods following the administration (i.v.) of ^{125}I-HFg at 30, 54 or 78 h post-challenge

Fig. 1b: The persistence of fibrin (·····) and oedema (- - -) during the inflammatory response.

For comparative purposes the results are expressed as percent of the 24 h value and are mean values (n=6) ± S.E.M. *$p < 0.05$ (Students modified 't' test) comparing results with the 24 h result.

subjected to thoracic duct lymph (TDL) drainage (22) to deplete the body pool of re-circulating T-lymphocytes (23).

Daily dosing of animals with CsA from the time of immunisation reduced e-v fibrin formation at all the time periods studied (Fig. 2). Oedema was also inhibited to a similar extent. TDL drainage preceding challenge also reduced e-v fibrin formation and oedema when measured at 24 h post-challenge (Fig. 3).

These data indicate that T-lymphocytes play a role in e-v fibrin formation. As histological evidence shows that heavy fibrin deposits are seen around infiltrating mononuclear cells it seems likely that this is the result of the expression of procoagulant activity on the surface of these cells following lymphocyte/macrophage interaction (24). This aspect of e-v coagulation has been explored at the cellular level in these laboratories and is described and discussed elsewhere in these proceedings (25).

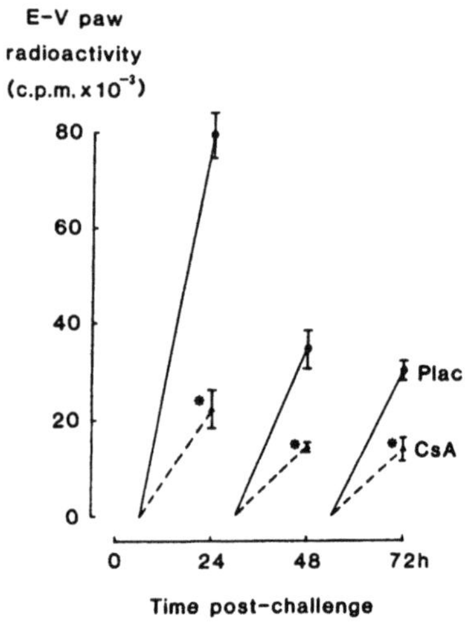

Fig. 2: The effect of CsA on e-v fibrin formation. ^{125}I-fibrin accumulation was measured over 18 h periods following administration of ^{125}I-HFg at 6, 30 or 54 h post-challenge. CsA was administered s.c. (20 mg/kg/day) commencing on the day of immunisation. Results are mean values (n=6) ± S.E.M. *p < 0.05 (Students modified 't' test) comparing CsA treated with placebo.

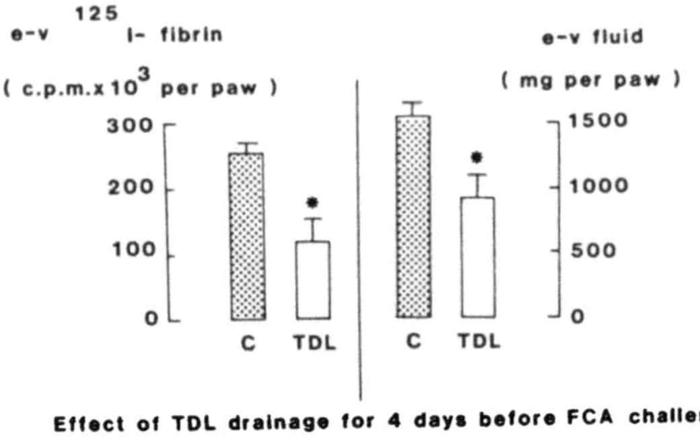

Fig. 3: Effect of TDL drainage on e-v fibrin formation and oedema at 24 h post-challenge. TDL drainage (22) was continued for 4 days following immunisation. ^{125}I-HFg was administered (i.v.) at 6 h post-challenge. Results are mean values (n=5) ± S.E.M. *p < 0.05 (Students modified 't' test) comparing TDL with control animals.

Extravascular fibrinolysis

Preliminary studies have been carried out on the involvement of plasminogen activator(s) and plasminogen in the fibrinolytic processes accompanying chronic inflammation in the rat model of cellular hypersensitivity. SDS PAGE electrophoresis and fibrin autography of extracts of control (non-inflamed) tissue showed no evidence of plasminogen activators (Fig. 4), but extracts of inflamed tissue 24 h after challenge showed two main bands of activity. A low molecular weight band running between high and low molecular weight urokinase standard and a double band corresponding to mtPA standard. At 48 h the

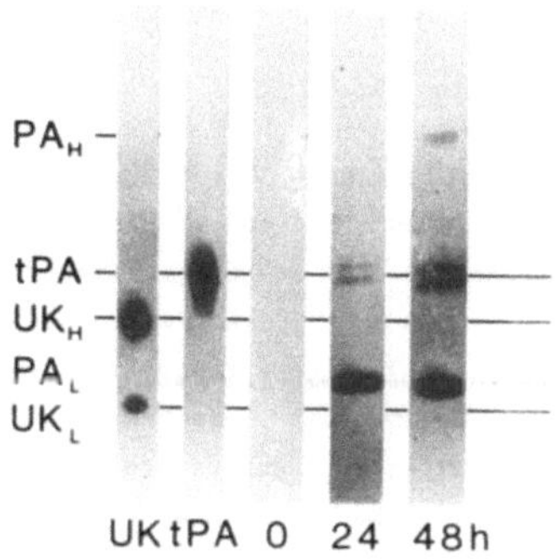

Fig. 4: Plasminogen activator(s) in inflamed tissues. SDS PAGE/fibrin autography was performed on extracts of inflamed paw tissue (see methods).

activity of both bands had increased and an additional high molecular weight band was also visible. This was almost certainly an inhibitor-activator complex. Thus it seems that as the response develops the level of plasminogen activator(s) at the inflammatory site increases; however, these results do not indicate whether this increase has occurred intravascularly, extravasculary or both. It is known that fibrinolysis is regulated by molecular interactions between fibrin-bound tPA and plasminogen and that effective clot dissolution *in vivo* requires continuous replacement at the fibrin surface of inactivated plasmin molecules by plasminogen (15). The fact that, in inflamed tissue, fibrin deposition is seen only in the e-v compartment suggests that the increased levels of plasminogen activator(s) occur extravascularly. This hypothesis was investigated by studying the accumulation at the site of inflammation of intravenously administered ^{125}I-mtPA and ^{125}I-Plg.

Initially paw accumulation of ^{125}I-mtPA was measured at various time intervals up to 120 mins after its administration; however, interpretation of the data was complicated by the very short biological half-life of tPA *in vivo*. This has been reported previously in the rabbit (26) in the mouse (27) and in man (28) and our studies showed a circulating half-life of approximately 2 mins in the rat. In an attempt to overcome this problem ^{125}I-mtPA was administered intravenously using an implanted slow release osmotic mini-pump (Alzet Corporation) and its accumulation in the paw compared with similarly administered ^{131}I-albumin (Fig. 5). In the non-inflamed (L) paw the accumulation of each tracer was the same at 24 h and at 72 h post-challenge, indicating that exchange between the intravascular and extravascular compartments were the same at both times. A similar situation appeared to exist in the inflamed (R) paw for ^{131}I-albumin, the accumulation of which, while 5-6 times greater than that in the non-inflamed paw, was also the same at

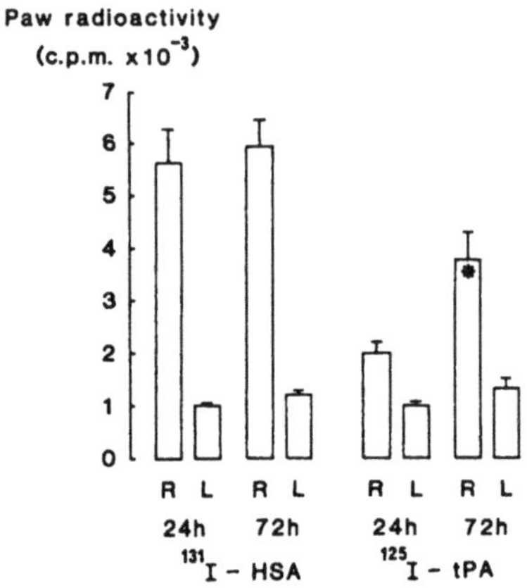

Fig. 5: Accumulation of ^{125}I-tPA and ^{131}I-HSA at 24 h and 72 h post-challenge in the inflamed paw (R) and non-inflamed paw (L). ^{125}I-tPA and ^{131}I-HSA were administered (i.v.) using a controlled release osmotic mimi-pump implanted s.c. 18 h before challenge. Results are mean values (n=5) ± S.E.M. * $p < 0.05$ (Students modified 't' test) comparing 72 h and 24 h results.

24 h and at 72 h. In contrast the accumulation of ^{125}I-tPA at 72 h was nearly twice that at 24 h. We have already shown that fibrin deposits persist in the e-v compartment as a result of their continuous formation and removal and the above data is consistent with the continuous selective binding of ^{125}I-tPA to e-v fibrin.

Unlike tPA, studies of ^{125}I-plasminogen accumulation are not complicated by a short circulating half-life (15). Hence, the initial paw accumulation of an itravenous bolus dose of ^{125}I-Plg could be measured and compared with that of similarly administered ^{125}I-fibrinogen and ^{131}I-albumin. The data in Fig. 6 show that, when expressed as percent of administered dose, ^{125}I-Plg accumulated in the inflamed paw to a greater extent than either ^{125}I-fibrinogen or ^{131}I-albumin. It can be assumed that the exudation rate of all three proteins

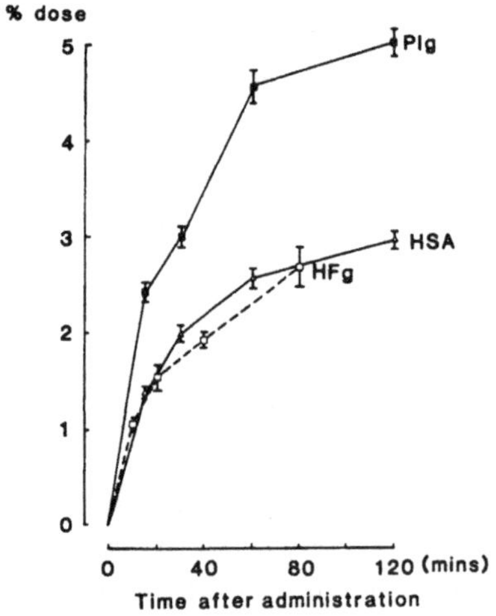

Fig. 6: Initial accumulation of ^{125}I-Plg, ^{125}I-HFg and ^{131}I-HSA in the inflamed paw at 24 h post-challenge. ^{125}I-Plg, ^{125}I-HFg and ^{131}I-HSA were administered i.v. at 0 time. Results are percent of administered dose (c.p.m.) and are the mean values (n=6) ± S.E.M.

was the same in these circumstances and hence this difference could also represent selective binding of Plg to e-v fibrin.

The relative contributions of exudation rate and e-v fibrin to the accumulation of ^{125}I-Plg at the inflammatory site was explored using agents known to affect one or both of these parameters in this model of cellular hypersensitivity.

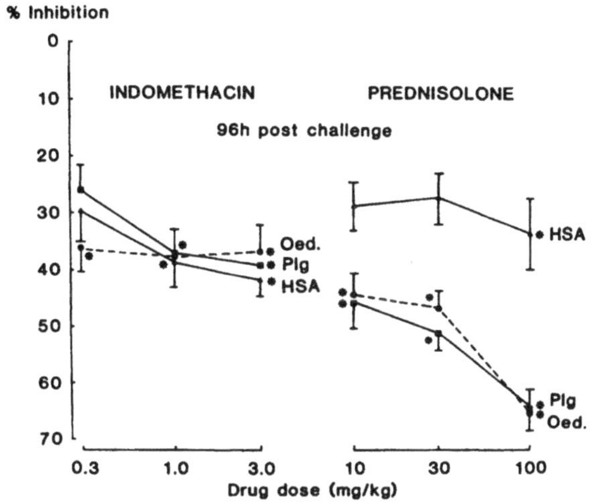

Fig. 7: The effects of indomethacin and prednisolone on oedema and ^{125}I-Plg and ^{131}I-HSA accumulation in the inflamed paw at 96 h post-challenge. ^{125}I-Plg and ^{131}I-HSA were administered i.v. 3 h before measurements were made. Indomethacin and prednisolone were administered p.o. daily in polyethylene glycol 400 commencing 6 h post-challenge. Results are mean percent inhibition (± S.E.M.) compared with placebo treated animals (n=6). *$p < 0.05$ (Students modified 't' test) comparing drug treated with placebo.

Animals were treated with either indomethacin, which has been shown to be both anti-exudative and anti-fibrinolytic, or with prednisolone, which has been shown to inhibit fibrin formation but have little effect on exudation or fibrinolysis (17). The initial accumulation of ^{125}I-Plg and ^{131}I-albumin were measured over a 3 h period at 96 post-challenge and compared with the effect of the two drugs on the inflammatory response measured as the formation of paw oedema (Fig. 7). As expected, indomethacin inhibited oedema at all three doses and inhibited exudation of ^{131}I-albumin at 1 and 3 mg/kg. The accumulation of ^{125}I-Plg was also inhibited to the same extent as albumin. Prednisolone, on the other hand, did not inhibit exudation at 10 and 30 mg/kg but caused considerable inhibition of both Plg accumulation and oedema. At 100 mg/kg exudation was significantly inhibited and was accompanied by a greater inhibition of Plg accumulation and oedema. These data suggest that, in the case of indomethacin, which causes limited inhibition of e-v fibrin formation (17), the inhibition of Plg accumulation was the result of the reduction in the exudation rate. However, in the case of prednisolone, the inhibition of Plg accumulation was not related to inhibition of exudation. We have previously shown that prednisolone causes a marked reduction in e-v fibrin formation in this model (17) and therefore the inhibition of Plg accumulation by prednisolone could be a reflection of the reduction in the level of e-v fibrin.

Conclusions

Using a model of cellular hypersensitivity to M.tuberculosis in the rat the data presented in this report show that:

1. Extravascular fibrin formation involves a role for T-lymphocytes
2. After their initial formation e-v fibrin deposits persist, as fibrinolysis is balanced by further fibrin formation
3. Both tPA and plasminogen are implicated in e-v fibrinolysis.

Acknowledgements

The authors would like to thank Dr. Ian McGregor (S.E. Scotland Blood Transfusion Service, Edinburgh) for the supply of ^{125}I-mtPA, Dr. Désiré Collen (University of Leuven, Belgium) for the generous gift of mtPA and Dr. Stephen Christmas for TDL surgery.

References

1. Colvin, R.B. and Dvorak, H.F. 1975. J. Immunol., 114, 377-387.
2. Dvorak, H.F., Galli, S.J. and Dvorak, A.M. 1980. Int. Rev. Exp. Pathol., 21, 119-194.
3. Hopper, K.E., Geczy, C.L. and Davies, W.A. 1981. J. Immunol., 126, 1052-1058.
4. Dvorak, H.F., Mihm, M.C., Dvorak, A.M., Johnson, R.A., Manseau, B.A., Morgan, E. and Colvin, R.B. 1974. Lab. Invest., 31, 111-130.
5. Colvin, R.B., Johnson, R.A., Mihm, M.C. and Dvorak, H.F. 1973. J. Exp. Med., 138, 686-696.
6. Barnhart, M.I., Riddle, J.M., Bluhm, G.B. and Quintana, C. 1967. Ann. Rheum. Dis., 26, 206-218.

7. Jasani, M.K. 1979. In: Immunopathogenesis of Rheumatoid Arthritis (G.S. Panayi and P.M. Johnson, eds.). Reedbooks Ltd., Chertsey, U.K. pp. 137-146.

8. Dvorak, H.F., Mihm, M.C., Dvorak, A.M., Barnes, B.A., Manseau, E.J. and Galli, S.J. 1979. J. Exp. Med., 150, 322-337.

9. Bullock, G.R., Jasani, M.K., Roberts, J.M. and Williamson, I.H.M. 1985. Histochem. J., 17, 143-151.

10. Zvaifler, N.J. 1973. Adv. Immunol., 16, 265-336.

11. Bullock, G.R., Jasani, M.K. and Lewis, G.P. 1977. Cell. Biol. Int. Rep., 1, 123-135.

12. Platt, J.L., Grant, B.W., Eddy, A.E. and Michael, A.F. 1983. J. Exp. Med., 158, 1227-1242.

13. Bach, C.S. and Jasani, M.K. 1976. Brit. J. Pharmacol., 58, 292P.

14. Bullock, G.R., Christmas, S.E., Jasani, M.K., Jayson, M.I.V., Kemmenoe, B.H. and Sibbons, P.D. 1984. Brit. J. Pharmacol., 81, 92P.

15. Lijnen, H.R. and Collen, D. 1982. Sem. Thromb. Haemost., 8, 2-10.

16. Bullock, G.R., Christmas, S., Jasani, M.K., Peters, R.F., Tweed, M.F. and Williamson, I.H.M. 1983. Brit. J. Pharmacol., 79, 240P.

17. Jasani, M.K., Peters, R.F. and Tweed, M.F. 1983. Brit. J. Pharmacol., 80, 444P.

18. Eriksson, E., Eriksson, B., Teger-Nilsson, A.-C., Thorsen, S. and Risberg, B. 1983. In: Clinical Aspects of Fibrinolysis and Thrombolysis (J. Jespersen, C. Kluft and O. Korsgaards, eds.). S. Jultand Univ. Pres, Esbjerg, Denmark. pp. 59-70.

19. Loskutoff, D.J., van Mourik, J.A., Erickson, L.A. and Lawrence, D. 1983. Proc. Nat. Acad. Sci., 80, 2956-2960.

20. Holland, C.D., Rennie, J.A.N., Hassan, I.F., Jasani, M.K. and Jayson, M.I.V. 1982. Ann. Rheum. Dis., 41, 311.

21. Thomson, A.W., Whiting, P.H. and Simpson, J.G. 1984. Agents and Actions, 15, 306-327.

22. Ford, W.L. 1978. In: Handbook of Experimental Immunology (D.M. Weir, ed.). Blackwell Scientific Publications, London, U.K. pp. 23.2-23.6.

23. Hall, B.M., Dorsch, S. and Roser, B. 1978. J. Exp. Med., 148, 878-888.

24. Geczy, C.L. 1984. Haemost., 14, 400-411.

25. Talbot, M.D., Peters, R.F., Tweed, M.F. and Jasani, M.K. 1985. (this volume).

26. Korninger, C., Stassen, J.M. and Collen, D. 1981. Thromb. Haemost., 46, 658-661.

27. Fuchs, H.E., Berger H. and Pizzo, S.V. 1985. Blood, 65, 539-544.

28. Nilsson, T., Wallen, P. and Mellbring, G. 1984. Scand. J. Haematol., 33, 49-53.

EXTRA-VASCULAR FIBRIN DEPOSITION IN CELLULAR HYPERSENSITIVITY - THE ROLE OF T LYMPHOCYTE-MACROPHAGE INTERACTIONS

M.D. Talbot, R.F. Peters, M.F. Tweed, M.K. Jasani
Ciba-Geigy Pharmaceuticals, Wimblehurst Road, Horsham, West Sussex RH12 4AB

Introduction

As discussed in the previous contribution to these proceedings extra-vascular fibrin deposition is characteristic of many cell-mediated immune responses including delayed-type hypersensitivity and graft rejection. Mononuclear cell infiltration into the inflamed site is a consistent accompanying feature of these responses. A direct link between these events is suggested by in vitro findings which demonstrate the enhanced expression of monocyte/macrophage procoagulant activity as a result of an interaction with activated T lymphocytes (see review (1)). Furthermore, in vivo depletion of lymphocytes by thoracic duct drainage has been shown to lead to a marked reduction in intra-lesional fibrin deposition in rejecting rat cardiac allografts (2) and in the inflamed footpad of previously immunised rats challenged with M.tuberculosis (3). In addition treatment with the T lymphocyte-active immunosuppressant cyclosporin A also brought about a similar reduction in the latter model.

The studies described were designed to investigate the possibility that extra-vascular fibrin deposition in a model of rat footpad inflammation is a result of the expression of procoagulant activity by mononuclear cells infiltrating the inflamed site and that this expression is mediated by interaction at the site between activated T lymphocytes and cells of the monocyte/macrophage series.

Methods

Rats were immunised by an injection, in the scruff, of M.tuberculosis suspended in liquid paraffin B.P.. Six days later the animals were challenged with a further injection into the right hind paw (4).

Fibrinogen - Fibrin Formation and Fibrinolysis, Vol. 4
© 1986 Walter de Gruyter & Co., Berlin · New York - Printed in Germany.

Inflammatory exudate cells were isolated from the inflamed footpad of rats at various times after challenge. These cells were then washed extensively and their procoagulant activity measured as the ability of the whole cells to shorten the recalcification time of citrated rat plasma. Clotting times were compared with those obtained with dilutions of a purified 'standard' rabbit brain thromboplastin preparation (American Hospital Supplies U.K.) and units of procoagulant activity calculated.

Mononuclear leucocytes from spleen and peripheral blood were separated by differential centrifugation over Lymphopaque (Nyegaard, Norway).

Adherent macrophages were separated from mixed cell suspensions by adherence to 24-well plastic tissue culture clusters which had been pre-incubated overnight with heat-inactivated foetal calf serum (FCS). The serum was removed and the cells applied in medium containing 10% FCS (5×10^6 cells/well). After 2 h culture at 37°C non-adherent cells were removed by washing twice with pre-warmed medium. Ice-cold medium was then added and 30 min later the adherent cells removed with the aid of a rubber policeperson.

T lymphocytes were prepared from the non-adherent fraction obtained above by a further adherence procedure on nylon-wool columns. Cells (1×10^7) were loaded onto a nylon wool column, pre-incubated with medium containing 10% FCS, and incubated at 37°C for 1 h. The non-adherent cells were eluted with warm medium and applied to a second similar column for further purification. The resultant cells were shown to be T lymphocytes (> 90%) by immunofluorescence studies.

The degree of in vivo lymphocyte activation was measured by increased DNA polymerase α activity or by the accumulation of cells labelled with ^{125}I-iododeoxuridine. DNA polymerase α activity measurements were carried out on the homogenates of cells or tissue using a method modified from that of Bollum (5) . In vivo labelling of activated lymphocytes was carried out using intravenously administered ^{125}I-iododeoxyuridine (0.2 ml, 5 µCi per animal) and paw accumulation of ^{125}I was measured 18 h later.

Results and Discussion

1. Expression of procoagulant activity

Inflammatory exudate cells from the challenged footpad of immunised rats expressed substantial procoagulant activity (PCA) when freshly isolated, with a maximum expression found at 96 h post-challenge (Fig. 1). In contrast mononuclear cells isolated from the peripheral blood, spleen or regional popliteal lymph node of challenged rats expressed negligible PCA when freshly isolated, a finding in keeping with the localisation of fibrin deposition only at the site of inflammation. After overnight culture (Fig. 2) the level of PCA expressed by footpad cells from 24, 48 and 72 h post-challenge rats increased by approximately two-fold but no such increase was found with cells from 96 h post-challenge rats. Mononuclear cells from peripheral blood, spleen and popliteal lymph node of challenged rats also showed increased levels of PCA expression after overnight culture, with the maximum expression shown by cells from 72 h post-challenge animals (Fig. 2). The finding that PCA expression could be increased by culture of mixed mononuclear cells could be explained by the continued release of lymphokines from activated lymphocytes into the culture medium resulting in enhancement of monocyte/macrophage PCA, a possibility which is explored further in a later section. In the case of 96 h post-challenge footpad cells, PCA expression may be maximal when freshly isolated.

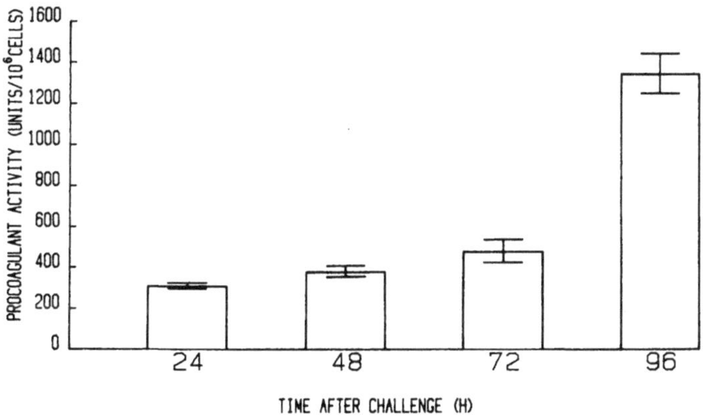

Fig. 1: Procoagulant activity of freshly isolated footpad inflammatory exudate cells at various times after challenge. Results are mean values ± S.E., n=6.

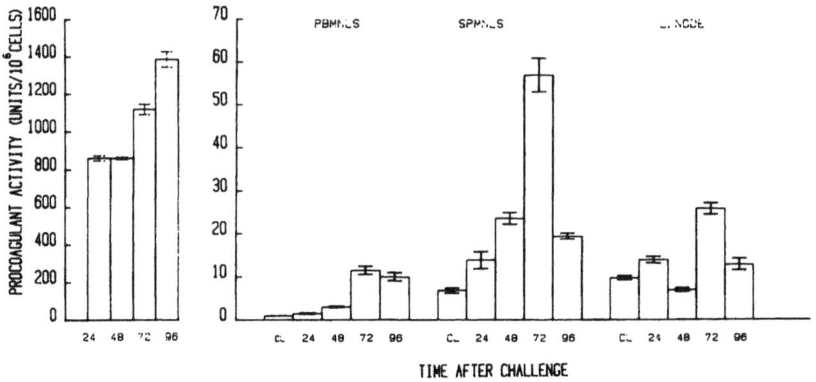

Fig. 2: Procoagulant activity of footpad inflammatory exudate cells (left-hand histogram) after unstimulated overnight culture, compared with cells from peripheral blood, spleen or regional lymph node.

The cell type responsible for the expression of PCA described above was investigated using splenocytes which had been separated on the basis of adherence to plastic (Fig. 3). The unseparated cells could be stimulated to higher PCA expression by the macrophage stimulant, muramyl dipeptide (MDP) and the plant lectin phytohaemagglutin (PHA) which is a polyclonal T lymphocyte activator but which can, at higher concentrations, stimulate PCA expression directly (6). After separation the majority of the PCA expressed was detected in the adherent macrophage cell population, in which MDP stimulation was augmented and PHA stimulation was absent, whereas the non-adherent population expressed barely detectable PCA. The nature of the PCA expressed by these cells and also by challenged footpad inflammatory exudate cells was found to resemble thromboplastin in two respects. Firstly, the activity was susceptible to inactivation by phospholipase C and secondly the procoagulant was largely inactive when assayed with Factor-VII deficient plasma.

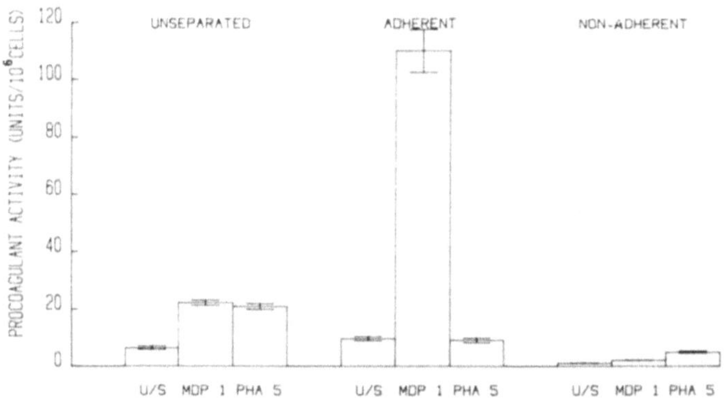

Fig. 3: The expression of procoagulant activity by splenocytes separated on the basis of their adherence to plastic.

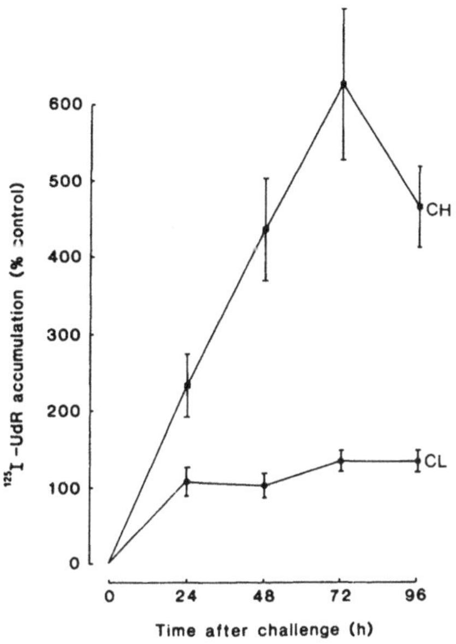

Fig. 4: The accumulation of activated lymphocytes in control and challenged paws 18 h after a pulse of ^{125}I-iododeoxyuridine (5 µCi per rat, i.v.).

However definitive characterisation as thromboplastin would require the demonstration of neutralisation of the PCA by an antibody to thromboplastin apoprotein III which is not yet available for the rat protein.

2. Lymphocyte activation

The accumulation of activated lymphocytes at the inflamed site was demonstrated using in vivo labelling with ^{125}I-iododeoxyuridine (Fig. 4). A clear difference in accumulation of label was found between the challenged and non-challenged paws at various times after challenge indicating the marked intralesional accumulation of activated lymphocytes with a peak at 72 h post-challenge. This finding was further confirmed using an alternative technique for estimating lymphocyte activation in vivo, based on the increase in activated lymphocytes of the activity of the replicative enzyme, DNA polymerase α (Fig. 5). The results using this method indicated a similar peak in activated lymphocytes within the inflamed footpad at 72 h post-challenge, a pattern of increase which was also reflected systemically by increased polymerase α activity in the spleen, although to a lesser extent. The relationship between the timings of peak in vivo lymphocyte activation and

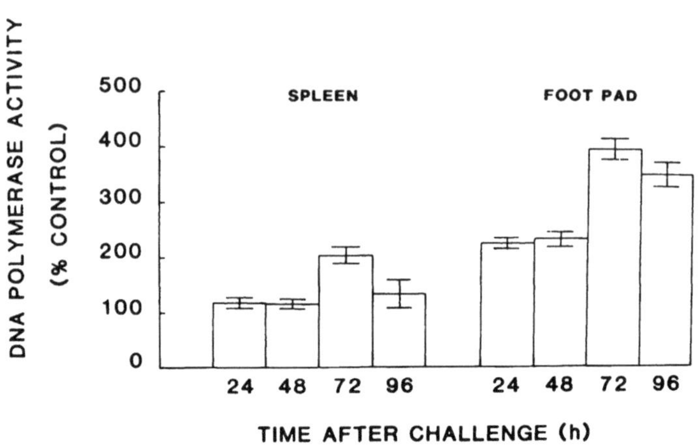

Fig. 5: DNA polymerase α activity of cells from spleen and footpad of challenged rats at various times after challenge.

procoagulant activity can be explained in terms of lymphokine-induced generation of monocyte/macrophage PCA. Since induction of thromboplastin has been shown to require transcription and translation (7) a delay between the peak times of lymphocyte activation (and hence lymphokine release) and the functional expression of thromboplastin could be expected. In vitro studies of PCA induction on mouse macrophages in the presence of added lymphokine indicating a steady increase in PCA over time of incubation, up to 20 h in these studies (8), support this hypothesis. Thus, in the ex vivo experiments described above (Fig. 2), the mixed mononuclear cells from 72 h post-challenge rats displayed greatest PCA expression after overnight culture, due to the optimal presence of activated lymphocytes, and hence presumably optimal lymphokine release in these cultures. Similarly the fact that the peak of footpad cell PCA in vivo was found at 96 h could be explained by the influence of lymphokines released by activated lymphocytes, which maximally accumulate at the inflamed site at 72 h post-challenge.

The importance of T lymphocytes in mediating the in vivo expression of PCA has been confirmed using the agent, cyclosporin A, which has been shown by many workers to inhibit T lymphocyte functions in vivo and in vitro, a subject recently reviewed (9). When rats were treated with this drug daily from the day of immunisation (15 mg/kg/day) and measurements made at 72 h post-challenge a dramatic inhibition of the activation and accumulation of lymphocytes within the lesion and also of the expression of PCA by footpad inflammatory exudate cells was found (Fig. 6).

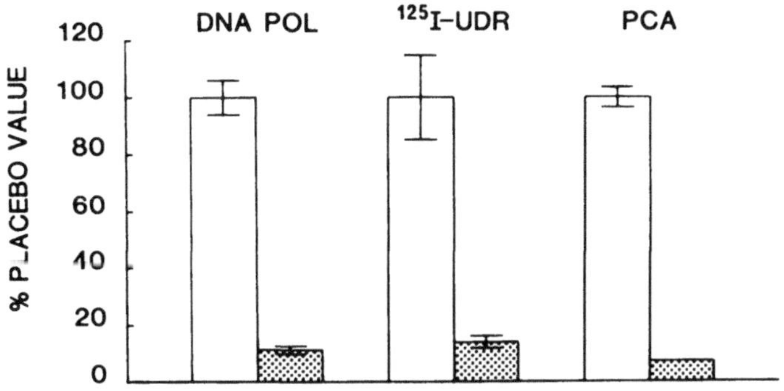

Fig. 6: Effect of cyclosporin A (15 mg/kg/day) (hatched bars) on lymphocyte activation and PCA expression in 72 h post-challenge rats compared with placebo values (open bars).

In order to provide further insight into the interaction between T lymphocytes and macrophages expressing PCA co-culture studies have been carried out, using separated cell populations obtained from challenged and control animals. After overnight culture T lymphocytes isolated by elution from nylon wool columns, were shown to express negligible activity whether obtained from either control or challenged rats (Fig. 7). In contrast adherent macrophages from control rats expressed some PCA after unstimulated overnight culture but this expression was unaltered by co-culture with T lymphocytes from control animals in a 1:1 ratio. However when co-cultured with T cells from challenged animals there was a significant enhancement of the expression of PCA by control macrophages.

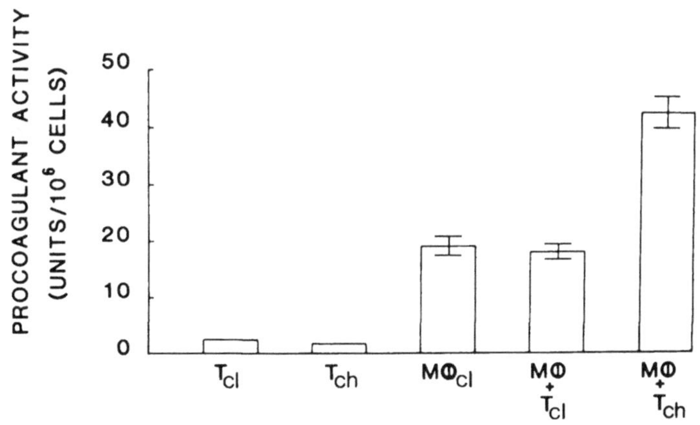

Fig. 7: Expression of PCA by isolated T lymphocytes and macrophages and in co-cultures of these cells.

Summary

In summary the studies reported above indicate that:

1. macrophages, but not T lymphocytes, express substantial procoagulant activity when isolated from the site of inflammation,
2. activated lymphocytes accumulate at the inflamed site,
3. inhibition of T lymphocyte function with cyclosporin A leads to marked inhibition of footpad exudate cell PCA in vivo, and finally
4. T lymphocytes isolated from challenged rats can stimulate the increased expression of PCA by control macrophages in vitro.

These findings suggest that the extra-vascular fibrin deposition seen in this model of cellular hypersensitivity is the result of interaction between T lymphocytes and monocyte/macrophages infiltrating the site of inflammation as depicted in the schematic diagram (Fig. 8).

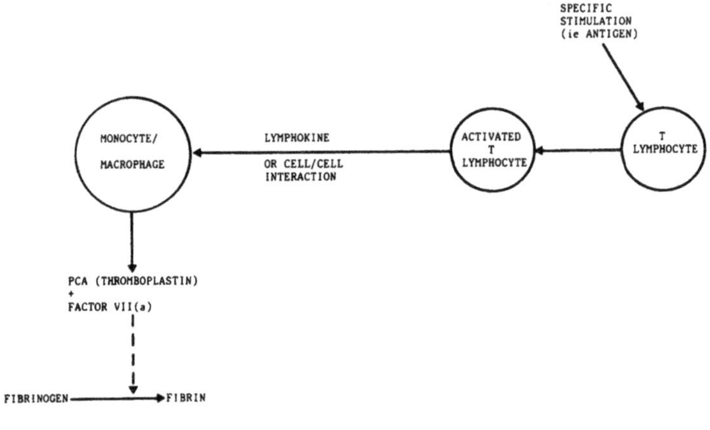

Fig. 8: Schematic diagram of the mechanism of extravascular fibrin deposition in inflammation.

References

1. Bullock, G.R., Christmas, S.E., Jasani, M.K., Jayson, M.I.V., Kemmenoe, B.H., Sibbons, P.D. 1984. Brit. J. Pharmacol., 81, 92 P.
2. Geczy, C.L. 1984. Haemostasis, 14, 400.
3. Peters, R.F., Jasani, M.K., Tweed, M.F., Knight, I. and Lane, D.A. 1985. (this volume).

4. Bullock, G.R., Christmas, S., Jasani, M.K., Peters, R.F., Tweed, M.F. and Williamson, I.H.M. 1983. Brit. J. Pharmacol., 79, 140P.

5. Bollum, F.J. 1959. J. Biol. Chem., 234, 2733.

6. Prydz, H., Lyberg, T., Deteix, P. and Allison, A.C. 1979. Thromb. Res., 15, 465.

7. Lyberg, T. 1984. Haemostasis, 14, 393.

8. Geczy, C.L., Farram, E., Moon, D.K., Meyer, P.A. and McKenzie, I.F.C. 1983. J. Immunol., 130, 2743.

9. Thomson, A. 1984. Agents and Actions, 15, 306.

FIBRINOLYTIC STUDIES IN DISORDERS OF CONNECTIVE TISSUE

A. Keegan, M.I.V. Jayson, I. Tomlinson, R. Million, G. Pountain
Rheumatic Diseases Centre, University of Manchester, Hope Hospital, Salford

Introduction

Chronic inflammation and fibrosis is the hallmark of a wide range of connective tissue diseases. Microscopic examination of inflamed tissues not only shows the presence of chronic inflammatory cells such as lymphocytes, monocytes and macrophages, but also the presence of fibrin. Fibrin may develop as a result of the chronic inflammatory process but failure to clear the fibrin could lead to perpetuation and chronicity of the inflammatory change and to the progressive development of fibrosis. Dumonde and Glynn (1952) have shown that in the sensitised rabbit intra-articular injection of fibrin will produce a chronic inflammatory reaction which bears many of the features of rheumatoid arthritis. Browse (1983) has suggested that persistence of fibrin in tissues, particularly around small blood vessels, may lead to poor diffusion of oxygen and anoxia of the tissues. In turn this could be responsible for the perpetuation of chronic tissue damage. In view of these findings we have conducted detailed studies of fibrinolytic parameters in patients with systemic sclerosis and with chronic back pain syndromes.

Systemic Sclerosis

This is a multisystem disorder which is characterised by fibrosis of the tissues, chronic inflammatory cell infiltration, vascular obstruction and ischaemic atrophy. These features are present in varying degrees in the body tissues. The characteristic clinical features seen in the hands include fibrosis of the skin and subcutaneous structures with progressive contractures and loss of joint

Fibrinogen - Fibrin Formation and Fibrinolysis, Vol. 4
© 1986 Walter de Gruyter & Co., Berlin · New York - Printed in Germany.

function. Raynaud's phenomenon is a hallmark of systemic sclerosis and is experienced by virtually all patients. This is a reversible peripheral ischaemia which particularly develops on exposure to cold. Progressive ischaemic atrophy may occur at the finger tips and may be followed by areas of infarction or even gangrene. Some patients may lose digits.

The vascular phenomena are mediated by progressive obstruction of the digital blood vessels. Histological examination shows gross intimal thickening and eventually complete obstruction. On histochemical staining deposits of fibrin may be seen lining the vessel walls. It is believed that defective fibrinolytic activity may be responsible for the persistence of fibrin and so be one of the factors playing a pathogenic role in this process.

Several studies (Goyle and Dormandy, 1976; McGrath *et al.*, 1977) have shown evidence of hyperviscosity of the blood in systemic sclerosis. This is most marked at low shear rates and at low temperatures when the relative viscosity of the blood can show quite marked increases. These are the conditions which apertain in the periphery and particularly in the fingers where the microcirculatory blood flow is necessarily slow and where the hands are exposed to cold. This may explain the reason why these vascular phenomena are most marked in the extremities.

With these observations we have undertaken detailed studies of fibrinolytic activity in patients with systemic sclerosis and with matched controls. We have been able to demonstrate a significant reduction in the fibrin plate lysis area and elevation of fibrinogen levels in systemic sclerosis patients compared with controls. We also undertook a test of fibrinolytic reserve by a venous occlusion test. The standard test involves 20 minutes venous occlusion but we have found that this could not be tolerated by patients who already have problems of digital ischaemia. For these reasons we use a 5 minute venous occlusion test. We found that this could produce an increase in fibrinolytic activity. In some of the systemic sclerosis patients there was apparently no fibrinolytic reserve with no increase in activity, but the differences between the systemic sclerosis and controls failed to reach statistical significance.

We have also been able to demonstrate that there is normally a diurnal variation in fibrinolytic activity with increased levels in blood taken in the afternoon compared with the morning. In a matched series of systemic sclerosis patients, however, this diurnal variation was lacking. To determine whether the reduced physical activity that may be associated with disabled patients could be responsible for this alteration we therefore repeated these diurnal measurements on normal control subjects who rested throughout the day. In these subjects, however, the diurnal variation was preserved with a normal increase detected in the afternoons. It therefore appears that the failure to increase levels of fibrinolytic activity does represent a specific defect associated with systemic sclerosis.

These observations have led us to undertake a controlled trial of fibrinolytic enhancement therapy. The agent that we used is Stanozolol which is a non-virilising anabolic steroid, in a dose of 5 mg bd. Currently we are conducting a double blind controlled cross-over trial in patients receiving six months of placebo and Stanozolol in random order. Patients receive detailed assessments of objective vascular problems, clinical findings, measurements of peripheral blood flow, as well as fibrinolytic measurements before and after each course of therapy.

The study is still on going but an interim analysis of the data does suggest that this form of treatment is effective, not only in normalising the fibrinolytic parameters, but also in reducing the frequency and severity of Raynaud's phenomenon and in improving peripheral blood flow.

Back Pain

Chronic inflammation and scarring may occur in the spine following myelography (particularly if oil based), laminectomy and other invasive procedures. It may also develop in association with lumbar spondylosis and spinal stenosis and may be the cause of chronic back pain. Chronic inflammation and scar tissue may develop around the nerve roots and in the arachnoid and may be responsible for persistence of severe pain in the back and referred into the lower limb. From histological examination of tissue removed at surgery it is possible to see dense scar tissue which is intimately blended with fibrin. These observations have led us to undertake detailed studies of fibrinolytic activity in patients with chronic back pain syndromes.

Eighteen patients with severe chronic back pain of mechanical cause (conditions such as ankylosing spondylitis had been excluded), were assessed and their fibrinolytic measurements were compared with a series of age and sex matched control subjects. The patients had chronic back pain for a mean of 11.6 (± S.D. 8.1) years. Of these two had previous laminectomies and four previous myelographies. Patients with psychological problems were excluded. The details of the patients are shown in Table 1.

Measurements of the fibrinolytic parameters were performed on subjects at the same time each morning, the subjects had rested for at least an hour and had not eaten or smoked for the previous 12 hours. Measurements were made of fibrin plate lysis area, euglobulin clot lysis time, plasma fibrinogen, plasminogen, α_2-antiplasmin and α_2-macroglobulin.

The results are shown in Table 2. They demonstrate significant decrease of fibrin plate lysis area, increase of the euglobulin clot lysis time, reduction of the plasminogen and increase of the inhibitors α_2-antiplasmin and α_2-macroglobulin.

We are now extending these observations to a much larger series of patients and the results are similar to those which we have demonstrated.

These results have prompted us to undertake fibrinolytic enhancement therapy for such patients. In a pilot study we have demonstrated that Stanozolol can normalise the fibrinolytic parameters with apparent clinical improvement (Table 3). However, the assessment of treatment for back pain is notoriously difficult and a

Table 1. Back Pain Study

	Patients	Controls
Age	45.7 ± 13.2 years	41.1 ± 9.5 years
Sex	5M: 13F	6M: 12F
Duration of back pain	11.6 ± 8.1 years	
Nerve root symptoms	8	
Myelography	4	
Spinal surgery	2	
ESR	5.5 ± 4.3 mm/hr	
Smokers	3	2

Table 2. Results of Tests of Fibrinolysis

Variable	Controls (n = 18)	Patients (n = 18)	p*
ELT (min)	125.2± 57	265.5±135.4	0.01
FPLA (mm^2)	103.4± 25.7	78.2± 36.8	0.01
Fg (mm/dl)	278.1±100.5	263.3±123.0	N.S.
Pg (%)	108.8± 18.4	99.0± 16.5	0.05
α_2-Antiplasmin (%)	110.8± 12.7	124.1± 23.5	0.05
α_2-Macroglobulin (%)	101.0± 15.2	125.3± 32.8	0.05

double blind controlled trial is currently in progress.

In summary, we suggest that a variety of insults to the spine such as myelography, laminectomy, lumbar spondylosis, spinal stenosis, etc. can all produce damage and give rise to chronic inflammation and fibrosis associated with fibrin deposition. The patients show evidence of defective fibrinolytic activity which may occur in response to the damage or may be caused by other factors. These other factors may include smoking and ischaemic heart disease, both of which are known to be associated with back pain and with

Table 3. Fibrinolytic Enhancement in Low Back Pain

36-year-old female with low back pain for 10 years.
All spine assessments limited.
ESR 2 mm/hr. HLA B27 negative.
X-ray: lumbar spondylosis.
Treated with Stanozolol 5 mg bd with gradual improvement.

	Initial	1 Month	2 Months	3 Months
ELT	177	74	67	62
FPLA	86	144	147	143
Fg	225	200	92	125
Pg	72	98	100	119
α_2-Antiplasmin	95	95	116	115
α_2-Macroglobulin	158	95	105	81

depressed fibrinoloysis. Because of the defective fibrinolytic activity the fibrin persists and this is associated with perpetuation of the chronic inflammation and fibrosis and persistence of the back pain problem.

References

Browse, N.L. 1983. Br.Med.J. 283, 1920.

Dumonde, D.C., L.E. Glynn. 1962. Br.J.Exp.Pathol. 43, 373.

Goyle, K.B., J.A. Dormandy. 1976. Lancet 1, 1317.

McGrath, M.A., R. Peek, R. Penny. 1977. Ann.Rheum.Dis. 36, 569.

SOLUBLE FIBRIN/FIBRINOGEN RELATED ANTIGEN IN HUMAN INTIMA IN RELATION TO ATHEROGENESIS

Elspeth B. Smith, Joyce E. Walker
Department of Chemical Pathology, University of Aberdeen, Foresterhill, Aberdeen AB9 2ZD, Scotland

Introduction

There is increasing evidence that fibrinogen or fibrin may be involved in atherogenesis as well as thrombotic occlusion (1,2). Soluble fibrin/fibrinogen related antigen (FRA) is present in all intimal samples and fibrin is a major component of many atherosclerotic lesions (3), where it may be present as an encrustation on, or immediately below, the endothelium, in discrete bands or patches at all levels in the plaque, or diffusely distributed. It may stimulate atherogenesis in several ways; a fibrin thrombus provides a scaffold along which smooth muscle cells (SMC) migrate, 'modified' fibrin may be involved in binding of low density lipoprotein, some fibrin degradation products (FDP) are chemotactic for SMCs and leukocytes, and some may stimulate mitosis and collagen synthesis (1,3,4).

It is not known if the fibrin in lesions is derived from incorporation of mural thrombus or from 'clotting' of fibrinogen within the intima, but recent studies suggest that fibrinogen leaking into the extravascular space is rapidly clotted (5). It is also not known if the soluble FRA in intima is mainly native fibrinogen; Shainoff & Page (6) suggested that it is cryoprofibrin, and on isoelectric focussing we observed peak broadening, and in some samples of intima a component that appeared to be D-dimer-E (7). In the present study we have extracted the soluble FRA from normal intima and atherosclerotic lesions of different types, and attempted to characterize its components by gradient SDS-polyacrylamide gel electrophoresis.

Fibrinogen - Fibrin Formation and Fibrinolysis, Vol. 4
© 1986 Walter de Gruyter & Co., Berlin · New York - Printed in Germany.

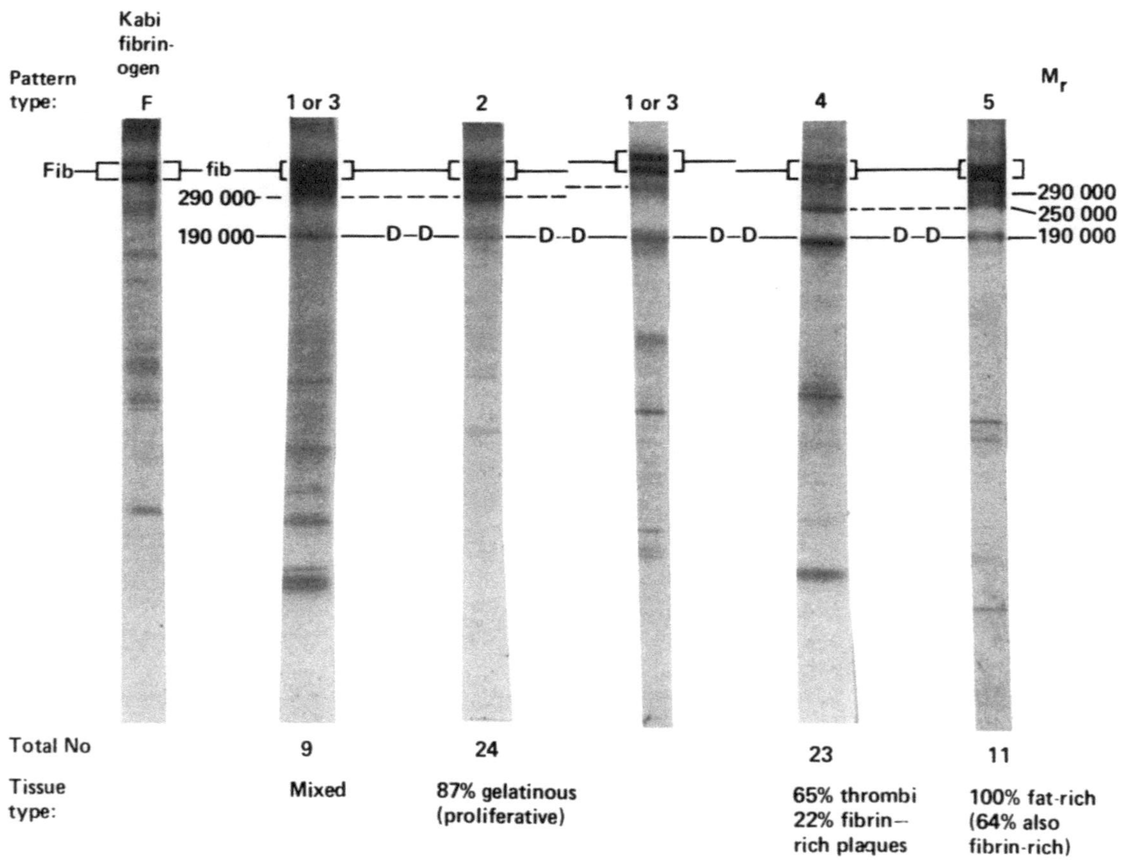

Figure 1 Soluble FRA separated by SDS-polyacrylamide gel electrophoresis using a 3% to 20% gradient. Most samples gave one of the four clearly defined types of pattern shown.

Materials and Methods

Aortas were obtained at autopsy within 24 hours of death, and segments of arteries were obtained within a few minutes of excision during reconstructive vascular surgery. Samples of normal intima or individual lesions were dissected off the media, weighed, and scissor minced with 100µl of 2% EDTA per 100mg wet tissue. The minces were then extracted with citrate buffered saline, pH 7.0 containing EDTA and e-aminocaproic acid; FRA were isolated from the extracts on sepharose-antifibrinogen affinity columns. The bound FRA were eluted with 8M urea, the eluate desalted and concentrated to about 400µl volume for electrophoresis on 4-20% SDS-gradient polyacrylamide gels, using the discontinuous system of Leamlli (8). Gels were stained with Coomasie brilliant blue, or silver.

Results

High molecular mass bands

The two bands of fibrinogen were present in virtually all samples, and accounted for about 30-60% of total staining. In addition, three other high molecular mass (HMr) bands were regularly observed, with approximate Mr 290000, 250000 and 190000 (Fig. 1). Fibrinogen and these three bands accounted for 70-85% of total staining; the band with Mr 190000 exactly co-migrated with D-dimer derived from plasmin digestion of cross-linked fibrin.

Band patterns and type of tissue sample

Visual inspection of the gels suggested that the HMr bands formed a limited number of distinctive patterns (Fig. 1). The width and intensity of staining of each band was scored visually, and expressed as per cent of total (fibrinogen & fragments) HMr band staining score; the identity of the samples was not known to the assessor. The samples were then grouped according to the relative proportions of the Mr 190000, 250000 and 290000 bands into four pattern types. Of necessity, arbitrary cut-off points were selected, and the definitions of each pattern type are summarized in Table 1.

Table 1

Characteristics used to Define Different HMr Pattern Types

HMr band	Percent of total HMr (fibrinogen & fragments) bands Type 1&3	Type 2	Type 4	Type 5
290 KD	-	-	<10	Bands approx. equal
250 KD	<5	<5	> twice 290 KD level	
190 KD	>25	<25	-	-

The Type 1 patterns (n=9) showed the greatest heterogeneity; the predominant band was Mr 190000 (mean level 35%) and the 250000 band was virtually absent (mean level 2%). The mean level of the 290000 band was 18%, but it covered a continuous distribution between 6% and 32%.

The Type 2 pattern was defined as <25% of the 190000 band and <5% of the 250000 band and the characteristics of the 25 patterns are shown in Fig. 2a. In Type 4 patterns the 290000 band was low (<10%) and the 250000 band at least twice its level (Fig. 2b). In Type 5 patterns the 290000 and 250000 bands were of approximately equal intensity (Fig. 2c).

The gross and microscopic characteristics of the tissue samples were then correlated with type of pattern. The Type 1 patterns were not associated with any specific tissue type, and included normal intima, fibrous and fatty plaques and two atypical thrombi. Initially it appeared that high levels of the 290000 band were associated with normal intima whereas a sub-group with lower levels (Type 3, Fig. 1) was associated with fibrous plaques. However, with larger numbers the distribution became continuous and normal intima and lesions were found throughout the range.

TYPE 2 PATTERN HMW = 83% of Total n = 24

	% of HMW Fraction	
Fibrinogen	Mean	Range
F1	27	10–50
F2	36	17–50
Fragments		
M_r 290 000	22	9–40
M_r 250 000	1.5	0–5
M_r 190 000 (DD)	13	3–25

COR. COEF. - 0.5035

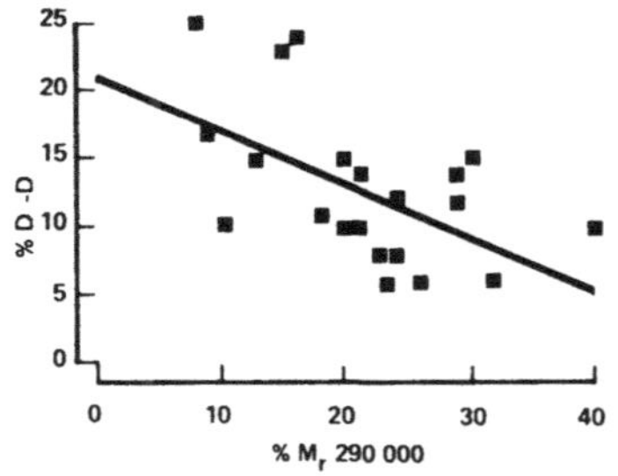

TYPE 4 PATTERNS HMW = 70% of Total n = 23

	% of HMW Fraction	
Fibrinogen	Mean	Range
F 1	21	6–32
F 2	21	6–32
Fragments		
M_r 290 000	5	0–9
M_r 250 000	22	8–35
M_r 190 000 (DD)	34	15–54

COR. COEF. = –0.8037

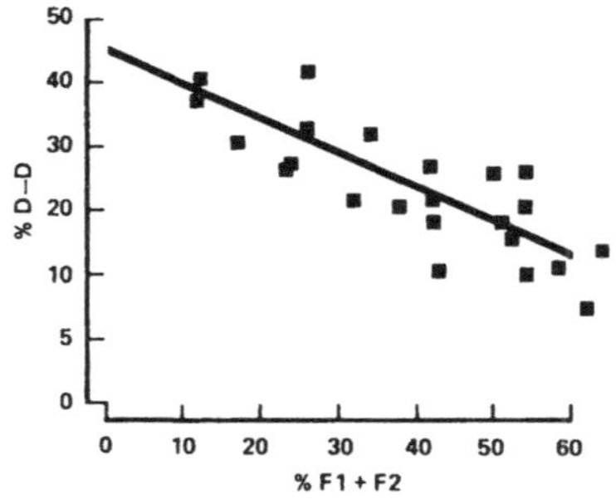

TYPE 5 PATTERN HMW = 78% of Total n = 11

	% of HMW Fraction	
Fibrinogen	Mean	Range
F1	19	4–34
F2	22	11–34
Fragments		
M_r 290 000	17	7–26
M_r 250 000	16	7–26
M_r 190 000 (DD)	25	7–57

COR.COEF. = -0.7659

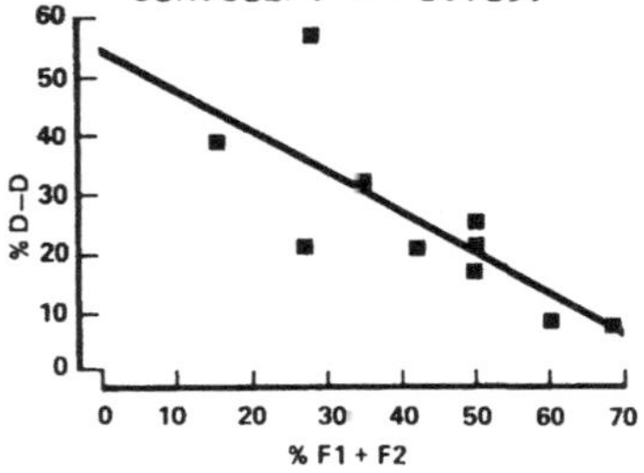

Figure 2 Distribution of high molecular mass bands in samples grouped according to the criteria shown in Table 1. Significant correlations ($p<0.01$) between components are shown in the graphs.

By contrast, 21 of the 24 samples giving Type 2 patterns were the proliferative, oedematous thickenings (gelatinous lesions (9)) that appear to be the precursors of fibrous plaques. In a sub-group that just fell outside the arbitrary definition of the Type 2 pattern because they contained 6 or 7% of the 250000 band, six of the seven samples were also gelatinous. Thus gelatinous lesions comprised 27 of the 31 samples (87%) with Type 2 or 2b patterns. In the strikingly different Type 4 pattern, 14 of the 23 samples were occlusive or mural thrombi and six were plaques containing large amounts of histologically visible fibrin; four patterns fell into a sub-group (4b) with 10-20% of the 290000 band, and three of these were derived from thrombi. All samples giving Type 5 patterns (n=11) were lipid-rich plaques, and seven of them also contained abundant fibrin. No particular characteristics could be assigned to normal intima, which gave Types 1, 2 and 4b patterns.

Discussion

There are three surprising features in these findings; the sharp definition of the HMr band pattern - very few intermediate bands were encountered; the invariable occurrence of a band that appeared to be D-dimer (both in terms of molecular mass markers and co-migration with D-dimer in plasmin digests) suggesting degradation of cross-linked fibrin; the low level and extreme variability of smaller fragments, including the absence of a band with Mr 90000 (D-monomer) from more than half the samples.

The Mr 290000 band might be fibrinogen from which the exposed carboxy terminal portion of only one Aα chain had been cleaved, or the Y-Y fragment derived from cross-linked fibrin (10). The low level of this band in the Type 4 pattern, which is characteristic of mural and occlusive thrombi, suggests that it is more likely to be the former. However, in patterns of Types 1 and 2 there were significant <u>inverse</u> correlations between D-dimer and the Mr 290000 band (Fig. 2a) suggesting that it may be a precursor, whereas its weak inverse correlation with fibrinogen was not significant. The Mr 250000 band might be fragment X derived from fibrinogen, or an X-D fragment derived from cross-linked fibrin, and its characteristically high level in thrombi (Type 4 pattern, Fig. 2b) supports this latter idea. However, again the internal correlations are confusing because it showed no correlation with levels of D-dimer; significant inverse correlations were found between fibrinogen and D-dimer in both Type 4 and Type 5 patterns.

It is possible that some fragments result from catheptic rather than plasmic degradation. In a high proportion of intimal samples we have failed to recover plasminogen, or to generate D-dimer-E on incubation of the intima at pH 7.0, but large amounts of D-dimer-E were generated in all samples of intima incubated at pH 4.0 (7).

The low levels and extremely variable patterns of fragments with Mr lower than D-dimer are difficult to understand. Fragments with Mr <20000 may not be retained by the antifibrinogen column, but the antiserum reacts strongly with both fragments D and E. Release of D-dimer should be accompanied by release of fragment E (11) but we failed to detect it in about one third of samples in which D-dimer was a prominent component.

References

1. Niewiarowski, S. and Rao, A.K. 1983. Contribution of thrombogenic factors to the pathogenesis of atherosclerosis. Prog. Cardiovasc. Dis. 26, 197-222.

2. Wilhelmsen, L., Svardsudd, K., et al 1984. Fibrinogen as a risk factor for stroke and myocardial infarction. N. Engl. J. Med. 311, 501-505.

3. Smith, E.B. and Staples, E.M. 1981. Haemostatic factors in human aortic intima. Lancet i, 1171-1174.

4. Thompson, W.D., Campbell, R. and Evans, I. 1985. Fibrin degradation and angiogenesis. J. Path. 145, 27-37.

5. Dvorak, H.F.,Senger, D.R., Dvorak, A.M., Harvey, V.S. and McDonagh,J. 1985. Regulation of extravascular coagulation by microvascular permeability. Science 227, 1059-1061.

6. Shainoff, J.R. and Page, I.H. 1972. Deposition of modified fibrinogen within the aortic intima. Atherosclerosis 16, 287-305.

7. Smith, E.B. and Ashall, C. 1985. Fibrinolysis and plasminogen concentration in aortic intima in relation to death following myocardial infarction. Atherosclerosis 55, 171-186.

8. Laemlli, Y.K. 1970. Cleavage of structural proteins during assembly of the head of bacteriophage T4. Nature (London) 277, 680-685.

9. Smith, E.B. 1982. Indentification of the gelatinous lesion. In: Atherosclerosis VI (G. Schettler, A.M. Gotto, G. Middelhoff, A.J.R. Habenicht and K.R. Jurutka, eds.) Springer-Verlag, Berlin, New York pp. 170-173.

10. Francis, C.W. and Marder, V.J. 1982. A molecular model of plasmic degradation of crosslinked fibrin. Seminars in Thrombosis and Haemostasis 8, 25-35.

11. Gaffney, P.J. and Joe, F. 1979. The lysis of human crosslinked fibrin by plasmin yields initially a single molecular complex, D-dimer-E. Thromb. Res. 15, 673-687.

FIBRINOGEN AS A POSSIBLE RISK FACTOR FOR IHD IN THE CAERPHILLY STUDY

J.W.G. Yarnell, P.M. Sweetnam, P.C. Elwood

MRC Epidemiology Unit, 4 Richmond Road, Cardiff CF2 3AS, United Kingdom

R. Eastham, R.A. Gilmour

Frenchay Hospital, Bristol BS16 1LE, United Kingdom

J.R. O'Brien, M.D. Etherington

Central Laboratory, St. Mary's Hospital, Portsmouth PO3 6AG, United Kingdom

Introduction

The long-term objective of the Caerphilly Prospective study of ischaemic heart disease (IHD) is to determine the predictive value of tests of haemostatic function for future IHD. The present data from this community study are cross-sectional; they describe levels of possible risk factors in subjects with IHD, either by history or by electrocardiography (ECG), and in subjects without any evidence of IHD. Haemostatic and epidemiological factors which are significantly associated with plasma fibrinogen are also examined.

Methods

Population and clinical methods: Two samples of men from the town and surrounding villages of Caerphilly, South Wales were selected: a random sample of men aged 30 to 69 years (final sample 711; 89% of those eligible); and a total sample of men aged 45 to 59 years (final sample 2512; 85% of those eligible). Recruitment began in September 1979 and was completed in 1983.

Fibrinogen - Fibrin Formation and Fibrinolysis, Vol. 4
© 1986 Walter de Gruyter & Co., Berlin · New York - Printed in Germany.

Each man was screened for evidence of IHD at an evening clinic by the use of standardized questionnaires and a twelve-lead ECG. ECG tracings were coded by two experienced observers by the Minnesota convention. Subjects were classified into three main classes for subsequent data analysis: those free of disease; those with a history of angina, myocardial infarction or major Q waves (probable IHD); and those with ECG changes only (possible IHD). A more complete description of the epidemiological methods is to be found elsewhere (1).

Laboratory methods: Each subject was asked to attend subsequently at a morning clinic. A venous blood sample was taken with minimum stasis after an overnight fast (minimum 8 hours, average 12 hours). Fibrinogen was estimated by two methods; a nephelometric determination following heat precipitation in buffered saline (2) (Fibrinogen N), and a clotting assay (3) (Fibrinogen C). Plasma viscosity was estimated on EDTA plasma by the method of Harkness (4). The heparin neutralizing activity of platelet-poor plasma was measured by the use of the heparin-thrombin clotting time (5) (HTCT). A dilute thrombin clotting time (5) was also carried out and this test was used in part to screen out subjects with abnormally long clotting times which would significantly influence the clotting in the HTCT.

A full blood count which included a white cell (WBC) and platelet count was carried out by the use of a Coulter model S-plus Cell Counter in whole blood anticoagulated with EDTA. Cell counts were carried out within four to ten hours after venepuncture (average six hours) and the nephelometric fibrinogen and plasma viscosity usually within 12 hours of collection. The assays on platelet-poor plasma (the HTCT, thrombin-time and clottable fibrinogen) were carried out after a standard delay overnight in a cooled container (during warm weather) of between 28 to 32 hours.

A five per cent sample of duplicate samples were presented 'blindly' to each laboratory during the course of the study. The coefficients of variation of the duplicate pairs for fibrinogen N, fibrinogen C, viscosity, HTCT, WBC and platelet count were 7%, 11%, 2%, 3%, 24% and 7% respectively. A second blood sample was taken from a small group of men (n = 8 to 12) some four to 12 weeks after the initial sample. Coefficients of variation for these pairs of results for fibrinogen N, fibrinogen C, viscosity, WBC and HTCT are as follows: 10%, 18%, 2%, 11% and 21%.

Results

Table 1 shows the distribution of subjects with IHD by age in the sample of 711 men. Overall 8% of subjects had only ECG evidence of IHD (possible IHD) and 10% of subjects had a history or had symptoms of IHD.

Table 1: Prevalence of IHD by Age

Age	30-44		45-54		55-69		All Ages	
IHD Category	n	%	n	%	n	%	n	%
None	297	90%	141	78%	143	71%	581	82%
Possible	18	5%	17	9%	25	12%	60	8%
Probable	15	5%	22	12%	33	16%	70	10%

Table 2 shows the mean plasma levels of fibrinogen N in subjects with and without evidence of IHD.

Table 2: Mean Fibrinogen Levels (g/l) by IHD Category

Age	30-44	45-54	55-69
IHD Category			
None	3.21	3.56	3.78
Possible	3.61	3.94	4.27
Probable	3.56	3.77	3.88

Standard deviations range from 0.7 to 1.0

Mean levels of fibrinogen tend to increase with age and are higher in subjects with IHD.

Table 3 shows the clotting activity attributable to fibrinogen (Fibrinogen C) in subjects with and without evidence of IHD. In general the clotting activity (seconds) is increased or shorter in subjects with IHD and tends to be shorter with increased age.

Table 3: Fibrinogen Clotting Activity (secs) by IHD Category

Age	30-44	45-54	55-69
IHD Category			
None	14.7	13.8	13.0
Possible	13.6	13.4	12.0
Probable	13.5	13.9	12.3

Standard deviations range from 2.3 to 3.8

In the course of analysis strong interrelationships between clotting factors were noticed. Multivariate analyses were then carried out by a series of logistic regression analyses and a preliminary analysis is shown in Table 4.

Table 4: Association of Factors with IHD by Logit Risk Function

	t-value*
Age	4.55
Fibrinogen N	2.30
HTCT (log)	-2.05

* Values in excess of 1.98 are significant at 5% level

In these preliminary data among 711 men, fibrinogen was also treated as a dependent variable and the influence of various factors on its plasma level was determined. Table 5 shows the results of a series of stepwise regression analyses which examine these associations. Only variables which are associated at conventional levels of statistical significance are listed.

Table 5: Accumulative Percentage of Variance in Fibrinogen Levels Explained by Certain Factors

	Accumulative percentage explained	Direction of association
Fibrinogen N		
Age	12.8	+
Smoking habit	21.3	+
Body mass index	22.8	+
Alcohol consumption	23.5	-
Cereal fibre consumption	24.2	-
Fibrinogen C		
Age	10.2	+
Smoking habit	15.4	+

Finally we have the first results from the analysis of our main cohort of 2512 male subjects aged 45 to 59 years. Table 6 shows the prevalence of IHD in this sample.

Table 6: Prevalence of IHD by Age

Age	45-49		50-54		55-59	
IHD Category	n	%	n	%	n	%
None	669	81%	600	74%	612	70%
Possible	43	5%	74	9%	76	9%
Probable	116	14%	137	17%	185	21%

The prevalence of probable IHD is somewhat higher in this sample because a conventional epidemiological criterion (severe chest pain for 30 minutes or more) has been used in place of a stricter clinical definition of myocardial infarction used for Table 1.

Table 7 shows the mean levels of Fibrinogen N and Fibrinogen C by IHD category.

Table 7: Mean Levels of Fibrinogen N and Fibrinogen C by IHD Category

IHD Category	Fibrinogen N (g/l)	Fibrinogen C (sec)
None	3.73	13.1
Possible	3.91	13.0
Probable	3.99	12.8
Standard deviations	(0.82 to 0.91)	(2.3 to 2.8)

Multivariate analyses have not yet been carried out but correlations between clotting factors have been examined. Table 8 shows these results.

Table 8: Correlation Matrix of Clotting Factors in 2512 Subjects

	Fibrinogen N	Fibrinogen C+	Viscosity	HTCT*	WBC*
Fibrinogen C	0.53				
Viscosity	0.56	0.44			
HTCT	-0.39	-0.82	-0.36		
WBC	0.32	0.27	0.27	-0.27	
Age	0.18	0.12	0.11	-0.08	0.01

* logarithmic transformation

\+ 100/Fibrinogen C

These variables are highly intercorrelated. The correlation of each with age is small in comparison with the correlations between the other variables.

Discussion

Preliminary data from the Caerphilly study show several haemostatic variables, which include fibrinogen, show univariate associations with IHD. However several of these variables show strong intercorrelations. In a multivariate analysis which included both fibrinogen and white cell count the latter replaced the former in a formal statistical association with IHD (6). The present data relate only to associations with prevalent IHD, and factors such as cessation of smoking may modify these associations in symptomatic subjects.

Prospective studies provide data not affected by such uncertainties and two studies which examine the predictive power of plasma fibrinogen levels for future IHD in men have been reported. Among 1500 men from London, United Kingdom, Meade et al (7) reported fibrinogen to be independently related to future IHD in an early report. From Sweden Wilhelmsen et al (8) reported that, among 792 men followed on average for 13.5 years, fibrinogen levels showed univariate associations for both myocardial infarction and stroke. But in a multivariate analysis these associations were significant only for stroke. The combined cohorts of the Caerphilly and Speedwell samples number some 4,800 men; prospective data will be available during the next four years to provide further evidence about the relationship between fibrinogen and IHD.

References

1. Caerphilly and Speedwell Collaborative Group. 1984. The Caerphilly and Speedwell collaborative heart disease studies. J. Epidemiol. Community Health 38, 259-62.

2. Thorp, J.M., G.B. Horsfall, M.C. Stone. 1967. A new red-sensitive micronephelometer. Medical and Biological Engineering 5, 51-6.

3. Clauss, A. 1957. Gerrinnungephysiologische Schnellmethode sur Bestimmung des Fibrinogens. Acta Haematol. 17, 237-46.

4. Harkness, J. 1971. The viscosity of human blood plasma; its measurement in health and disease. Biorheology 8, 171-93.

5. O'Brien, J.R., M. Etherington, S. Jamieson, P. Lawford, J. Sussex, S.V. Lincoln. Heparin neutralizing activity test in the diagnosis of acute myocardial infarction. J. Clin. Pathol. 28, 975-9.

6. Yarnell, J.W.G., P.M. Sweetnam, P.C. Elwood, et al. 1985. Haemostatic factors and ischaemic heart disease: the Caerphilly study. Brit. Heart J. 53, 483-7.

7. Meade, T.W., R. Chakrabarti, A.P. Haines, W.R.S. North, Y. Stirling, S.G. Thompson. 1980. Haemostatic function and cardiovascular death; early results of a prospective study. Lancet i, 1050-4.

8. Wilhelmsen, L., K. Svardsudd, K. Korsan-Bengtsen, B. Larsson, L. Welin, G. Tibblin. 1984. Fibrinogen as a risk factor for stroke and myocardial infarction. N. Engl. J. Med. 311, 501-5.

VIII. Appendix: Data on Fibrinogen

Fibrinogen Aα-chain, human

										10											20										30
1	A	D	S	G	E	G	D	F	L	A	E	G	G	G	V	R↓	G	P	R	V	V	E	R	H	Q	S	A	C	K	D
31	S	D	W	P	F	C	S	D	E	D	W	N	Y	K	C	P	S	G	C	R	M	K	G	L	I	D	E	V	N	Q
61	D	F	T	N	R	I	N	K	L	K	N	S	L	F	E	Y	Q	K	N	N	K	D	S	H	S	L	T	T	N	I
91	M	E	I	L	R	G	D	F	S	S	A	N	N	R	D	N	T	Y	N	R	V	S	E	D	L	R	S	R	I	E
121	V	L	K	R	K	V	I	E	K	V	Q	H	I	Q	L	L	Q	K	N	V	R	A	Q	L	V	D	M	K	R	L
151	E	V	D	I	D	I	K	I	R	S	C	R	G	S	C	S	R	A	L	A	R	E	V	D	L	K	D	Y	E	D
181	Q	Q	K	Q	L	E	Q	V	I	A	K	D	L	L	P	S	R	D	R	Q	H	L	P	L	I	K	M	K	P	V
211	P	D	L	V	P	G	N	F	K	S	Q	L	Q	K	V	P	P	E	W	K	A	L	T	D	M	P	Q	M	R	M
241	E	L	E	R	P	G	G	N	E	I	T	R	G	G	S	T	S	Y	G	T	G	S	E	T	E	S	P	R	N	P
271	S	S	A	G	S	W	N	S	G	S	S	G	P	G	S	T	G	N	R	N	P	G	S	S	G	T	G	G	T	A
301	T	W	K	P	G	S	S	G	P	G	S	T	G	S	W	N	S	G	S	S	G	T	G	S	T	G	N	Q	N	P
331	G	S	P	R	P	G	S	T	G	T	W	N	P	G	S	S	E	R	G	S	A	G	H	W	T	S	E	S	S	V
361	S	G	S	T	G	Q	W	H	S	E	S	G	S	F	R	P	D	S	P	G	S	G	N	A	R	P	N	N	P	D
391	W	G	T	F	E	E	V	S	G	N	V	S	P	G	T	R	R	E	Y	H	T	E	K	L	V	T	S	K	G	D
421	K	E	L	R	T	G	K	E	K	V	T	S	G	S	T	T	T	T	R	R	S	C	S	K	T	V	T	K	T	V
451	I	G	P	D	G	H	K	E	V	T	K	E	V	V	T	S	E	D	G	S	D	C	P	E	A	M	D	L	G	T
481	L	S	G	I	G	T	L	D	G	F	R	H	R	H	P	D	E	A	A	F	F	D	T	A	S	T	G	K	T	F
511	P	G	F	F	S	P	M	L	G	E	F	V	S	E	T	E	S	R	G	S	E	S	G	I	F	T	N	T	K	E
541	S	S	S	H	H	P	G	I	A	E	F	P	S	R	G	K	S	S	S	Y	S	K	Q	F	T	S	S	T	S	Y
571	N	R	G	D	S	T	F	E	S	K	S	Y	K	M	A	D	E	A	G	S	E	A	D	H	E	G	T	H	S	T
601	K	R	G	H	A	K	S	R	P	V																				

↓ denotes thrombin cleavage site.

References

Blombäck,B., Hessel,B., Iwanaga,S., Reuterby,J., Blombäck,M.: J. Biol. Chem., 247, 1496-1512 (1972).

Doolittle, R.F., Watt, K.W.K., Cottrell, B.A., Strong, D.D., Riley, M.: Nature 280, 464-468 (1979).

Henschen, A., Lottspeich, F., Hessel, B.: Hoppe-Seyler's Z. Physiol. Chem., 360, 1951-1956 (1979).

Rixon, M.W., Chan, W.Y., Davie, E.W., Chung, D.W.: Biochem. 22, 3237-3244 (1983).

Fibrinogen Aα-chain, rat

10 20 30

1 A D T G T T S E F I E A G G D I R ↓ G P R I V E R Q P S Q C K

31 E T D W P F C S D E D W N H K C P S G C R M K G L I D E A N

61 Q D F T N R I N K L K N S L F D F Q K N N K D S N S L T R N

91 I M E Y L R G D F A N A N N F D N T F G Q V S E D L R R R I

121 E I L K R K V I E K A Q Q I Q V L Q X X X X D Q L I D M K R

151 L E V D I D I K I R S C K G S C S R S V S R E I N L K D Y E

181 G Q Q K Q L E Q V I A K E L L P A K D R Q Y L P A I K M S P

211 V P D L V P G S F K S Q L Q E G P P E W K A L T E M R Q M R

241 M E L E R P G K D G L R E E I Y Q G D S R G D S A T R G P G

271 S K I E N P M T P G H G G S G Y W R P G S S G S G S D G N W

301 G S G T T G S D D T G T W G A G S S R P S S G S G N L K P S

331 N P D W G E F S E F G G S S S P S T R K E Y H T G K L V T S

361 K G D K E L L I G N E K V T S T G T S T T R R S C S K T I T

391 K T V L G N D G H R E V V K E V V T S D D G S D C G D G M D

421 L G L T H S F S G R L D E L S R M H P E L G S F Y D S R F G

451 S L T S N F K E F G S K T S D S D I F T D I E N P S S H V P

481 E F S S S S K T S T V R K Q V T K S Y K M A D E A A S E A H

511 Q E G D T R T T K R G R A R T M R G I H A

↓ denotes thrombin cleavage site.

References

Kehl, M., Henschen, A.: In Fibrinogen - recent biochemical and medical aspects. Henschen, A., Graeff, H., Lottspeich, F., Eds., 1, 109-114 (1982).

Crabtree, G.R., Comeau, C.M., Fowlkes, D.M., Fornace, A.J., Malley, J.D., Kant, J.A.: J. Mol. Biol. 185, 1-19 (1985).

Fibrinogen Bβ-chain, human

```
                              10                            20                            30
  1 Z G V N D N E E G F F S A R↓G H R P L D K K R E E A P S L R
 31 P A P P P I S G G G Y R A R P A K A A A T Q K K V E R K A P
 61 D A G G C L H A D P D L G V L C P T G C Q L Q E A L L Q Q E
 91 R P I R N S V D E L N N N V E A V S Q T S S S S F Q Y M Y L
121 L K D L W Q K R Q K Q V K D N E N V V N E Y S S E L E K H Q
151 L Y I D E T V N S N I P T N L R V L R S I L E N L R S K I Q
181 K L E S D V S A Q M E Y C R T P C T V S C N I P V V S G K E
211 C E E I I R K G G E T S E M Y L I Q P D S S V K P Y R V Y C
241 D M N T E N G G W T V I Q N R Q D G S V D F G R K W D P Y K
271 Q G F G N V A T N T D G K N Y C G L P G E Y W L G N D K I S
301 Q L T R M G P T E L L I E M E D W K G D K V K A H Y G G F T
331 V Q N E A N K Y Q I S V N K Y R G T A G N A L M D G A S Q L
361 M G E N⁺R T M T I H N G M F F S T Y D R D N D G W L T S D P
391 R K Q C S K E D G G G W W Y N R C H A A N P N G R Y Y W G G
421 Q Y T W D M A K H G T D D G V V W M N W K G S W Y S M R K M
451 S M K I R P F F P Q Q
```

Z denotes pyroglutamic acid and ↓ thrombin cleavage site.

References

Henschen, A., Lottspeich, F.: Hoppe-Seyler's Z. Physiol. Chem. 358, 1643-1646 (1977).

Hessel, B., Makino, M., Iwanaga, S., Blombäck, B.: Eur. J. Biochem. 98, 521-534 (1979).

Watt, K.W.K., Takagi, T., Doolittle, R.F.: Biochem. 18, 68-76 (1979).

Chung, D.W., Que, B.G., Rixon, M.W., Mace, M., Davie, E.W.: Biochem. 22, 3244-3250 (1983).

Fibrinogen Bβ-chain, bovine

										10										20										30
1	Z	F	P	T	D	Y	D	E	G	Q	D	D	R	P	K	V	G	L	G	A	R ↓	G	H	R	P	Y	D	K	K	K
31	E	E	A	P	S	L	R	P	V	P	P	P	I	S	G	G	G	Y	R	A	R	P	A	T	A	T	V	G	Q	K
61	K	V	E	R	K	P	P	D	A	D	G	C	L	H	A	D	P	D	L	G	V	L	C	P	T	G	C	K	L	Q
91	D	T	L	V	R	Q	E	R	P	I	R	K	S	I	E	D	L	R	N	T	V	D	S	V	S	R	T	S	S	S
121	T	F	Q	Y	I	T	L	L	K	N	M	W	K	G	R	Q	N	Q	V	Q	D	N	E	N	V	V	N	E	Y	S
151	S	H	L	E	K	H	Q	L	Y	I	D	E	T	V	K	N	N	I	P	T	K	L	R	V	L	R	S	I	L	E
181	N	L	R	S	K	I	Q	K	L	E	S	D	V	S	T	Q	M	E	Y	C	R	T	P	C	T	V	T	C	N	I
211	P	V	V	S	G	K	E	C	E	K	I	I	R	N	E	G	E	T	S	E	M	Y	L	I	Q	P	E	D	S	S
241	K	P	Y	R	V	Y	C	D	M	K	T	E	K	G	G	W	T	V	I	Q	N	R	Q	D	G	S	V	D	F	G
271	R	K	W	D	P	Y	K	Q	G	F	G	N	I	A	T	N	A	E	G	K	K	Y	C	G	V	P	G	E	Y	W
301	L	G	N	D	R	I	S	Q	L	T	N	M	G	P	T	K	L	L	I	E	M	E	D	W	K	G	D	K	V	T
331	A	L	Y	E	G	F	T	V	Q	N	E	A	N	K	Y	Q	L	S	V	S	K	Y	K	G	T	A	G	N	A	L
361	I	E	G	A	S	Q	L	V	G	E	N	R	T	M	T	I	H	N	S	M	F	F	S	T	Y	D	R	D	N	D
391	G	W	K	T	T	D	P	R	K	Q	C	S	K	E	D	G	G	G	W	W	Y	N	R	C	H	A	A	N	P	N
421	G	R	Y	Y	W	G	G	A	Y	T	W	D	M	A	K	H	G	T	D	D	G	V	V	W	M	N	W	Q	G	S
451	W	Y	S	M	K	K	M	S	M	K	I	R	P	Y	F	P	E	Q												

Z denotes pyroglutamic acid and ↓ thrombin cleavage site.

Reference

Chung, D.W., Rixon, M.W., MacGillivray, R.T.A., Davie, E.W.: Proc.Natl.Acad.Sci.USA,78, 1466-1470 (1981).

Fibrinogen γ-chain, human

										10										20										30
1	Y	V	A	T	R	D	N	C	C	I	L	D	E	R	F	G	S	Y	C	P	T	T	C	G	I	A	D	F	L	S
31	T	Y	Q	T	K	V	D	K	D	L	Q	S	L	E	D	I	L	H	Q	V	E	N^{+}	K	T	S	E	V	K	Q	L
61	I	K	A	I	Q	L	T	Y	N	P	D	E	S	S	K	P	N	M	I	D	A	A	T	L	K	S	R	K	M	L
91	E	E	I	M	K	Y	E	A	S	I	L	T	H	D	S	S	I	R	Y	L	Q	E	I	Y	N	S	N	N	Q	K
121	I	V	N	L	K	C	K	V	A	Q	L	E	A	Q	C	Q	E	P	C	K	D	T	V	Q	I	H	D	I	T	G
151	K	D	C	Q	D	I	A	N	K	G	A	K	Q	S	G	L	Y	F	I	K	P	L	K	A	N	Q	Q	F	L	V
181	Y	C	E	I	D	G	S	G	N	G	W	T	V	F	Q	K	R	L	D	G	S	V	D	F	K	K	N	W	I	Q
211	Y	K	E	G	F	G	H	L	S	P	T	G	T	T	E	F	W	L	G	N	E	K	I	H	L	I	S	T	Q	S
241	A	I	P	Y	A	L	R	V	E	L	E	D	W	N	G	R	T	S	T	A	D	Y	A	M	F	K	V	G	P	E
271	A	D	K	Y	R	L	T	Y	A	Y	F	A	G	G	D	A	G	D	A	F	D	G	F	D	F	G	D	D	P	S
301	D	K	F	F	T	S	H	N	G	M	Q	F	S	T	W	D	N	D	N	D	K	F	E	G	N	C	A	E	Q	D
331	G	S	G	W	W	M	N	K	C	H	A	G	H	L	N	G	V	Y	Y	Q	G	G	T	Y	S	K	A	S	T	P
361	N	G	Y	D	N	G	I	I	W	A	T	W	K	T	R	W	Y	S	M	K	K	T	T	M	K	I	I	P	F	N
391	R	L	T	I	G	E	G	Q	Q	H	H	L	G	G	A	K	Q	A	G	D	V									

$^{+}$ denotes carbohydrate binding site.

References

Blombäck, B., Gröndahl, N.J., Hessel, B., Iwanaga, S., Wallen, P.: J. Biol. Chem., 248, 5806-5820 (1973).

Lottspeich, F., Henschen, A.: Hoppe-Seyler's Z. Physiol.Chem., 358, 935-938 (1977).

Chung, D.W., Chan, W.Y., Davie, E.W.: Biochem. 22, 3250-3256 (1983).

Fibrinogen γ-chain, rat

```
                             10                            20                            30
  1 Z Y T A T R D N C C I L D E R F G S Y C P T T C G I S D F L
 31 N S Y Q T D V D T D L Q T L E N I L Q R A E N R T T E A K E
 61 L I K A I Q V Y Y N P D Q P P K P G M I E G A T Q K S K K M
 91 V E E I L K Y E A L L L T H E S S I R Y L Q D I Y T S N K Q
121 K I T N L K Q K V A Q L E A Q C K E P C K D S V R I Y D I T
151 G K D C Q D T A N K G A K E S G L Y S I R P L K A T Q Q S L
181 V Y C E T D G P G N G W T E F K K R L D G S V D F L K N W I
211 Q Y K E G F G H L S P T G T T E F W L G N E K N H L I S M Q
241 S T I P Y A L R I Q L K D W S G R T S T A D Y A M F R V G P
271 G S D K Y R L T Y A Y F I G G D A G D A F D G Y D F G D D P
301 S D K F F T S H N G M H F S T W D N D N D K F E G N C A E Q
331 D G S G W W M N K C H A G H L N G W Y Y Q G G T Y S K S S T
361 P N G Y D N G I I W A T W K T R W Y S M K E T T M K I I P F
391 N R L S I G D G Q Q H H M G G S K Q V G D M
```

Z denotes pyroglutamic acid.

References

Kehl, M., Henschen, A.: In Fibrinogen - recent biochemical and medical aspects. Henschen, A., Graeff, H., Lottspeich, F., Eds., 1, 109-114 (1982).

Crabtree, G.R., Kant, J.A.: Cell, 31, 159-166 (1982).

Fibrinogen γ-chain, lamprey

10 20 30

1 Z V R D L K Q C S N D P E F G R Y C P T T C G V A D V L S K

31 Y A K G V D E D S S F I D S V L T Q L A A K H G I V E G N V

61 N I V N E D V R I T R D E A Q I I K D S G Q K T V Q K I L E

91 E V R I L E Q I G V S H D A Q I Q E L S E M W R V N Q Q F V

121 T R L Q Q Q L V D I R Q T C S R P C Q D T T A N K I S P I T

151 G K D C Q Q V V D N G G K D S G L Y Y I K P L K A K Q P F L

181 V F C E I E N G N G W T V I Q H R H D G S V N F T R D W V S

211 Y R E G F G Y L A P T L T T E F W L G N E K I H L L T G Q Q

241 A Y R L R I D L T D W E N T H R Y A D Y G H F K L T P E S D

271 E Y R L F Y S M Y L D G D A G N A F D G F D F G D D P Q D K

301 F Y T T H L G M L F S T P E R D N D K Y E G S C A E Q D G S

331 G W W M N R C H A G H L N G K Y Y F G G N Y R K T D V E F P

361 Y D D G I I W A T W H D R W Y S L K M T T M K L L P M G R D

391 L S G H G G Q Q Q S K G N S R G D N

Z denotes pyroglutamic acid.

Reference

Strong, D.D., Moore, M., Cottrell, B.A., Bohonus, V.L., Pontes, M., Evans, B., Riley, M., Doolittle, R.F.: Biochem. 24, 92-101 (1985).

AUTHOR INDEX

SUBJECT INDEX

Fibrinogen

Recent Biochemical and Medical Aspects
Volume 1

Proceedings · International Symposium, Max-Planck-Institute for Biochemistry, February 17–18, 1981, Martinsried/Munich, Germany

Editors *A. Henschen · H. Graeff · F. Lottspeich*

1982. 17 x 24 cm. X, 400 pages. Numerous illustrations.
Hardcover. DM 135,–; approx. US $52.00 ISBN 3 11 008543 7

Fibrinogen

Structure – Functional Aspects – Metabolism
Volume 2

Proceedings · Workshop on Fibrinogen
May 12–14, 1982, Leiden, The Netherlands

Editors *F. Haverkate · A. Henschen · W. Nieuwenhuizen · P. W. Straub*

1983. 17 x 24 cm. XVI, 343 pages. Numerous illustrations.
Hardcover. DM 145,–; approx. US $55.75 ISBN 3 11 008986 6

Fibrinogen

Structural Variants and Interactions
Volume 3

Proceedings · Workshop on Fibrinogen
July 9–10, 1983, Stockholm, Sweden

Editors *A. Henschen · B. Hessel · J. McDonagh · T. Saldeen*

1985. 17 x 24 cm. XII, 418 pages. Numerous illustrations.
Hardcover. DM 270,–; approx. US $103.90 ISBN 3 11 009806 7

Fibrinogen

Fibrin Formation and Fibrinolysis · Volume 4

Proceedings · Workshop on Fibrinogen
April 2–3, 1985, London, England

Editors *D. A. Lane · A. Henschen · M. K. Jasani*

1986. 17 x 24 cm. XVIII, 398 pages. Numerous illustrations.
Hardcover. DM 250,–; approx. US $96.20 ISBN 3 11 010597 7

Prices are subject to change without notice

Walter de Gruyter · Berlin · New York

Protein C

Biochemical and Medical Aspects

Proceedings of the International Workshop, Titisee/Freiburg, Federal Republic of Germany, July 9–11, 1984

Editor *Irene Witt*

1985. 17 cm x 24 cm. XIII, 191 pages. Numerous illustrations.
Hardcover. DM 160,–; approx. US $61.50 ISBN 3 11 010222 6

The proceedings of the workshop reflect current knowledge on the **complex Protein C system** in biochemistry, physiology and pathophysiology. It furthermore includes reviews on several cases of hereditary Protein C and S deficiency as well as on conditions of acquired diminution of Protein C. The clinical pictures of Protein C and Protein S dificiency and methods for the immunological and functional determination of Protein C are described.

Heparin

New Biochemical and Medical Aspects

Proceedings of the Symposium of the Deutsche Gesellschaft für Klinische Chemie · Titisee, Breisgau, Germany · June 29th–July 1st, 1981

Editor *Irene Witt*

1983. 17 cm x 24 cm. XVI, 372 pages. Numerous illustrations.
Hardcover DM 155,–; approx. US $59.60 ISBN 3 11 008637 9

This book presents reviews on new aspects of heparin structure, its biosynthesis, mechanism of action and its medical usage. Each article is followed by a discussion which has been condensed in order to include only the most important aspects.

Contents (Main Chapters):
Heparin: Structure, Mechanism of Action, Biosynthesis and Catabolism · Methods for the Determination of Heparin · Clinical Usage of Heparin · Experience with "Monitoring of Heparin Therapy" · Concluding Discussion · Author Index · Subject Index.

Prices are subject to change without notice

Walter de Gruyter · Berlin · New York

Bei Fragen zur Produktsicherheit wenden Sie sich bitte an:
If you have any questions regarding product safety,
please contact:

Walter de Gruyter GmbH
Genthiner Straße 13
10785 Berlin
productsafety@degruyterbrill.com